A.M. Ehrly · W. Fleckenstein · J. Hauss · R. Huch (Eds.)

Clinical Oxygen Pressure Measurement II

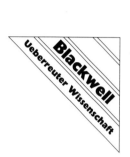

A. M. Ehrly · W. Fleckenstein
J. Hauss · R. Huch (Eds.)

Clinical Oxygen Pressure Measurement II

Tissue Oxygen Pressure and Transcutaneous Oxygen Pressure

Blackwell Ueberreuter Wissenschaft · Berlin 1990

Prof. Dr. med. A. M. Ehrly
Zentrum der Inneren Medizin
Klinikum der Johann Wolfgang Goethe-Universität
Theodor-Stern-Kai 7, D-6000 Frankfurt/Main

Dr. med. W. Fleckenstein
Transducer-Labor
Eiderweg 14, D-2301 Kiel/Mielkendorf

Prof. Dr. med. J. Hauss
Chirurgische Klinik/Poliklinik der Universität
Jungeboldtplatz 1, D-4400 Münster

Prof. Dr. med. Renate Huch
Universitätsfrauenklinik
Frauenklinikstraße 10, CH-8091 Zürich

English language advice:
David Paenson and Greg P. Twiss

ISBN 3-89412-082-7

CIP-Titelaufnahme der Deutschen Bibliothek

Clinical oxygen pressure measurement II : tissue oxygen
pressure and transcutaneous oxygen pressure / A. M. Ehrly …
(ed.). – Berlin : Blackwell Ueberreuter Wiss., 1990
  ISBN 3-89412-082-7
NE: Ehrly, Albrecht M. [Hrsg.]

© Blackwell Ueberreuter Wissenschafts-Verlag G.m.b.H. Berlin 1990
Printed in Germany

The use of general descriptive names, trade names, trade marks etc. in this publication, even if the former
are not especially identified, is not to be taken as a sign that such names, as understood by the Trade Marks
and Merchandise Marks Act, may accordingly be used freely by anyone.

Product Liability: The publisher can give no guarantee for information about drug dosage and application thereof contained in this book. In every individual case the respective user must check its accuracy
by consulting other pharmaceutical literature.

Cover design: R. Hübler, 1000 Berlin

Layout: Goldener Schnitt · Rainer Kusche, 7573 Sinzheim

Printing: Druckhaus Beltz, 6944 Hemsbach

Binding: J. Schäffer, 6718 Grünstadt

Preface

In recent years experimental and particularly clinical research in oxygen pressure measurement (tissue pO_2, trancutaneous pO_2 and others) has markedly increased. In parallel, progress in methodology and technique is obvious. After the symposia held in Frankfurt in 1980 and 1984 two scientific meetings took place in 1988. There was a Workshop on Theory and Practice of Tissue pO_2 Measurement in Lübeck March, 11 and 12, 1988, organized by Ch. Weiss followed by the 3rd Frankfurt Symposium on Clinical Oxygen Pressure Measurement organized by A. M. Ehrly. As can be concluded from the titles of both meetings the Lübeck meeting dealt more with theoretical and methodological topics whereas in Frankfurt predominantly clinical aspects of pO_2 measurements were discussed.

A great number of participants including so called pure microcirculationists and pure clinicians were attending. It became obvious that more and more groups are starting to discover the interdisciplinary relevance of microcirculation and the role of oxygen transport to tissue and thus oxygen pressure values for various organs. As expected, the application of oxygen pressure measurement has expanded considerably.

The organizers of both meetings agreed to join in publishing a proceedings book in order to bring together the many aspects of oxygen pressure measurement. We are proud that it was possible to bring together almost all groups working in this area. The organizers wish to thank all authors and the sponsors whose support made the symposia and the book possible.

Ch. Weiss   *A. M. Ehrly*

Contents

List of Contributors

Prof. Dr. med. H. Acker
Max-Planck-Institut
f. Systemphysiologie
Rheinlanddamm 201
D-4600 Dortmund

PD Dr. G. O. Bastian
Med. Universität Lübeck
Klinik f. Augenheilkunde
Ratzeburger Allee 160
D-2400 Lübeck

Dr. H. Baumgärtl
Max-Planck-Institut
f. Systemphysiologie
Rheinlanddamm 201
D-4600 Dortmund

Dr. G. I. J. M. Beerthuizen
Algemeene Chirurgie
Katholieke Universiteit
Postbus 9101
NL-6500 HB Nijmegen
Netherlands

Dr. E. Beinder
Universitäts-Frauenklinik
D-8520 Erlangen

Dr. med. P. Boekstegers
Med. Klinik I
Klinikum Großhadern
Marchinoninistr. 15
D-8000 München 70

Dr. H.-W. M. Breuer
Novesiastr. 28
D-4044 Kaarst/Büttgen

Dr. F. Carnochan
Ninewells Hospital and
Medical School
Tayside Health Board
DD1 9SY Dundee
U.K.

Dr. L. Caspary
Med. Hochschule Hannover
Abt. Angiologie
Konstanty-Gutschow-Str. 8
D-3000 Hannover

Prof. Dr. med. A. Creutzig
Universitätsklinikum
Abt. f. Angiologie
Konstanty-Gutschow-Str. 8
D-3000 Hannover

Prof. Dr. med. A. M. Ehrly
Universitätsklinikum
Abt. Angiologie
Theodor-Stern-Kai 7
D-6000 Frankfurt am Main 70

Dr. med. W. Fleckenstein
Transducer-Labor
Eiderweg 14
D-2301 Kiel/Mielkendorf

Prof. S. Forconi
  Universita degli studi di Siena
  Cattedra di Gerontologia
  e Geriatria
  Policlinico, Viale Bracci
  I-53100 Siena
  Italy

Dr. med. Ulrich K. Franzeck
  Universitätsspital
  Rämistraße 190
  CH-8091 Zürich
  Switzerland

Dr. K. Grossmann
  Med. Akademie Erfurt
  Abteilung Angiologie,
  Innere Medizin
  DDR Erfurt

Dipl.-Biol. M. Günderoth-Palmowski
  Fa. Eppendorf-Gerätebau
  Netheler-Hinz GmbH
  Postfach 650620
  D-2000 Hamburg 65

Dr. A. Hagendorff
  Universität Bonn
  Physiologisches Institut I
  Nußallee 11
  D-5300 Bonn

Prof. Dr. med. J. Hauss
  Med. Hochschule Hannover
  Klinik für Abdominal- und
  Transplantationschirurgie
  Konstanty Gutschow Straße 8
  D-3000 Hannover 61

PD Dr. R. Heinrich
  Geriatrische Universitätsklinik
  Marienhospital
  Widumerstr. 8
  D-4690 Herne 1

Dr. J. Hobbhahn
  Ludwigs-Maximilians-Universität
  Klinikum Großhadern
  Marchioninistr. 15
  D-8000 München 70

Dr. H.-G. Höffkes
  Universitätsklinik
  Abt. Angiologie
  Theodor-Stern-Kai 7
  D-6000 Frankfurt am Main

Prof. Dr. R. Huch
  Universitätsfrauenklinik
  Frauenklinikstraße 10
  CH-8091 Zürich
  Switzerland

Dr. med. F. Jung
  Universitätsklinikum
  Abt. Hämostaseologie
  D-6650 Homburg/Saar

Dr. N. Klause
  Universität Kiel
  Physiologisches Institut
  Olshausenstr. 40
  D-2300 Kiel

Dr. W. Kolepke
  Universitätsklinikum
  Abt. Hämostaseologie
  D-6650 Homburg/Saar

Dr. H. W. Krawzak
  Chirurgische Universitätsklinik
  Marienhospital
  Hölkeskampring 40
  D-4690 Herne 1

Dr. med. K. Krönert
  Universitätsklinik
  Med. Klinik Abt. IV
  Otfried-Müller-Str. 10
  D-7400 Tübingen

Dr. K. Ktenidis
  Krankenhaus Porz am Rhein
  Abt. Chirurgie
  Urbacherweg 19
  D-5000 Köln 90

Prof. Dr. med. H. Landgraf
  Universitätsklinik
  Abt. Angiologie
  Theodor-Stern-Kai 7
  D-6000 Frankfurt am Main 70

Dr. R. Leuwer
  Universität Bonn
  Neurochirurgische Klinik
  Sigmund-Freud-Str. 25
  D-5300 Bonn 1

M. D. Toshihiko Maeda
  St. George's Hospital
  Medical School
  Research Laboratoy,
  Dept. of Haematology
  Cranner Terrace Tooting
  SW17 London ORE
  U. K.

Prof. M. D. E. Mannarino
  Instituto II Clinica Medica
  Generale e Terpia
  Cattedra Angiologia
  Policlinico Monteluce
  I-6100 Perugia
  Italy

Dr. U. Martin
  Boehringer Mannheim GmbH
  Med. Forschung, Abt. MF-1H
  Sandhofer Str. 16
  D-6800 Mannheim 31

Dr. H. J. Meuer
  Medizinische Hochschule
  Zentrum Physiologie
  Konstanty-Gutschow-Str. 8
  D-3000 Hannover 61

M. D. P. A. Modesti
  University of Florence
  Clinica Medica I
  I-50123 Florence
  Italy

Dr. J. Roux
  Laboratoires Sarget
  Research Department
  Avenue President Kennedy,
  BP 100
  F-33701 Merignac Cedex
  France

Prof. Dr. med. M. E. Schlaefke
  Ruhr-Universität
  Arb. Gr. Physiologie
  Universitätsstraße 150
  D-4630 Bochum

Dr. med. André Schmidt
  Medizinische Universitätsklinik
  Baldingerstraße
  D-3550 Marburg

Prof. Dr. U. Schramm
  Medizinische Univ. Lübeck
  Institut f. Anatomie
  Ratzeburger Allee 160
  D-2400 Lübeck

PD Dr. med. G. Singbartl
  Knappschafts-Universitätsklinik
  Klinik für Anästhesie u.
  operative Intensivstation
  In der Schornau 23/25
  D-4630 Bochum7

Dr. Dipl. Ing. H. U. Spiegel
  Chirurg. Klinik/Poliklinik
  Universitätsklinikum
  Jungeblodtplatz 1
  D-4400 Münster

Dr. med. U. Staedt
  I. Med. Klinik
  Klinikum Mannheim
  Theodor-Kutzer-Ufer
  D-6800 Mannheim

Dr. J. M. Steinacker
  Universität Ulm
  Sportmedizinische
  Untersuchungsstelle
  Oberer Eselsberg M 25-336
  D-7900 Ulm

Dr. B. Steinberg
  Universitätskrankenhaus
  Eppendorf
  Abt. f. Anästhesiologie
  Martinistr. 52
  D-2000 Hamburg 20

Dr. R. Tenbrinck
  Erasmus Universiteit Rotterdam
  Dept. Anesthesiology
  Postbus 1738
  NL-3000 DR Rotterdam
  Netherlands

Dr. N. Weindorf
  St. Josef-Hospital,
  Ruhr-Universität
  Gudrunstr. 56
  D-4630 Bochum

Prof. Dr. S. Zapalski
  Institut of Surgery
  1 Dulaga Str.
  61-848 Poznan
  Poland

Methods of Measuring Tissue pO_2 in Clinical Medicine: The Multiwire Surface Electrode

H.U. Spiegel, A.M. Ehrly

History of pO_2 measurement

It is necessary to distinguish between *direct* and *indirect* methods for the measurement of pO_2 (see Fig. 1).
Kivasaari & Niinikoski [14] have described the *indirect* technique, the so-called perfusion method, whereby a permeable teflon tube is inserted into the tissue and is continuously perfused by an oxygen carrier solution. The pO_2 measurement is then performed polarographically or by means of a mass spectrometer.
As to the *direct* method, one can distinguish between the polarographic, potentiometric and optical measuring procedures.
Davies and Brink [4] reported experimental polarographic tissue pO_2 measurements in animals already in 1942. However, direct polarographic pO_2 measurements in blood or in protein-rich body fluids by means of an uncoated precious metal cathode proved problematic due to the development of an oxygen-poor convention-dependent diffusion zone [17] as a result of the oxygen consumption of the electrode itself.

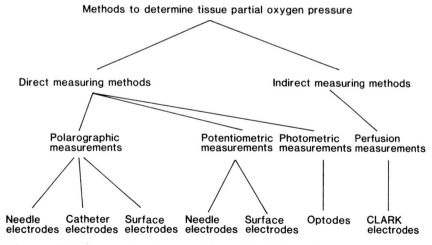

Fig. 1. Survey of techniques available for the determination of tissue PO_2

Clinical Oxygen Pressure Measurement II
A.M. Ehrly et al. (Eds.)
© Blackwell Ueberreuter Wissenschaft Berlin 1990

A substantial improvement in the measuring properties of polarographic electrodes was achieved with the introduction of an oxygen permeable electrolyte membrane covering only the cathode or both anode and cathode and thus separating them from direct contact with the surrounding medium (Clark's principle) [1].

The decisive technological breakthrough came in 1966, when Kessler and Lübbers [10] developed a Clark type multiwire surface electrode and established the basis for the later use of this technique in humans. However, it took a further 10 years before this method was applied to intensive care patients – by Schönleben et al. of the Surgical Hospital of Münster University, in 1975 [18].

In 1975 too, Ehrly and co-workers [5] published tissue pO_2-results of patients with chronic occlusive arterial disease using a micro platinum needle electrode technique.

Methodology of pO_2 measurements

1. Polarographic measuring principle

During polarographic measurement [3, 6, 9, 16], all oxygen molecules diffusing to the cathode are immediately reduced by applying an optimal polarization tension at polarization level:

$$O_2 + 4 \text{ e} \dashrightarrow 2 \text{ O}^- \text{ (total reduction)}$$

This means that within this range the oxygen tension on the platinum surface equals zero. Thus, the reduction current is solely determined by the *quantity* of subsequently diffusing oxygen. Assuming constant diffusion conditions between an oxygen permeated medium and the electrode surface, the oxygen partial pressure and the concentration of oxygen molecules in the medium can be determined by the measurement of the reduction current.

The polarographic measuring system consists of the tension generator, the current and voltage meters, and the gauge instrument (see Fig. 2). The tension generator **B** produces the polarization voltage **V**, which can be tapped at the resistor **R**. The polarization tension is switched to the gauge instrument **M**, which consists of a cathode (**Pt**), a silver/silver chloride anode, and a KCl electrolyte. The reduction current flowing through is indicated by the instrument **A**.

2. Polarogram and calibration curve

The correlation between the measured current and the applied voltage can be expressed by a current tension curve, the so-called *polarogram* (see Fig. 3). The curve of the polarogram characteristically flattens in the presence of oxygen, forming the so-called *polarographic plateau*, where an

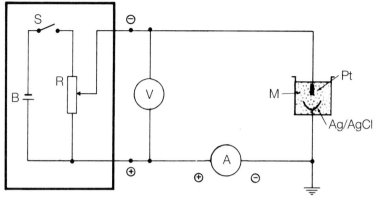

Fig. 2. Presentation of polarographic measuring circuit (after Lübbers)

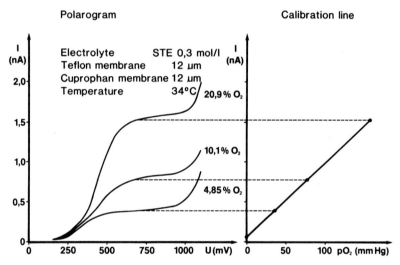

Fig. 3. Polarogram and calibration line of a multiwire surface electrode at 4.85, 10.1 and 20.9 percent oxygenation

increase in tension does not lead to an immediate increase in the current. The increase in current is delayed because other current-supplying electromechanical reactions are now interacting with the electrode. The plateau or characteristic diffusion level is achieved at a tension level of 600 to 800 mV, which was chosen as the operation voltage of the electrode. The calibration curve of the platinum electrode is obtained by plotting the amperage against the partial oxygen pressure. The greater the current intensity, the steeper this curve becomes.

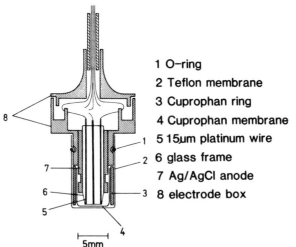

1 O-ring
2 Teflon membrane
3 Cuprophan ring
4 Cuprophan membrane
5 15µm platinum wire
6 glass frame
7 Ag/AgCl anode
8 electrode box

Fig. 4. Schematic set-up of the multiwire surface electrode

3. The multiwire surface electrode

The multiwire surface electrode for the clinical measurement of tissue pO_2 was specially developed by the Max-Planck-Institute for Systemic Physiology in Dortmund, West Germany [11, 12, 13, 18].

Fig. 4 shows the schematic set-up of this Clark-type [1, 2] 8-wire surface electrode. The 8 Pt-wire cathodes are sealed in glass and surrounded by a ring-type anode consisting of Ag/AgCl. The Pt-cathodes and the anode are separated from the measuring medium by an oxygen permeable teflon membrane. The inserted cuprophan 3 membrane [8] serves to stabilize the diffusion rate between the membrane and the Pt-wires. A sterile bromide-free 0.3 mol/l pH-buffered KCl solution served as electrolyte. The electrode, with its teflon cap reinforced by a rubber glove-ring, is so designed that it can be placed directly onto the moistened surface of the organ under study, whilst effectively preventing the access of ambient oxygen (see Fig. 5).

4. Technical data of the multiwire surface pO_2 electrode

Table 1. Specifications of the multiwire surface electrode

Cathode	15 µm platinum
Anode	Ag/AgCl
No. of wires	8
Membrane	12 µm Teflon
Membrane	12 µm Cuprophan
Electrolyte	sterile 0.3 mol/l KCl solution
Weight	2.1 g
Diameter	5 mm

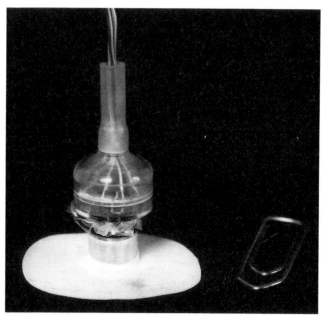

Fig. 5. The multiwire surface electrode can be adapted to the surface of the organ by fitting a positioning cap and a rubber ring

Table 2. Measurement parameters of the multiwire surface electrode

Polarization voltage	-700 mV
Sensitivity $\dfrac{I}{pO_2}$	0.6~1.4 · 10^{-11} A/mmHg
Sensitivity/100 mmHg in 0.9 % NaCl solution at 34°C, pH 6.0	0.6~1.4 · 10^{-9} A
N$_2$ value	<0.6 · 10^{-10} A
Response time t$_{90}$	<5.0 s
Electrode resistance	10^9 ~ 10^{10} Ohm
Drift (sensitivity)	max. ±8 %/h
Isolation resistance	>1 · 10^{12} Ohm

5. The measuring system

The schematic set-up of the pO$_2$ system, showing data acquisition, recording, processing and output, is displayed in Fig. 6. This compact electronic unit allows the simultaneous and continuous assessment of local tissue pO$_2$ at 8 different tissue sites. Immediate commuting and draft correction of the pO$_2$ values is performed by an integrated minicomputer. After on-line processing, the absolute pO$_2$ values are transformed graphically as a function of time.

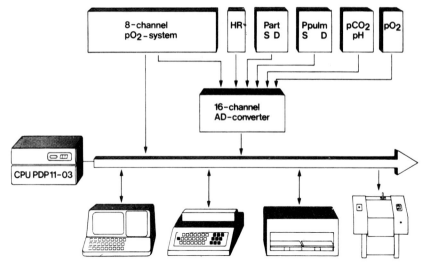

Fig. 6. Schematic set-up of the pO₂ measuring system showing data acquisition, integrated computer and data-output system

6. Calibration of the electrode

Pre- and post-calibration of the electrode is necessary for each measurement, since the stability of the electrode may be subject to alteration. The extent of the drift depends on the constancy of the polarization voltage applied, the cleanliness of the electrode surface and the presence of a specific boundary film on the platinum that stabilizes the process – possibly a mono-molecular Pt-O-layer [7].

The calibration of the electrode is performed before and after each measurement in a calibration container under standardized conditions. Generally, a two-step calibration is performed. Purified nitrogen is used to determined the O-value and the remaining current. The reference gas for measurement in tissue has to be selected in such a way that the calibration values correspond to the expected local oxygen tension. For clinical routine, a mixture of 5 % oxygen and 95 % nitrogen is used.

In hyperoxia conditions, with tissue values exceeding 50 mmHg, a calibration gas with adequate pO_2 should be introduced as a third reference gas. The calibration is performed after a 2 to 3 min adjustment period at 34 °C in a 0.9 % NaCl solution equilibrated with the calibration gases. The sensitivity/100 mmHg is then calculated, on the basis of the recorded currents and taking into consideration the air and steam pressures, using the following formula:

$$\frac{I}{100 \text{ mmHg}} = \frac{I_{5\% \text{ O2}} - I_{0\% \text{ O2}}}{pO_2 \text{ 5\% } O_2} \cdot 100$$

7. Sterilization

In order to rule out any risk of bacterial contamination, a sterilization procedure was developed which is compatible with the materials used [19, 20]. The electrode and electrode components are sterilized seperately in ethylene oxide 5 at a negative pressure of 600 to 700 mmHg and a working temperature of 45 °C. The electrolyte solution is prepared in a sterile bottle. The materials to be sterilized are packed and sealed in polythelene and polyamid foils. The assembly of the electrode in the intensive care unit or operation theater has to take place under sterile conditions.

References

1. Clark LC jr (1956) Monitor and control of blood and tissue oxygen tensions. Trans Am Soc Art Int Organ 2:41
2. Clark LC jr (1959) U.S. Patent 2, 913:386
3. Daneel H (1897) Über den durch diffundierende Gase hervorgerufenen Reststrom. Zeitschrift Elektrochemie 4:227
4. Davies PW, Brink F (1942) Microelectrodes for measuring local oxygen tensions in animal tissue. Rev Sc:Instrum 13:524
5. Ehrly AM, Köhler HJ, Schroeder W, Müller R (1975) Sauerstoffdruckwerte im isch-ämischen Muskelgewebe von Patienten mit chronischen peripheren arteriellen Ver-schlußkrankheiten. Klin. Wschr. 53, 687
6. Fatt I (1976) Polarographic oxygen sensors. CRC Press, Cleveland, Ohio
7. Feldberg SW, Enke CG, Bricker CE (1963) Formation and dissolution of platinum oxide film. Mechanism and kinetics. J Electrochem Soc 110:826
8. Gleichmann U, Lübbers DW (1960) Die Messung des Sauerstoffdruckes in Gasen und Flüssigkeiten mit der Pt-Elektrode unter besonderer Berücksichtigung der Messung im Blut. Plügers Arch Ges Physiol 271:431
9. Heyrovsky J (1948) Polarographisches Praktikum. Springer, Heidelberg
10. Kessler M, Lübbers DW (1966) Aufbau und Anwendungsmöglichkeiten verschiedener pO$_2$-Elektroden- Pflügers Arch Ges Physiol R 82:291
11. Kessler M (1968) Normale und kritische Sauerstoffversorgung der Leber bei Normo- und Hypothermie. Habilitationsschrift, Marburg
12. Kessler M, Grunewald W (1969) Possibilities of measuring oxygen pressure fields in tissue by multiwire platinum electrodes. Prog in Resp 3:147, Karger, Basel
13. Kessler M (1973) Problems with the use of platinum cathodes for the polarographic measurement of oxygen. In:Kessler M (ed) Oxygen supply. Urban & Schwarzenburg, München, p 81
14. Kivisaari J, Niinikoski J (1973) Use of siliastic tube and capillary sampling technic in the measurement of tissue pO$_2$ and pCO$_2$. Am J Surg Vol V, 125:623
15. Kolthoff IM, Lingane J (1952) Polarography. 2nd ed, Interscience Wiley, New York
16. Kolthoff IM, Jordan J (1952) Oxygen induced electroreduction of hydrogenperoxid and reduction of oxygen at the rotated gold wire electrode. J Am Chem Soc 74:4801
17. Nernst W (1904) Theorie der Reaktionsgeschwindigkeit in heterogenen Systemen. Z Physikal Chem 47:52
18. Schönleben K, Krimme BA, Bünte H, Kessler M (1976) Kontrolle der Intensivbehand-lung durch Messung von Mikrozirkulation und O$_2$-Versorgung. In: Junghanns H (ed) Chirurg Forum 76 für experimentelle und klinische Forschung. p 72 6
19. Spiegel HU, Hauss J, Schönleben K, Bösenberg H (1980) Platinum multiwire surface electrodes in clinical practice. Influence of low pressure ethylenoxide sterilisation on

measuring properties of the multiwire surface electrode (MDO). Arzneim Forsch Drug Res 30:2204

20. Spiegel HU, Hauss J, Schönleben K (1982) Einfluß der Unterdruck-Gassterilisation auf die Meßeigenschaften der Mehrdrahtoberflächenelektrode (MDO). Medizin Technik 101:103

The Effect of Hypercapnia on the Distribution of pO_2 Values in Resting Human Skeletal Muscle

P. Boekstegers, M. Weiss, W. Fleckenstein

Introduction

In order to study the effects of hypercapnia on the oxygen delivery to peripheral tissue in man, the distribution of local oxygen pressure values within the skeletal muscle was measured in healthy human volunteers during inhalation of a gas mixture containing 6.5 % carbon dioxide in air.
In order to be able to distinguish between the effects of hypercapnia on the pO_2 distribution due to the increased concentration of CO_2 and those due to the concomitant change in blood pH, the present study was performed with and without buffering blood pH during carbon dioxide inhalation.

Subjects and methods

For the measurements of the distribution of local oxygen pressure within the left m. biceps brachii, hypodermic polarographic needle electrodes with a tip diameter of 350 μm and a fast response time of t 90 < 500 ms were used in combination with a pO_2 histograph (Eppendorf, Hamburg, FRG) according to the method described by Fleckenstein and Weiss [3, 7]. The needle probe was guided into the muscle through the lumen of a previously inserted catheter (20 G Abbocath). Within the muscle, the needle probe was advanced in steps of 0.7 mm over a total distance of 17 mm. Local pO_2 was measured within less than one second after each step. At the end of each series of forward steps, the probe was swiftly retracted to the original position and its angle of insertion changed slightly for the next series of forward steps.
Thus, every single pO_2 value was taken at a topographically random location within a total muscle volume of approx. 2 to 3 cm³. Within 8 minutes 200 single pO_2 values in the m. biceps brachii were registered in this way and computed to calculate one pO_2 histogram. Three histograms per subject were obtained: one before CO_2 inhalation, one between the 10th and 20th minute and one between the 20th and 30th minute after start of CO_2 inhalation.

Clinical Oxygen Pressure Measurement II
A.M. Ehrly et al. (Eds.)
© Blackwell Ueberreuter Wissenschaft Berlin 1990

Measurements were performed on ten healthy non-smoking male volunteers aged between 21 and 32 years. All probands had a resting period of 20 min before measurements in the supine position were begun. The inspired gas consisted of 6.5 % carbon dioxide, 20 % oxygen and 73.5 % nitrogen in a water-vapour saturated gas mixture. The subjects breathed through a rubber mouth piece fitted with a non-rebreathing valve.

Prior to inhalation, blood samples were obtained from the ear and the cubital vein in order to determine the carbon dioxide partial pressure (pCO_2), the oxygen partial pressure (paO_2), the oxygen saturation of hemoglobin (saO_2), the pH (pH-a, pH-v), the base excess (BE-a, BE-v) and the hemoglobin concentration (Hgb) (ABL 3, Radiometer, Copenhagen; CO-Oximeter 2500, Corning, USA). Blood gases were measured 10, 20 and 30 min after begin of CO_2 inhalation (Table 1). Arterial oxygen saturation and heart rate were monitored throughout the experiments using a pulse oximeter (Nellcor N 100, Dräger, FRG).

Two weeks after this first series of experiments, five of the ten subjects were studied again. During this second session, a solution of 8.4 % sodiumbicarbonate was infused i.v. at a constant rate of 300 ml/h. In order to avoid pain due to the infusion of sodiumbicarbonate, 0.9 % saline was

Table 1. Summary of the data obtained from ten subjects before and during hypercapnia. Values are means (± SD). mpO_2 = mean muscle pO_2 within the m. biceps brachii; paO_2 = arterial pO_2; saO_2 = arterial oxygen saturation; $paCO_2$ = arterial pCO_2; Hb = venous hemoglobin content; pH-a = arterial pH; BE-a = arterial base excess; pH-v = venous pH; BE-v = venous base excess; h.r. = heart rate

	before CO_2 inhalation	10 min CO_2 inhalation	20 min CO_2 inhalation	30 min CO_2 inhalation
mpO_2 (mmHg)	33.3 (± 6.7)	45.5 (± 8.7)	46.9 (± 7.2)	
paO_2 (mmHg)	97.98 (± 12.80)	124.64 (± 10.28)	120.76 (± 6.82)	123.48 (± 4.44)
saO_2 (%)	97.20 (± 0.74)	98.26 (± 1.52)	98.01 (± 0.38)	98.13 (± 0.26)
$paCO_2$ (mmHg)	39.81 (± 2.16)	50.81 (± 3.88)	53.07 (± 3.21)	53.72 (± 1.47)
Hb (g/dl)	14.62 (± 1.41)			14.92 (± 1.04)
pH-a	7.40 (± 0.02)	7.33 (± 0.03)	7.32 (± 0.03)	7.32 (± 0.03)
BE-a (mmol/l)	− 0.07 (± 1.12)	− 0.38 (± 1.10)	0 (± 1.27)	− 0.75 (± 2.20)
pH-v	7.36 (± 0.03)			7.29 (± 0.05)
BE-v (mmol/l)	0.46 (± 0.98)			− 0.54 (± 0.87)
h.r. (1/min)	64 (± 6)	79 (± 6)	86 (± 7)	90 (± 10)

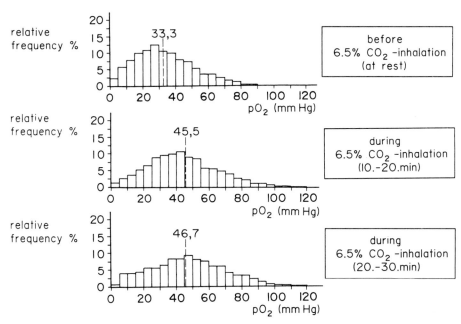

Fig. 1. Pooled pO$_2$ histograms of ten healthy subjects. Local pO$_2$ within m. biceps brachii (pO$_2$); relative frequency of local pO$_2$ values in pO$_2$ classes of 5 mmHg. Mean muscle pO$_2$ indicated by the dashed line

simultaneously given at a rate of 250 ml/h. Venous cannulation was performed at the right forearm, whereas pO$_2$ measurements were carried out in the left m. biceps brachii. All other measurements were repeated as in the first series of measurements.

From all local pO$_2$ values obtained in the ten (five) subjects during the pre-CO$_2$ inhalation period, so-called pooled pO$_2$ histograms (Fig. 1) were calculated. The data were statistically analyzed using the paired student's t-test. A difference was considered statistically significant if the p-value was < 0.01.

Results

1. CO$_2$ inhalation

Table 1 shows that 10 min after beginning of CO$_2$ inhalation, mean arterial pCO$_2$ in the ten subjects exceeded 50 mmHg. Mean arterial pCO$_2$ then remained almost stable between the 10th and 30th min.

pH decreased after beginning of inhalation, and remained fairly stable after that: pH after 10 min = 7.33, after 20 min = 7.32, after 30 min = 7.32.

During CO_2 inhalation arterial pO_2 increased from 98 to 125 mmHg. Before beginning inhalation, the calculated mean arterial oxygen content (caO_2) was 19.30 ml/100 ml. During inhalation, caO_2 climbed to 19.39 ml/100 ml after 10 min and was 19.38 ml/100 ml after 20 min. Mean muscle pO_2 (calculated on the basis of 2000 single pO_2 values) of the ten subjects increased significantly ($p<0.01$) by more than 35 % during CO_2 inhalation (Table 1). Mean muscle pO_2 variations between the 10 to 20 and the 20 to 30 min periods were not significant.

2. CO_2 inhalation at constant blood pH

Table 2 shows that buffering of respiratory acidosis by infusion of 8.4 % sodiumbicarbonate solution kept mean blood pH constant during inhalation. The increase in mean arterial pCO_2 and mean heart rate did not significantly differ from the first series of experiments. Fig. 2 shows that, just as in the experiments without buffering, mean muscle pO_2 (calculated from 1000 single pO_2 values) increased by more than 35 % in the 10 to 20 min period after beginning CO_2 inhalation. Although mean muscle pO_2 fell slightly again to 42 mmHg during the 20 to 30 min period after beginning inhalation, it was still significantly higher compared to the pre-inhalation level of 32 mmHg ($p<0.01$).

Table 2. Summary of the data obtained from the subjects before and during hypercapnia and buffering of blood pH. Values are means ($\pm$ SD). Abbreviations as in Table 1

	before CO_2 inhalation	10 min CO_2 inhalation	20 min CO_2 inhalation	30 min CO_2 inhalation
mpO_2 (mmHg)	32.4 ($\pm$ 6.1)	44.2 ($\pm$ 4.8)	41.6 ($\pm$ 4.4)	
paO_2 (mmHg)	91 ($\pm$ 3.95)	116.38 ($\pm$ 6.95)	119.66 ($\pm$ 6.15)	120.14 ($\pm$ 4.68)
saO_2 (%)	96.73 ($\pm$ 0.42)	97.30 ($\pm$ 1.48)	98.34 ($\pm$ 0.21)	98.42 ($\pm$ 0.15)
$paCO_2$ (mmHg)	39.78 ($\pm$ 1.5)	55.08 ($\pm$ 5.07)	53.72 ($\pm$ 2.88)	55.06 ($\pm$ 1.84)
Hb (g/dl)	15.79 ($\pm$ 1.23)			14.80 ($\pm$ 1.19)
pH-a	7.40 ($\pm$ 0.01)	7.37 ($\pm$ 0.01)	7.39 ($\pm$ 0.01)	7.41 ($\pm$ 0.01)
BE-a (mmol/l)	0.37 ($\pm$ 0.21)	3.78 ($\pm$ 0.79)	5.98 ($\pm$ 1.97)	7.48 ($\pm$ 1.54)
pH-v	7.37 ($\pm$ 0.03)			7.36 ($\pm$ 0.02)
BE-v (mmol/l)	0.35 ($\pm$ 0.57)			4.68 ($\pm$ 0.93)
h.r. (1/min)	68 ($\pm$ 10)	77 ($\pm$ 6)	87 ($\pm$ 7)	96 ($\pm$ 10)

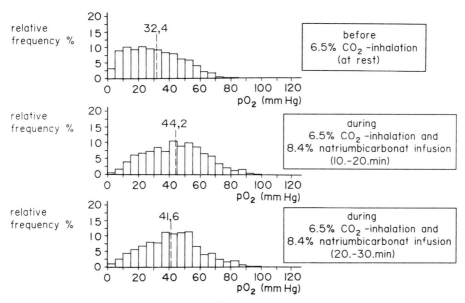

Fig. 2. Pooled pO₂ histograms of five healthy subjects. Local pO₂ within the m. biceps brachii (pO₂); relative frequency of local pO₂ values in pO₂ classes of 5 mmHg. Mean muscle pO₂ indicated by the dashed line

Discussion

CO₂ inhalation elicited a significant increase in mean muscle pO₂ (Table 1, Fig. 1), which remained constant during the first (10 to 20 min) and second (20 to 30 min) measuring periods. Buffering the blood pH did not eliminate this effect (Fig. 2). Thus, a decrease in peripheral blood pH cannot explain our results. As tentative explanation(s) for the observed increase in mean muscle pO₂ during hypercapnia, the following hypotheses might be considered:

1. a hypercapnia-induced decrease in the oxygen consumption of the muscle;
2. a hypercapnia-induced rise in the arterial oxygen content;
3. a hypercapnia-induced rise in the mean capillary blood flow within the muscle.

Re. 1: Since pO₂ measurements were performed in resting skeletal muscle in the supine position, it seems unlikely that a decrease in the oxygen consumption due to an altered muscle activity might explain the very large increase in mean muscular pO₂ observed.

Data on the oxygen consumption of the human skeletal muscle during hypercapnia could not be found in the literature. However, a decrease in whole body oxygen uptake (v̇O₂) was observed during hypercapnia [4].

Since in animal experiments no decrease in $\dot{v}O_2$ during hypercapnia occurred when blood pH was kept constant [2], the authors inferred that hypercapnia-elicited decrease in $\dot{v}O_2$ was largely mediated by a hypercapnia-induced decrease in blood pH. The magnitude of the increase in mean muscle pO_2 in our subjects was almost identical with and without buffering of blood pH (Figs. 1 and 2). Thus, a hypercapnia-induced decrease in muscular oxygen consumption could at best be responsible for only a small fraction of the increase in mean muscle pO_2 during hypercapnia.

Re. 2: During CO_2 inhalation, arterial pO_2 increased from 98 to 125 mmHg, apparently due to hyperventilation of our subjects. The arterial oxygen content increased only slightly by 0.09 ml/100 ml (see results). Though the increase in arterial pO_2 might have contributed to the observed increase in mean muscle pO_2, it seems unlikely that the quantitatively insignificant increase in arterial oxygen content could account for the more than 35 % increase in mean muscle pO_2 during hypercapnia.

Re. 3: Assuming that the observed increase in mean muscle pO_2 during hypercapnia was neither mainly induced by a decrease in the oxygen consumption nor by an increase in the arterial oxygen content, a plausible explanation for the results seems to be an increase in the mean capillary blood flow in the muscle. An increase in the mean capillary blood flow within the m. biceps brachii could be a result of the well documented increase in cardiac output during hypercapnia [5, 6].

Moreover, local vasodilation of muscular vessels due to a specific localized effect of carbon dioxide or a concomitant change in blood pH has been suggested [1, 5]. But since hypercapnia-induced increase in mean muscle pO_2 turned out to be similar both with and without buffering of blood pH, our results would be more consistent with a specific carbon dioxide mediated vasodilation. However, the precise mechanism underlying hypercapnia-induced increase in mean muscle pO_2 requires further investigation.

References

1. Daugherty RM, Scott JB, Dabney JM, Haddy FJ (1967) Local effects of O_2 and CO_2 on limb, renal, and coronary vascular resistance. Am J Physiol 213:1102
2. Cain SM (1970) Increased oxygen uptake with passive hyperventilation of dogs. J Appl Physiol 28:4
3. Fleckenstein W (1987) Die Entwicklung der Feinnadel-Gewebe-pO_2- Histographie zum klinisch eingesetzten Diagnoseverfahren. 2. Treffp. Medizintechnik. p 92
4. Karetzky MS, Cain MS (1970) Effect of carbon dioxide on oxygen uptake during hyperventilation in normal man. J Appl Physiol 28:8
5. Richardson DW, Wassermann AJ, Patterson JL (1962) General and regional circulatory responses to change in blood pH and carbon dioxide tension. J Clin Invest 40:31
6. Suutarinen T (1966) Cardiovascular response to changes in arterial carbon dioxide tension: An experimental study on thoracotomized dogs. Acta Physiol Scand 67:266
7. Weiss Ch, Fleckenstein W (1986) Local tissue pO_2 measured with "thick" needle probes. In: Funktionsanalyse biologischer Systeme. Steiner, Stuttgart 15:155

Intramuscular Oxygen Partial Pressure in the Tibialis Anterior Muscle of Apparently Healthy Subjects

F. Jung, M. Bock, R. Heinrich, W. Kolepke, H.W. Krawzak, H. Kiesewetter, E. Wenzel

Introduction

In order to be able to estimate the intramuscular oxygen supply in patients it is essential to know the physiologic oxygen pressure histogram under standard test conditions. For this reason we measured the local oxygen distribution in the tibialis anterior muscle in 71 apparently healthy subjects using a macro-pO_2-puncture electrode. The results were analyzed so as to highlight age and sex dependence as well as the influence of behavior-induced cardiovascular risk factors such as smoking and hypokinesia.

Since measurements of oxygen partial pressure at the angiologic out patient department are carried out between eight o'clock in the morning and about half past four in the afternoon and since it is known from experimental data in mammalians that there is a circadian rhythm of mean muscle pO_2 [4] we had to ascertain if time-dependent reference values needed to be taken so as to be better able to judge the results.

Therefore, the circadian rhythm of oxygen supply was investigated in a group of 14 subjects. Furthermore, we investigated the day-to-day variation in the test results.

Subjects

In all, 71 apparently healthy subjects aged between 19 and 80 years were examined at two different locations. The younger subjects between 19 and 50 years of age (n=58) were examined at the Angiologic Outpatient Department of the University of Saarland, the older ones between 60 and 80 years (n=13) at the Medical-Geriatric Hospital of the "Ruhruniversität Bochum". Methods, application and criteria for inclusion were fixed in advance and carried out identically in both centres. So as to exclude concomitant diseases all subjects underwent a medical examination including laboratory analysis and doppler sonography and their case histories were checked. Some demographic and clinical data are given in Table 1.

Clinical Oxygen Pressure Measurement II
A.M. Ehrly et al. (Eds.)
© Blackwell Ueberreuter Wissenschaft Berlin 1990

Table 1. Demographic and clinical data

Entire group	n=71
Sex (m/f)	50/21
Age (yrs)	38.3 ± 18.7
Height (cm)	176 ± 7.4
Weight (kg)	71.2 ± 10.1
Blood pressure, systolic (mmHg)	123 ± 13
Blood pressure, diastolic (mmHg)	78 ± 6
Heart rate (1/min)	72 ± 8

17 subjects were smokers and 7 were overweight. Drugs were not taken during the examination. 13 out of the healthy subjects practised sports at least 2 hours per week (about 4.9 ± 1.6 hrs/week), 21 participants had no sporting activities.

Test method

Intramuscular oxygen histograms were measured using the "Makroelektrode, Typ pO_2-Histograph KIMOC (Eppendorf Gerätebau GmbH, Hamburg)" according to the method developed by Fleckenstein et al. [2] [see also in this volume: Kolepke W et al.: Measurement of the intramuscular oxygen partial pressure in the tibialis anterior muscle of patients with stage I-III hypertension according to WHO].

Statistics

In order to compare the relative frequency (cathectic numbers of the categories of the oxygen partial pressure histogram) the Kolmogoroff-Smirnow test was applied [11]
Multiple-sample comparisons for the examination of both the circadian and the day-to-day variation were carried out as global test according to Friedman [12].
Differences below the 5 % level were considered to be significant, below the 10 % level to be according to tendency.

Results

The oxygen partial pressure histogram of the entire group of healthy subjects is shown in Fig. 1a. The sample displays a normal distribution (Kolmogoroff-Smirnow test), the mean oxygen partial pressure in healthy subjects is 27.2 mmHg, the median value 25.2 mmHg. The distribution of the relative frequency of mean oxygen partial pressure values is illustrated in Fig. 1b. Mean oxygen partial pressures below 12 mmHg were not found in healthy subjects, the most frequent mean oxygen partial pressure being about 28 mmHg (between 24 and 32 mmHg). The highest mean value ranges between 48 and 56 mmHg. The reference range (by definition 95 % of the range [3]) for the mean oxygen partial pressure is between 16.4

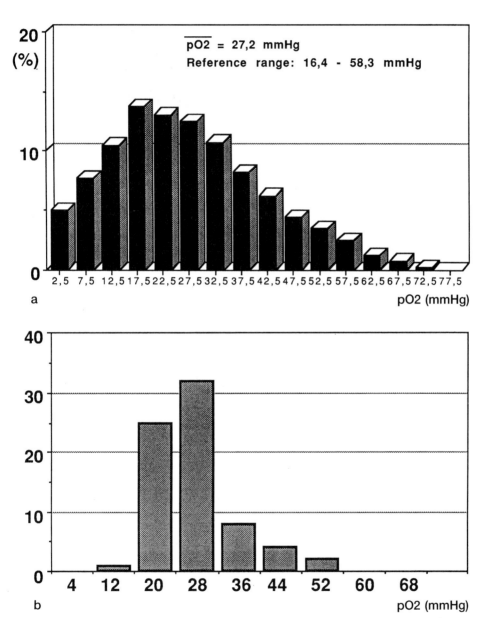

Fig. 1 a, b. a) Mean oxygen partial pressure histogram of healthy subjects. **b)** Distribution of mean oxygen partial pressure values

and 58.3 mmHg. The intramuscular oxygen partial pressure does not seem to be age dependent. Fig. 2a shows the correlation between the mean oxygen partial pressure and age, the coefficient of correlation is r=-0.09.

In a few cases oxygen supply seems to vary according to sex, but this cannot be substantiated by the statistics. The mean value of the females (n=21) with 30.1 mmHg (median 28.0 mmHg) is somewhat higher than that of the males (n=50) with 25.7 mmHg (median 24.0 mmHg). The pool distributions of the oxygen partial pressures are given in Fig. 2b.

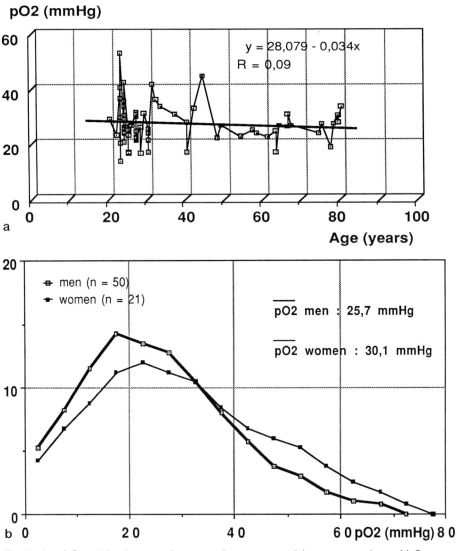

Fig. 2a,b. a) Correlation between intramuscular oxygen partial pressure and age. **b)** Oxygen pressure distribution for males and females

The mean oxygen partial pressure histogram of the younger healthy subjects (up to an age of 40 years) practising sports regularly is shown as line histogram in Fig. 3a. The non-athletes displayed oxygen partial pressure values below 25 mmHg more often than the athletes; above this value it was the other way round. The mean oxygen supply of athletes is on a somewhat higher level. This difference, however, is only according to tendency ($p < 0.09$, Kolmogoroff-Smirnow test).

Fig. 3b shows the line histograms of smokers and non-smokers in two age groups. The pooled oxygen pressure histograms of smokers (n=12) and non-smokers (n=28) up to the age of 40 are nearly identical, smokers presenting a mean pO_2 of 27.5 mmHg and non-smokers of 27.0 mmHg. Smokers (n=5) between the ages of 60 and 80 presented a mean oxygen partial pressure of 24.9 mmHg, but non-smokers of the same age group (n=8) almost the same value as the younger non-smokers. However, this result is not significant.

In order to judge the circadian rhythm, the oxygen partial pressure histogram in the tibialis anterior muscle of 14 subjects was measured at eight and eleven o'clock in the morning and four o'clock in the afternoon. The median values of each measurement for each subject at the three measuring times are shown in Fig. 4a, the mean course in Fig. 4b.

Significant differences between the measuring times could not be ascertained. The three samples with the mean oxygen partial pressure values are taken from the same parent population (Friedman test). The variation in the test results for repeated measurements in the course of the same day yields a coefficient of variation CV = 22.5 %.

Further, the variation in the test results over a period of three days was investigated in n=13 subjects. Measurements were done always at the same time, 8 o'clock in the morning, on a Monday, Tuesday and Wednesday. The results of each measurement – as median values – are to be seen in Fig. 5a, the mean results in Fig. 5b.

There was no significant change in the muscular oxygen partial pressures measured over this three-day period. The samples of the pO_2 mean values of the first three days are taken from the same parent population (Friedman test). The variation in the test results upon repeating the experiment the next day is CV = 18.3 %.

Finally, the reproducibility of the test method was investigated in n=30 subjects. To this effect, two measurements were made successively in an adjacent vascular region. One participant had a variation in the mean pO_2 of more than 50 % (increase). Variations between 40 and 50 % were not observed. In 5 participants the variation was between 30 and 40 % (3 increases, 2 decreases), in 4 between 20 and 30 % (2 increases, 2 decreases), and in 9 between 10 and 20 % (7 increases, 2 decreases). 11 healthy patients showed variations below 10 % (4 increases, 5 decreases, 2 constant). The coefficient of variation for repeated experiments is 13.5 %.

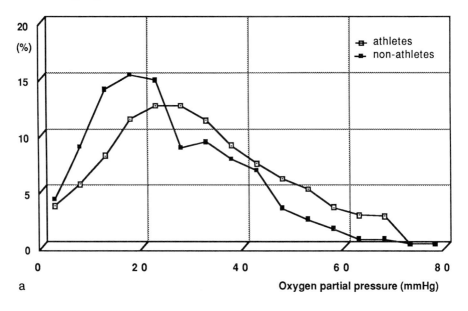

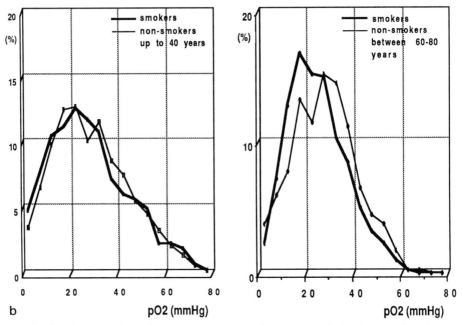

Fig. 3a, b. a) Comparison of the mean oxygen partial pressure of athletes (n=13) and non-athletes (n=8). **b)** Comparison of the mean oxygen partial pressure of smokers (n=14) and non-smokers (n=30)

pO2 (mmHg)

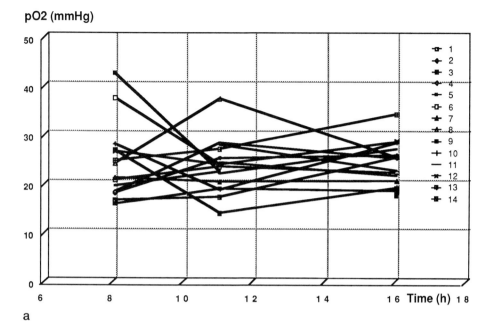

a

Mean pO2 (mmHg)

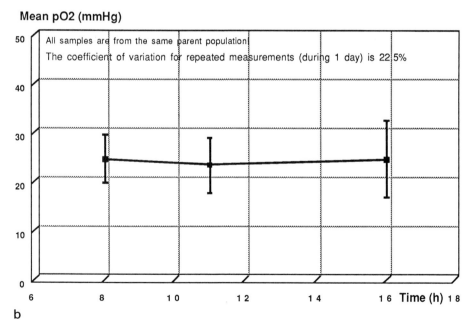

All samples are from the same parent population.
The coefficient of variation for repeated measurements (during 1 day) is 22.5%

b

Fig. 4a, b. a) Median values of the oxygen partial pressure for 14 subjects during one day.
b) Mean oxygen partial pressure values of 14 subjects at 8 and 11 a.m. and 4 p.m.

Discussion

The mean oxygen partial pressure of apparently healthy subjects between 19 and 80 years of age is 27.2 mmHg (median 25.2 mmHg), the reference range varying between 16.4 and 58.3 mmHg. The distribution of the pooled single values is shown in Fig. 1. The median value of 25.2 mmHg

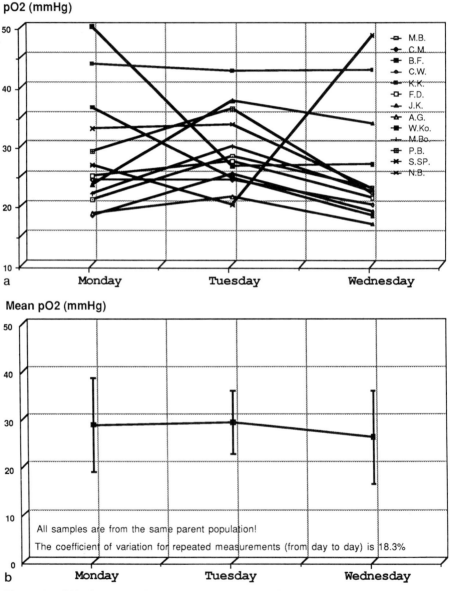

Fig. 5 a, b. a) Median values of the oxygen partial pressure for 13 subjects for three days running. b) Mean partial oxygen pressure values of 13 subjects for three days

determined here is comparable with the value of 27.0 mmHg found by Kersting et al. [9] in n=9 healthy subjects.

The comparison of age and intramuscular pO_2 mean values yielded no age dependence of the intramuscular partial oxygen pressure (Fig. 2). The slight decrease in the mean pO_2 with increasing age might be due to some very athletic younger participants (practising regularly more than 7 hours sports per week) with an extraordinarily high oxygen pressure level (measurements on 3 patients with approx. 50 mmHg were repeated one week later, but the same high values were again obtained). This result agrees well with rheologic results and with results determined by vital capillaroscopy. We were able to demonstrate that the capillary blood flow as well as the vasomotor reserve remain nearly constant with increasing age (in healthy subjects) [6]. Also blood fluidity turned out to be age independent in healthy subjects [8].

The oxygen supply seems to be marginally sex dependent, the mean oxygen pressure for the females being 30.1 mmHg (median 28.0 mmHg) and thus somewhat higher than for the males with 25.7 mmHg (median 24.0 mmHg). The number of female participants examined (n=21) is, however, too small to make a reliable statement.

Also the statements concerning the behavior-induced risk factors are to be considered only as preliminary results. Anyhow, sports seems to have a positive influence on the muscular supply. The 13 participants practising sports regularly displayed a mean oxygen partial pressure of 30.4 mmHg, which was 19.7 % higher than the 24.4 mmHg of the non-athletes.

Between smokers (n=17) and non-smokers (n=36) there was no difference up to the age of 40, the pool distributions of the oxygen partial pressure being nearly identical (see Fig. 3). However, apart from the small case number, the relatively moderate mean consumption of 18 cigarettes a day as well as the relatively limited number of years the subjects had been smoking must also be taken into consideration. Besides, it must be assumed that the vascular regulation in these young healthy subjects is very efficient and that the hematocrit, which is slightly increased in smokers, is only of subordinate importance for the capillary system [1]. As for the older participants, smokers have a mean pO_2 value which is aprrox. 9 % lower than that of the non-smokers. This might – besides the gradual loss of arterial elasticity [10] - also be due to a chronic bronchitis with markedly elevated plasma viscosity [7] in patients who have been smoking for many years.

The coefficients of variation for measuring the oxygen partial pressure (22.5 % for repeated measurements during the course of one day and 18.3 % for measurements between days) are within the usual range for biological measurements (under resting conditions) [6]. The circadian variation in oxygen supply of the individuals, however, is accidental and does not lead to a change in the mean values of the groups under the test conditions described here. This also applies to the measurements between days, there being no significant differences observable here either. Nevertheless, important variations may occur in individual cases.

In summary, it can be concluded that valid judgements of the intramuscular oxygen partial pressure can be effected by means of the test method presented. The reference range of the oxygen pressure in the tibialis anterior muscle is between 16.4 and 58.3 mmHg with a mean value of 27.2 mmHg. But to confirm these results further investigations are needed. There is no age dependence of the intramuscular oxygen partial pressure. While sports tends to produce a shift to the right of the oxygen histogram, a shift to the left can be observed in patients who have been smoking for many years.

Acknowledgements. We thank Ms G. Natterer for her skilful technical assistance.

References

1. Dintenfass L (1975) Elevation of blood viscosity, aggregation of red cells, hematocrit and fibrinogen levels in cigarette smokers. Med J Aust 1:617
2. Fleckenstein W, Heinrich R, Kersting Th, Schomerus H, Weiss Ch (1984) A new method for the bed-side recording of tissue pO₂ histograms. Verh Dtsch Ges Inn Med 90:439
3. Galen RS, Gambino SR (1979) Norm und Normabweichung klinischer Daten. Fischer, Stuttgart
4. Günderoth-Palmowski M, Heinrich R, Palmowski P, Dette S, Daiss B, Grauer W, Egberts EH (1988) Circadian course of pO₂ oscillations in skeletal muscle of intact and portocaval shunted (PCA) rats. Adv Exp Med Biol 222:603
5. Heinrich R, Günderoth-Palmowski M, Grauer W, Machac N, Dette S, Egberts EH (1987) Gewebe pO₂ im Muskel tibialis anterior gesunder Probanden bei normovolämischer Hämodilution mit 10 % HES 200. VASA 16:318
6. Jung F, Berthold R, Wappler M, Konze R, Kiesewetter H, Wenzel E (1987) Referenzbereich der reaktiven Hyperämie anscheinend gesunder Probanden im Alter zwischen 6 und 65 Jahren. In: 6. gemeinsame Tagung der Angiologischen Gesellschaft der Bundesrepublik Deutschland, der Schweiz und Österreichs, Wien
7. Jung F, Roggenkamp HG, Ringelstein EB, Leipniz G, Schneider R, Kiesewetter H, Zeller H (1986) Effect of sex, age, body height and smoking on plasma viscosity. Klin Wochenschr 64:1076
8. Jung F, Kiesewetter H, Roggenkamp HG, Nüttgens HP, Ringelstein EB, Gerhards M, Kotitschke G, Wenzel E, Zeller H (1986) Bestimmung der Referenzbereiche rheologischer Parameter. Klin Wochenschr 64:375
9. Kersting T, Reinhart K, Fleckenstein W, Dennhardt R, Eyrich K, Weiss Ch (1985) The effect of dopamin on muscle pO₂ in healthy volunteers and intensive care patients. Eur J Anaesthesiol 2:143
10. Korkuschko OW, Iwanow LA, Sarkissow KG (1984) Über die Gefäßveränderungen der unteren Extremitäten und ihre Bedeutung für die Sauerstoffversorgung der Gewebe im höheren und hohen Lebensalter. Z Gerontol 17:39
11. Kreyszig E (1979) Statistische Methoden und ihre Anwendung. Vandehoeck & Ruprecht, Göttingen
12. Sachs L (1984) Angewandte Statistik. Springer, Berlin

Investigation on the Reproducibility of Intramuscular pO$_2$ Measurement in Patients by means of the Tissue pO$_2$-Histograph KIMOC/Sigma

G. Singbartl, G. Metzger, G. Beister, R. Stögbauer

Introduction

Tissue pO$_2$ (tpO$_2$) measurements with polarographic needles enable clinicians to determine tpO$_2$ in patients as a routine procedure with only minimal invasiveness [1]. Measurements are influenced by the physical and clinical properties of the polarographic needle and the tissue as well as by the variability of the probe signal due to histological damage when introducing the needle into tissue [2]. Therefore, both the judgement of local oxygen supply and the monitoring of the therapeutic measures applied make it important to know just how reliable the method is. Accuracy and reproducibility of the single tpO$_2$-measurement by means of the tissue pO$_2$-Histograph KIMOC were examined under a variety of clinical conditions by comparing a first measurement succeeded immediately by a second one, in order to allow a precise judgement and interpretation of tpO$_2$ measurements and changes.

Methods

The investigation was performed in 60 persons (5 healthy persons, 38 patients with arterial occlusive disease of the lower limb, 17 intensive care patients). All measurements were made in the resting tibial anterior muscle after a period of equilibration of at least 30 minutes. The second measurement followed immediately after the first one within 15 minutes. Experimental conditions (room temperature, patients' position, FIO$_2$, ventilation, pharmacological therapy) were held constant during the study. The investigation was carried out with the Sigma-pO$_2$-Histograph/KIMOC (Sigma Instrumente GmbH, Berlin, FRG) using polarographic needle probes with recessed and membranized gold wire ($\varnothing 12.5\mu m$) microcathodes as described by Fleckenstein et al. [1]. The diameter of the probe shaft was 350μm. Every single measurement was the result of the recording of 200 individual local pO$_2$ values. After every single value the stepwise movement of the needle consisted of a rapid forward movement of 1.0 mm followed by a rapid backward movement of 0.3 mm. After

Clinical Oxygen Pressure Measurement II
A.M. Ehrly et al. (Eds.)
© Blackwell Ueberreuter Wissenschaft Berlin 1990

proceeding into the muscle to a maximum depth of 3.0 cm the needle was withdrawn automatically and inserted by hand again in a slightly changed direction so as to obtain local values from fresh tissue. The 200 local values were recorded and computed by the integrated computer and displayed on a monitor screen. The resulting tpO₂ histogram of the probe was established as well as the mean value and the values of the 10%, 50% and 90% percentiles. The statistical significance of the results was calculated using student's t-test for paired observations ($p \leq 0.05$).

Results

The mean values of the first set of measurements are scattered over a wide range (7.4 – 43.5 mmHg) because of the inhomogenity of the group of patients. The pooled histograms of the first and second sets of measurements are identical with regard both to configuration and position (Fig. 1). This is reflected by the mean values of the first (18.9 mmHg) and the second set of measurements (18.7 mmHg) and the likewise small differences in the 10%, 50% and 90% percentiles (for values see Fig. 1). The second set of measurements yielded higher tpO₂ values in comparison to the first set in 32 cases ($\bar{x} = +2.0$ mmHg) and lower tpO₂ values in 28 other cases ($\bar{x} = -2.1$ mmHg) (Fig. 2). This adds up to a deviation of + 11.4% and − 11.6% in either direction. The deviations obtained reveal a normal distribution. Figure 3 compares the absolute values (mmHg) of the corresponding mean values and the percentiles of the first and the second set

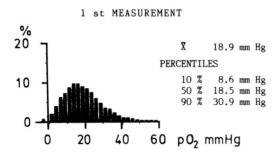

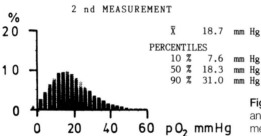

Fig. 1. Pooled histograms of the 60 first and 60 second measurements. Values of mean, 10%, 50% and 90% percentiles

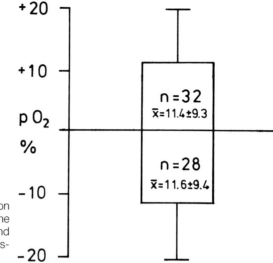

Fig. 2. Mean value ±SD of the deviation of the second measurement from the first one. n = 60 for both the first and second set of measurements. Abscissa: percentage of deviation

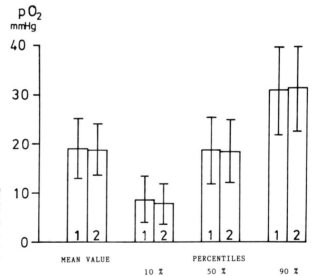

Fig. 3. Mean values ±SD of the first (1) and second (2) set of measurements of the tpO₂ mean value (x) and the 10%, 50% and 90% percentiles. n = 60 for both the first and second set of measurements.

of measurements. A statistically significant difference cannot be found either for the mean values or for the percentiles (p ≤ 0.05). The group of patients investigated showed a large variation in the tpO₂ values obtained in the first set of measurements. For this reason we established three groups according to the height of the first tpO₂ value (I. <15 mmHg, II. ≥15 ≤25 mmHg, III. >25 mmHg), in order to find out whether there was a difference in the deviation pattern of the second set of measurements correlating with the height of the first tpO₂ values (Table 1). The resulting

Table 1

	1st Measurement $\bar{x} \pm SD$ (mmHg)	2nd Measurement $\bar{x} \pm SD$ (mmHg)	absol. $\bar{x} \pm SD$ (mmHg)	% 2 vs 1 $\bar{x} \pm SD$ (%)
Entire Group n = 60	18.9 ± 6.3	18.7 ± 5.7	2.1 ± 1.8	11.5 ± 9.3
Group I n = 17	12.3 ± 1.9	13.5 ± 2.8	2.0 ± 1.3	15.8 ± 10.2
Group II n = 33	19.1 ± 2.5	18.6 ± 3.2	1.8 ± 1.5	9.7 ± 8.5
Group III n = 10	29.4 ± 5.3	27.9 ± 4.6	3.1 ± 2.7	10.3 ± 8.9

mean values of the deviations (9.7% – 15.8%) are in the same range as for the entire group (x = 11.5%), so there was no statistically significant difference in the deviation pattern for groups I, II and III.

Discussion

The method applied for tissue pO_2 measurement is impaired by systematic and accidental errors in measurement [2]. Oxygen consumption, stirring effect and temperature effect of the electrode are some of the error sources that have to be mentioned [1]. The degree of error of the O_2-electrode under standardized in-vitro-conditions amounts to about ±1 % [3]. In contrast to these errors in measurement the influence of histological damages when introducing and advancing the needle are very difficult to estimate [2]. It can be assumed that this error is much smaller than the deviation between the first and the second set of measurements demonstrated in this paper. However, the physiological variability of perfusion, arterio-venous-difference for oxygen, and O_2-consumption in the resting muscle [4] could be at least one reason leading to the deviation obtained – besides a certain error in measurement caused by the method itself. According to the normal distribution, the expression $\bar{x} \pm 2$ SD describes the field in which we find more than 95% of all deviations; this leads to an in-vivo-reproducibility of about ± 25 to ± 30% (11.5 ± 2 x 9.3%). These findings are in agreement with the variability of pO_2-values in the tibial anterior muscle in healthy people [5].

References

1. Fleckenstein W, Heinrich R, Kersting T, Schomerus H, Weiss C (1984) A new method for the bedside recordings of tissue-pO_2- histograms. Verh Dtsch Ges Inn Med 90:439

2. Baumgärtl H (1985) Systematische Untersuchungen der Meßeigenschaften von Nadel-elektroden bei polarographischer Messung der lokalen pO$_2$ im Gewebe. In: Ehrly AM, Hauss, Huch (eds) Klinische Sauerstoffdruckmessung. Münchner Wissenschaftliche Publikationen, München
3. Kunze K (1969) Das Sauerstoffdruckfeld im normalen und pathologisch veränderten Muskel. Schriftenreihe Neurologie, Springer, Berlin, p 14
4. Golenhofen K (1971) Skeletmuskel. In: Lehrbuch der Physiologie in Einzeldarstellungen. Vol. 1, Springer, Berlin, p 385
5. Kunze K (1966) Sauerstoffdruck und Durchblutung in der menschlichen Muskulatur. Pflügers Arch Ges Physiol 298:59

Effects of Hemodilution with Middle Molecular HES Solution on Muscle Tissue pO$_2$ in Healthy Volunteers

R. Heinrich, M. Günderoth-Palmowski, N. Machac

Introduction

The main area indicated for use of hydroxyethyl starch preparations (HES: 10 % HES 200/0.5; Pfrimmer & Co. GmbH, Erlangen, FRG, in cooperation with Laevosan, Linz, Austria) is normovolemic hemodilution in the treatment of peripheral arterial occlusive diseases. Extensive investigations in patients and healthy subjects are available in the literature demonstrating that the infusion of low molecular HES preparations both changes blood flow properties and, at the same time, improves the oxygen supply to the extremity muscles [Ehrly et al., 1979 and 1987; Kopp et al., 1982). The studies on the effect of HES infusion or hemodilution on tissue pO$_2$ in the skeletal muscles were performed either with microneedle electrodes or with multi-wire surface electrodes [Ehrly et al., 1979; survey in Kiesewetter et al., 1986]. Both methods can be used clinically only to a limited extent: microneedle probes have the disadvantage of mechanical instability, and measurement with the multi-wire surface electrode requires the surgical exposure of the organ. A technically new method for measuring tissue pO$_2$ in the muscle with fast reacting macro-electrodes (probe diameter 0.35 mm; pO$_2$-Histograph, KIMOC®, GMS Kiel-Mielkendorf, FRG) yields data comparable to the results obtained with the microneedle electrode or multi-wire surface electrode [Fleckenstein et al., 1984]. The clinical applicability of this pO$_2$ measuring method is warranted by the following features: mechanical and electrical stability of the measuring probes and reusability after sterilization.

The aim of the present study was to examine the changes in tissue pO$_2$ in the M. tibialis anterior of healthy subjects during isovolemic hemodilution with infusion of 500 ml of HES 200.

Subjects and methods

The study was performed in 7 healthy male subjects, non-smokers, aged between 40 and 57 years (average age: 45.7 years). The study protocol had previously been approved by the Ethics Commission of Tuebingen University.

Clinical Oxygen Pressure Measurement II
A. M. Ehrly et al. (Eds.)
© Blackwell Ueberreuter Wissenschaft Berlin 1990

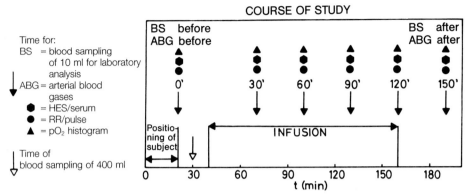

Fig. 1. Experimental design

Hemodilution

A sample of 400 ml of venous blood was taken over a period of 15 min from each subject for the purpose of normovolemic hemodilution. For the determination of laboratory parameters, blood samples of 10 ml were taken at defined times during the course of the study, i.e. also during HES infusion (Fig. 1). The total blood volume collected amounted to about 500 ml, which was substituted within 2 hours by infusion of 500 ml of a 100% HES solution (MW 200,000; degree of substitution 0.5).

Clinico-chemical parameters

Before, during and after isovolemic hemodilution, the following laboratory parameters were determined together with the pO_2 measurements: Hb, Hct, hemogram, serum electrolytes, sodium and potassium, serum protein, serum HES concentration, arterial blood gases. Determination of the serum concentration of HES 200 was performed according to Foerster et al. [1981]. In addition, close meshed controls of blood pressure and heart rate were performed.

pO_2 measurement

For measurement of tissue pO_2, local anaesthesia with 2 ml of Meaverin was strictly limited to the skin. The pO_2 needle probes (diameter 0.35 mm, steel-sheated) were gradually inserted into the M. tibialis ant. by a micromanipulator through a catheter (20 G Abbocath) serving as guide. Further details of this method have already been published [Fleckenstein 1982, 1984].

Experimental Design

Histograms were recorded at intervals of 30 minutes before, during and after hemodilution (Fig. 1). For each histogram, 200 individual pO_2 values were recorded (measuring time 5 minutes). After each histogram, an intermediate calibration for calculating the probe drift was performed. The individual histograms of the subjects were pooled to corresponding sum histograms per measuring time, a usual procedure for comparing test results.

Results

In none of the 7 cases under observation infusion of 500 ml of 10% HES 200 per subject did cause any allergic reactions. Measurement of tissue pO_2 was without complications in all subjects so that all investigations could be carried through to the end. Evaluation of blood pressure, heart rate, and measurements of arterial blood gases before, during and after hemodilution yielded values which were all within the normal range; they are therefore not taken into consideration in the presentation of results.

Laboratory Parameters

Hemodilution led to an average decrease in the Hb concentration from 14.7g % ±0.4 to 12.6g % ±0.4 and of the hematocrit (Hct) from 43.5 % ±2.2 to 37.4 % ±1.5. Total protein dropped from 7.33g % ±0.3 to 5.9g % ±0.2. Serum values of sodium (Na^+) and potassium (K^+) remained unaffected by HES infusion. Table 1 shows the individual values of the subjects.

Fig. 2 shows the average course of the serum HES concentration in the subjects during and after infusion. As expected, serum HES values increased during infusion.

Tissue pO_2

Mean tissue pO_2 in the muscle examined was 16.2 ±3.5 mmHg before hemodilution (t=0). As expected, the sum histogram shows an almost bell-shaped configuration. 30 minutes after the start of infusion (t=30) of HES 200, the mean tissue pO_2 rose to 19.1 ±6.6 mmHg. 60 minutes after the start of infusion (t=60), a further rise of the tissue pO_2 to 27.3 ±9.3 mmHg was observed. The rise of mean tissue pO_2 is paralleled by an increased saturation of pO_2 values classed above 40 mmHg so that the homogenous, i.e. bell-shaped, distribution of the pO_2 classes within the sum histogram is lost. After 90 minutes (t=90), mean muscle pO_2 has

Table 1. Age and laboratory parameters of the test subjects before and after normovolemic hemodilution (*p < 0.005; n.m. not measured)

Successive no.	1	2	3	4	5	6	7	x̄ ± SD	Normal value
Age	41	41	57	42	39	48	52	45.7 ± 6.8	
before Hb (g %)	14.8	15.1	14.2	14.0	15.1	15.0	14.7	14.7 ± 0.4	14.0−18.0
after	12.9	13.0	12.3	12.5	11.9	13.0	12.9	12.6 ± 0.4*	
before Hct %	44.5	43.4	40.4	40.9	43.8	46.6	45.1	43.5 ± 2.2	42−52
after	38.8	38.2	38.4	36.2	36.2	39.5	37.6	37.4 ± 1.5*	
before Total protein (g %)	7.4	7.7	6.9	7.2	7.0	7.0	7.5	7.3 ± 0.3	6.5 −8.5
after	6.1	6.0	5.5	6.0	5.6	5.9	n.m.	5.9 ± 0.2*	
before Sodium (mEq/l)	142	145	140	138	139	140	142	142 ± 3.8	130−150
after	140	145	134	135	145	146	136	140 ± 5.2	
before Potassium (mEq/l)	3.9	3.6	4.4	4.2	4.0	4.6	4.0	4.1 ± 0.3	3.6−5.2
after	3.9	3.6	4.7	3.9	4.3	4.2	3.7	4.0 ± 0.4	

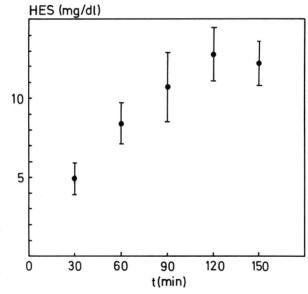

Fig. 2. Average course of the serum HES concentration (mg/dl) in the subjects (n=7) during and after infusion of a 10 % HES 200 solution

slightly dropped to 24.8 ±7.1 mmHg. After 120 minutes (t=120), the volume has been restored, but a mean tissue pO$_2$ of 26.4 ±8.4 mmHg was found, i.e. no further significant change of the mean tissue pO$_2$ as compared to that at time t=90 was demonstrable.

Thirty minutes after the end of infusion (t=150), mean tissue pO₂ remained at 27.1 ±7.8 mmHg, thus showing no further marked change. The configuration of sum histograms at times t=90 and t=120 essentially corresponds to the sum histogram at time t=60, showing an increased saturation of the pO₂ classes above 40 mmHg and concomitant inhomogenous histogram configuration. The configuration of the sum histogram

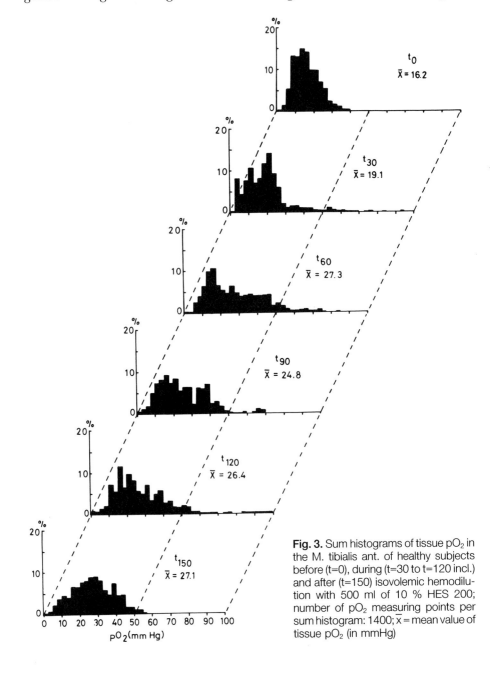

Fig. 3. Sum histograms of tissue pO₂ in the M. tibialis ant. of healthy subjects before (t=0), during (t=30 to t=120 incl.) and after (t=150) isovolemic hemodilution with 500 ml of 10 % HES 200; number of pO₂ measuring points per sum histogram: 1400; x̄ = mean value of tissue pO₂ (in mmHg)

Table 2. Mean tissue pO$_2$ in the M. tibialis ant. of the subjects before (t=0), during (t= 30 to t=120 incl.) and after (t=150) normovolemic hemodilution with 10 % HES 200

Successive no.	1	2	3	4	5	6	7	$\bar{x} \pm$ SD
t = 0	20.6	17.9	14.7	17.0	19.0	13.4	10.5	16.2 ± 3.5
t = 30	25.9	19.7	22.0	20.4	19.6	6.7	11.3	19.1 ± 6.6
t = 60	42.4	27.7	23.7	33.7	21.4	28.8	13.8	27.3 ± 9.3
t = 90	30.0	29.6	17.1	21.7	17.4	35.6	21.1	24.8 ± 7.1
t = 120	37.3	23.8	26.2	33.8	18.2	31.6	14.2	26.4 ± 8.4
t = 150	27.2	33.0	15.9	19.3	24.3	37.2	32.9	27.1 = 7.8

at time t=150 shows an almost bell-shaped distribution as compared to the histograms described above.

The values of the mean muscle pO$_2$ (in mmHg) of the individual subjects at the different measuring times are listed in Table 2 and Fig. 3).

Discussion

The main clinical field of application of hydroxyethyl starch (HES) with a molecular weight of 200,000 and a degree of substitution of 0.5 is volume deficiency of various origins. In addition, it is administered for therapeutic hemodilution. This principle of reducing the relative volume portion of blood cells, i.e. lowering of the hematocrit value, as a simple therapeutic measure, for example within the scope of stage-adapted therapy of peripheral arterial occlusive disease, is called isovolemic hemodilution. An important therapeutic effect of isovolemic hemodilution with colloidal substances is their positive influence on the flow properties of blood [Ehrly et al., 1979; Landgraf et al., 1981], which leads to an improvement in oxygen supply to the tissue, as direct measurements of tissue pO$_2$ show. Since the studies by Rudofsky et al. [1981, 1982] it is known that hemodilution leads furthermore to an increase in blood flow which, under normovolemic conditions, can be demonstrated over a period of several weeks. This increase in blood flow is explained by a decrease in peripheral resistance (cardiac afterload) accompanied by an increase in cardiac output without any increase in heart rate. The expected reduction in the oxygen transport capacity of the blood can thus be compensated for [Rieger, 1982]. Sunder- Plassmann was able to demonstrate in animal experiments not only that collateral perfusion is increased by 100%, but also that homogenization of the blood flow pattern occurs throughout the capillary system [Sunder-Plassmann et al., 1982].

The aim of the present study was to investigate the effect of isovolemic hemodilution, using a middle molecular HES solution, on oxygen supply and pO$_2$ pressure distribution in the extremity muscles of healthy male subjects. In addition to a significant reduction in the hematocrit (Hct) within the scope of isovolemic hemodilution from about 44% to about 37% and unchanged arterial blood gas values, an increase in the mean muscle pO_2 from about 16 mmHg (before hemodilution) to about 27 mmHg (30 minutes after having reached isovolemia) was observed. The increase in mean tissue pO_2 is demonstrable already 30 minutes after the start of infusion (t=30) of 10% HES 200 (see table 2). The markedly raised level of tissue pO_2 in the M. tibialis anterior as compared to the initial value is demonstrable both during and after isovolemic hemodilution. In addition to this dilution-related increase in mean tissue pO_2, a marked change in the configuration of the pO_2 histograms is found. There is an increased saturation of the pO_2 classes in the pressure ranges above 40 mmHg, which can be interpreted as an increased perfusion of certain areas of the muscular capillary system. In our opinion, the results clearly show that middle molecular HES solutions, too, lead to an improvement of muscular perfusion and to an increase in mean tissue pO_2 if used within the scope of isovolemic hemodilution.

Summary

The aim of the present study was to investigate the effect of normovolemic hemodilution, using a middle molecular HES solution, on oxygen supply and pO_2 pressure distribution in the extremity muscles of healthy male subjects. In addition to a significant reduction in hematocrit (Hct) by hemodilution from about 44% to about 37% and unchanged arterial blood gas values, an increase in mean muscle pO_2 from about 16 mmHg (before hemodilution) to about 27 mmHg (30 minutes after having reached normovolemia) was observed. The increase in mean tissue pO_2 is demonstrable already 30 minutes after the start of infusion (t=30) (see Table 2). The markedly raised level of tissue pO_2 in the M. tibialis anterior as compared to the initial value is demonstrable both during and after normovolemic hemodilution. In addition to this dilution- related increase in mean tissue pO_2, a marked change in the configuration of the pO_2 histograms is found. There is an increased saturation of the pO_2 classes in the pressure ranges above 40 mmHg. The conspicuous increase in the intra-individual dispersion of pO_2 mean values during and after infusion of HES 200 cannot be interpreted for the moment. Similar observations were, for example, reported by Landgraf and Ehrly [1985] when measuring the muscular tissue oxygen pressure in patients with intermittent claudication before, during and after infusion of 0.9% saline solution. This could be interpreted as an increased perfusion of certain areas of the muscular capillary system.
In our opinion, the results clearly show that the middle molecular HES solution tested leads to an improvement in muscular perfusion and to an increase in mean tissue pO_2 if used within the scope of normovolemic hemodilution.

Acknowledgements. Supported by Deutsche Forschungsgemeinschaft (He 1293/1-2)

References

1. Ehrly AM, Landgraf H, Saeger-Lorenz K, Sasse S (1979) Verbesserung der Fliesseigenschaften des Blutes nach Infusion von niedermolekularer Hydroxyaethylstaerke (Expafusin) bei gesunden Probanden. Infusionstherapie 6:331
2. Ehrly AM, Landgraf H, Moschner P-V, Saeger-Lorenz K (1987) Verhalten des Gewebesauerstoffdruckes und der Fliesseigenschaften des Blutes bei Patienten mit Claudicatio intermittens nach Infusion von 500 ml 6%iger Hydroxyaethylstaerkelösung im Vergleich zu physiologischer Kochsalzlösung. VASA 16:103
3. Fleckenstein W, Weiss Ch (1982) Evaluation of pO$_2$-histograms obtained by hypodermic needle electrodes. In: Bleifeld, Hardess, Leetz (eds) Proceedings of the World Congress on Medical Physics and Biomedical Engineering. Schaldach. Kuenzel, Goettingen.
4. Fleckenstein W, Heinrich R, Kersting Th, Schomerus H, Weiss Ch (1984) A new method for the bedside recording of tissue pO$_2$ histograms. Verh Dtsch Ges Inn Med 90:666
5. Fleckenstein W, Weiss Ch (1984) A comparison of pO$_2$-histograms from rabbit hind limb muscle obtained by simultaneous measurements with hypodermic needle electrodes and with surface electrodes. Adv Exp Med Biol 169:447
6. Foerster H, Wicarkcyk, C, Dudziak R (1981) Bestimmung der Plasmaelimination von Hydroxyaethylstaerke und von Dextran mittels verbesserter analytischer Methodik. Infusionstherapie 2:88
7. Kiesewetter H, Jung F (1986) Rheologische Therapie der peripheren arteriellen Verschlusskrankheit im Stadium IIb. Angio 8:21
8. Kopp KH, Sinagowitz E, Kaeshammer B, Weidmann H (1981) Methodische Probleme bei Sauerstoffpartialdruckmessung im Gewebe von Intensivpatienten. In: Ehrly (ed) Messung des Gewebesauerstoffdruckes bei Patienten. Witzstrock, Baden- Baden, Koeln, p 61
9. Kopp KH, Kieser M, Sinagowitz E, Lund M (1982) Der Einfluss von niedermolekularer Hydroxyaethylstaerke und Dextran 60 auf die Muskelsauerstoffversorgung bei Intensivpatienten. Infusionstherapie 9:44-51
10. Landgraf H, Ehrly AM, Saeger-Lorenz K, Vogel V (1981) Untersuchung ueber den Einfluss mittelmolekularer HES auf die Fliesseigenschaften des Blutes gesunder Probanden. Infusionstherapie 8:200
11. Rieger H (1982) Induzierte Blutverduennung (Haemodilution) als neues Konzept in der Therapie peripherer Durchblutungsstoerungen. Internist 23:375
12. Rudofsky G, Strohmenger HG, Trexler S, Brock FE (1981) Isovolaemische Haemodilution bei Patienten mit arterieller Verschlusskrankheit im Stadium II. In: Breddin K. (ed) Thrombose und Atherogenese. G. Witzstrock, Baden-Baden
13. Rudofsky G, Meyer P, Strohmenger HG (1982) Effects of hemodilution on resting flow and reactive hyperemia in lower limbs. Bibl Haematol 47:157
14. Sunder-Plassmann L, von Hessler F, Endrich B, Messmer K (1982) Improvement of collateral circulation in chronic vascular occlusive disease of the lower extremity. Bibl. Haematol. 47:43

Morphological Assessment of Skeletal Muscular Injury Caused by pO$_2$ Measurements with Hypodermic Needle Probes

U. Schramm, W. Fleckenstein, C. Weber

Introduction

It is well accepted that tissue pO$_2$ data, obtained by polarographic micro-wire needle probes of only a few µm in tip- diameter, are not falsified by artifacts which result from reactions of the tissue around the needle (Ehrly 1981, Lübbers 1981, Kunze 1966, Whalen et al. 1967). It was supposed that local pO$_2$ readings would not be influenced by the low O$_2$ consumption of membranised recessed microwire needle probes, and that micro-circulation would not be disturbed because of their tapering tip (Baum-gärtl and Lübbers 1983, Schneidermann and Goldstick 1978). Micro-needle probes sealed in glass are rather fragile. Hence, for application in man, these microneedle probes were inserted deeply into muscle tissue within the plastic tube of a previously inserted vein catheter; after the needle probes' tip was advanced to the end of the plastic tube, the tube was then withdrawn over the shaft of the needle; in this way, the probe was brought into contact with the tissue. In order to determine a continuous pO$_2$ profile, the needle was then drawn slowly backwards.

For clinical measurements, hypodermic needle probes of a diameter of between 400 µm and 600 µm were also drawn slowly backwards within muscle, in order to determine pO$_2$ profiles (van der Kleij et al. 1984; van der Kleij and de Koning 1981). However, it was doubted (Lübbers 1981; Fleckenstein 1982; Fleckenstein et al. 1983; Fleckenstein and Weiss 1984; Weiss and Fleckenstein 1986) whether local pO$_2$ values measured with hypodermic needle probes correspond to the local tissue pO$_2$ values of undisturbed tissue.

The pO$_2$ signal of a fast responding (T$_{90}$ < 500 ms) hypodermic needle probe, inserted in muscle, starts to decrease markedly 1.5 sec after a stepwise displacement into a part of muscle tissue which was not pre-viously in contact with the probe (Fleckenstein 1982; Fleckenstein 1985); at a minimal percentage of probe tip positions, an increase of local pO$_2$ readings, also starting about 1.5 sec after sensor-tissue contact, was ob-served. We concluded that only a local pO$_2$ value determined immediately after a step movement of the pO$_2$ sensitive probe tip into "virgin" tissue, represents the local pO$_2$ value which was present there under the pre-

Clinical Oxygen Pressure Measurement II
A.M. Ehrly et al. (Eds.)
© Blackwell Ueberreuter Wissenschaft Berlin 1990

viously undisturbed conditions. In resting muscle tissue, the time span after a forward step, during which "undisturbed" pO_2 measurements are possible was empirically determined to be 1.5 sec (Fleckenstein and Weiss 1984). The pO_2 decrease, after contact between the sensor tip and "virgin" tissue, could not be explained by the O_2 consumption of the polarographic pO_2 sensitive site of the probe, since its polarographic current lay at only 6 ± 1.5 pA / mmHg pO_2 (37°C); also, within agar jelly, prepared with 2 M KCl solution (with O_2 diffusion properties nearly equivalent to muscle tissue), the decrease in pO_2 reading after a forward step was practically absent (Fleckenstein 1987). Finally, probe poisoning was also ruled out. Hence, we explained the decrease in the local pO_2 signal within muscle tissue by a local reduction of O_2 delivery to a tissue layer surrounding the needle probe. It was plausible to assume that the hypothesized local reduction of O_2 delivery was due to a compression of capillaries in course of the volume displacement caused by the insertion of the hypodermic needle probe itself.

In this study, we examined the histological changes within the muscle tissue surrounding the needle probe during the later phase of pO_2 decrease after probe-tissue contact (15-120 sec after insertion). The gracilis and the tibialis anterior muscles of 30 rats were punctured by hypodermic needle probes 15 to 120 sec before fixation. The probes had a diameter of 350 µm. The examinations were performed by light microscopy, transmission electron microscopy, scanning electron microscopy, and morphometry. We were interested to find out the following in detail: the position of the probe in the muscle tissue during pO_2 measurements, the tissue compression due to penetration of the probe, the occurrence of muscle fibre necrosis and of vascular changes in the vicinity of the electrode track.

Materials and Methods

Procedures were carried out on 30 Wistar-rats. The gracilis and tibialis anterior muscles of both legs were used. The legs were dissected free and an incision was made into the overlying fascia. A hypodermic pO_2 needle probe was inserted through the incision at an angle of 20° and about 1.5 cm deep into the muscle. The needle probe with a shaft diameter of 350 µm and a lancet- formed tip was inserted either by hand or with a KIMOC®-micromanipulator in a stepwise manner, as previously described (Fleckenstein 1985). The muscle was then grasped with a clamp of two straight hemostats which were fixed parallel to each other by means of an interposed piece of aluminium. The process from insertion of the probe to immersion into the fixative took 15 – 120 sec. The contralateral leg which served as control, was treated in a similar fashion, but no probe was inserted.

In order to get paraffin-sections for light transmission microscopy, the tissue was fixed in formalin, then dehydrated and embedded in paraffin, and then cut into serial sections. The sections were stained with haematoxylin and eosin, Masson's trichrome, PAS, toluidine-blue and alcianeblue.

For transmission electron microscopy, the preparations were fixed in 2.5% glutaraldehyde (O.1 M cacodylate buffer, pH 7.2), postfixed in 2% buffered OsO_4, dehydrated in ascending alcohols and embedded in Epon with propylene oxide as an intermedium. Semithin sections were stained with Methylenblue-Azure II. Ultrathin sections were stained with uranylacetate and lead citrate and were examined with a Zeiss EM 109.

In order to obtain corrosion casts of blood vessels, at first the external iliac artery was exposed and a cannula was inserted; the vessels of the hind limb were then flushed with physiological saline and subsequently filled with MERCOX. After maceration, the corrosion casts were mounted on a microscope specimen plate. The probe track was exposed using a pulsed excimer laser and the specimen was then sputtered with gold-paladium and observed in a Philips 505 scanning electron microscope.

Cross-sections of microvessels were morphologically measured using a Zeiss EM 109 with projecting mirrors. The following parameters were planimetrically determined using a MOP- KONTRON: total vessel circumference, luminal circumference, circumference of endothelial nuclei and minimum vessel diameter. The total vessel, luminal, endothelial and nuclear cross-sectional areas were calculated. Form factors for the total vessel and the lumen were determined as follows: a deviation from an ideal circular form, characterized by a "form factor" of 1, resulted in factors of less than 1.

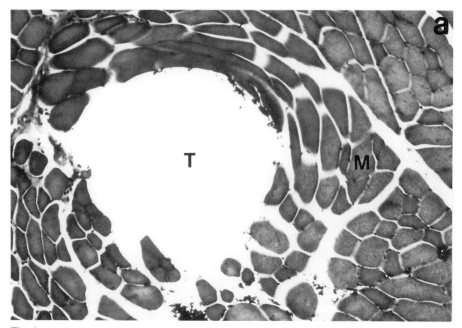

Fig. 1a

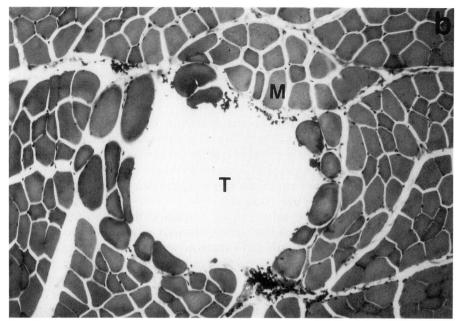

Fig. 1b

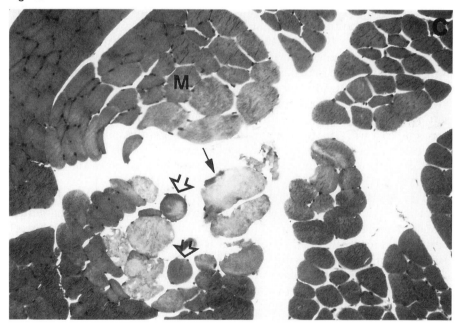

Fig. 1c

Fig. 1a–c. Cross-section of an electrode track and the surrounding muscle tissue: **a)** near the insertion of the needle- electrode; **b)** near the electrode tip; **c)** region of the lancet- formed probe tip. a, b and c – same electrode track. T = electrode track; M = muscle fibre cross-section; → muscle fibre necrosis; ⇒ segmental contraction, rounding of muscle fibres. Paraffin section, 140 x

Results

As determined from serial sections, the probe took an almost linear course through the muscle tissue. The connective tissue of the perimysium influenced the direction of the probe only slightly. However, major connective tissue septa, e.g. epimysium and fasciae, could divert the axial propagation of the probe.

The tissue displacement, due to the insertion of the probe, lead to a compression of the surrounding tissue structures. In smaller connective tissue septa there were more muscle fibres in the compression zone than in bigger septa. Vessels lying within the compression zone were always affected. In Fig.1a-c these compression zones, stained with Toluidine-blue and Masson's trichrome, are shown.

Muscle fibres which were squeezed or sustained injury to their sarcolemma by the progression of the probe, showed morphological changes which were already seen by the light microscope (Fig.1c). These changes ranged from segmental fibre lesions, as a minimum sign of damage, up to characteristic fibre necrosis. From electron microscopy, it was seen that the sarcolemma were damaged or lost in some of the slightly altered fibres, whereas their basal lamina appeared to be normally shaped and did not show any morphological signs of damage. The extent of morphological changes was dependent on the time span between insertion of the probe and chemical fixation of the tissue.

The probes' track always contained extravasated erythrocytes. Single or smaller groups of erythrocytes stemming from microvessels ruptured along the shaft of the probe, were seen. Only one out of 30 examined cases showed the rupture of a larger arteriole resulting in hemorrhage.

Due to the density of microvessels in rat muscles, as seen by corrosion casts, it is not surprising that the probe destroys them. Fig.2 shows such a corrosion cast with the pO_2 probe in- situ; muscle fibres, connective tissue and vessel walls are macerated away. The vessels are pressed together in front of the probe tip. If these vessels cannot be pushed aside they rupture.

From transmission electron microscopy, alterations of vasculature around the probes' track could be seen, e.g. relatively small vessel lumina which were confined by broad endothelia (Fig.3a; compare with Fig.3b – control specimen). However, at a greater distance from the probe, dilated vessel lumina and normal appearing endothelia occurred. To confirm and quantitate these observations, planimetry of microvascular cross-sections in an area 200 µm around the probe tip was performed and morphometrically analysed; ruptured vessels which could not be measured were numerically registered. For planimetry the 200 µm range around the probe tip was divided into an inner and an outer zone. The inner zone reached to a distance of 70 µm from the surface of the probe into the surrounding tissue. The outer zone included the area between 70 and 200 µm from the probe surface. Comparing the frequency distributions of vessel diameters from the inner zone, (Fig.4a, tissue 0 to 70 µm distant to probe surface),

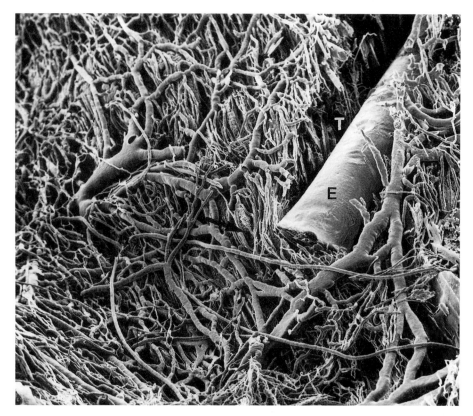

Fig. 2. Corrosion cast of vessel lumina. pO_2-electrode (E) and electrode track (T); → Vessels pressed together by forward movement of the probe. SEM, 90 x

the outer zone (Fig 4b, tissue 70 to 200 μm distant to probe surface) and randomly selected control tissue (Fig.4c), the following became apparent. Average vessel diameter, determined from the control tissue was 25.1 ± 7.8 rel. units, determined from the tissue of the inner zone 20 ± 10.2 rel. units and from tissue of the outer zone 28.6 ± 9.4. In histograms the vessel diameters within control tissue were symmetrically distributed, near the probe the distribution was skewed to the left side of the histogram, and in the outer zone to the right side. The mean vessel diameter of 25 rel. units within control tissue is equivalent to an absolute value of 3 μm. This is less than what would be expected from capillary diameters of vital tissue. We suppose that the smaller diameters found in our material are an artifact of tissue processing or of preparation under arterial occlusion that was induced some seconds before fixation. However, since control tissue and tissue containing the electrode track underwent the same processing procedures, a comparison of data seemed justified.

Fig.5 shows mean values of luminal, nuclear and endothelial cross- sectional areas as a percentage of mean total cross-sectional area (CSA) of the

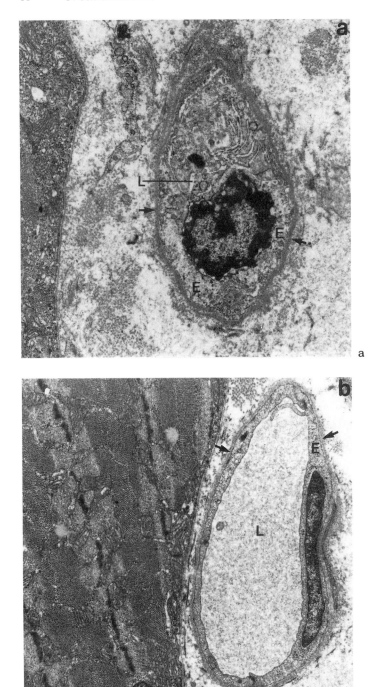

Fig. 3a, b. Cross-section of capillary. **a)** in the 70 μm-zone of the electrode track; **b)** in control specimen. **E** = endothelium; **L** = vessel lumen; → base of the endothelium. TEM, 15 000 x

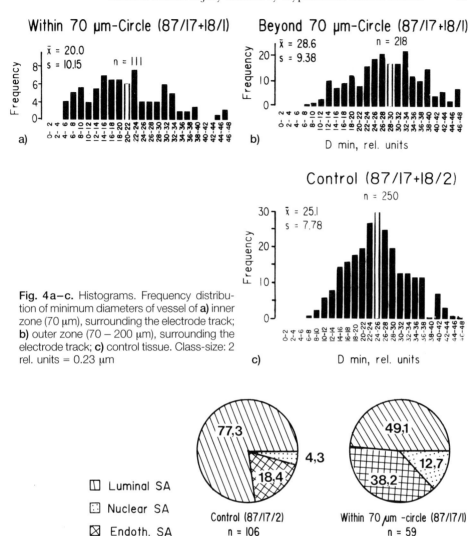

Fig. 4a–c. Histograms. Frequency distribution of minimum diameters of vessel of a) inner zone (70 μm), surrounding the electrode track; b) outer zone (70 – 200 μm), surrounding the electrode track; c) control tissue. Class-size: 2 rel. units = 0.23 μm

Fig. 5. Mean luminal, nuclear and endothelial CSA (cross-sectional area) as a percentage of mean total CSA of control tissue and inner zone

vessels. Within control tissue, on average 77% of the mean cross-sectional area of tissue was allotted to the vascular lumen; within the inner 70 μm zone in direct adjacency to the needle, on average only 45% of the total capillary cross-sectional areas were luminal areas. Hence, here not only the absolute vessel diameter (Fig.5), but also the fractional diameter was significantly reduced. The lumina of vessels of the outer zone took on average 70% of the total cross-sectional area.

Looking at the luminal form factor of the vessels in the two respective zones around the probe track, a change of vessel lumina in the inner zone

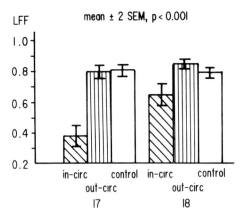

Fig. 6. Mean luminal form factors (± SEM) of the two vessel groups related to the electrode track, and of the control group. Numbers 17 and 18 refer to the respective tissue specimens. Maximum ordinate is '1', designating the form of an ideal circle

again becomes apparent (Fig.6). In the two specimens under investigation, within the 70 µm-zone luminal form factors (LFF) of 0.38 and 0.65 on average were respectively found, indicating that the vessels here were flattened. These values of the luminal form factor differed significantly from the mean values of about 0.8 that were found in the control tissue. In one specimen the vessels in the outer zone had a slightly increased mean luminal form factor.

Discussion

The findings illustrate that tissue compression in the vicinity of a needle probe not only involves alteration of muscle fibres but, in particular, of blood vessels. The most markedly compressed tissue lies immediately next to the probe surface within a layer of a thickness of 70 µm. Compared to control tissue, within the inner 70 µm-zone, the absolute and the relative mean luminal areas of capillaries were significantly reduced (-20% and -26% respectively) resulting in a reduction of the functional capillary lumen by 49.2%. But in addition to this, the marked flattening of these capillaries (Fig.6) is a finding of functional significance, since the vessels' perfusion resistance for the corpuscular erythrocytes is highly dependent on the luminal form factor (Gaehtgens 1981). Considering that the capillaries' lumina are reduced by half and markedly flattened within the inner 70 µm zone, it can be assumed that near the probe, only plasma (of low O_2 capacity) but nearly no erythrocytes can pass the vessels. Our hypothesis, of a reduction of local oxygen delivery in the nearest vicinity of the pO_2 sensitive probe tip, as was derived from evidence of tissue oxygen measurements (Fleckenstein and Weiss 1984; Weiss and Fleckenstein 1986), is impressively supported by the histological findings of this study.

The histological findings further show that within an outer tissue layer, at a distance of more than 70 µm and less than 200 µm around the needle, the local O_2 delivery is possibly increased. But the radius of the pO_2 catchment field of the pO_2 sensitive recessed microcathode lies far below 70 µm, if the low sensitive (6 ± 1.5 pA / mmHg pO_2 at 37°C) polarographic KIMOC® probe type (Fleckenstein 1987), or if low sensitive probes according to de Koning and van der Kleij (1980) or Whalen (1980) are used. So it is reasonable to assume that only pO_2 values of the inner 70 µm tissue layer, of reduced O_2 delivery, exert their influence on the pO_2 reading of low sensitive hypodermic needle probes. However, as shown by Meuer (this book), in resting skeletal muscle the local muscular pO_2 is only slightly reduced during the first second after a sudden change of the balance between local O_2 consumption and delivery (capillary compression respectively). This delay is due to O_2 storage in hemoglobin and myoglobin, and to O_2 diffusion conditions within muscle tissue. Hence, it can be explained that the pO_2 reading of a fast responding hypodermic needle probe does not decrease during the first second of the probe-tissue contact, although it is reasonable to assume that the capillaries are compressed at the same moment of the positioning of the needle. In any case, we conclude that local tissue pO_2 should be measured as soon as possible after contact of a pO_2 sensitive probe's cathode with previously uncompressed tissue. The only technical limitation to this is the speed of the probe's response to changes of the pO_2 after a step movement. Probes of a T_{90} of below 500 ms seem to be fast enough for measurements in resting muscle tissue; probes of KIMOC® type and Whalen type (1980) fulfil the condition. Other types of hypodermic needle pO_2 probes which we know, are much too slow in response to pO_2.

According to our technique of pO_2 measurement, probes with a diameter of 350 µm are moved forward from one measuring site to the next in steps of at least 700 µm in length. This is necessary in order to leave the previously compressed tissue area with each step; the histological findings show that a step length of 700 µm, as empirically determined (Fleckenstein 1982, Fleckenstein et al. 1984), is sufficiently large.

Our histological findings show that pO_2 measuring with hypodermic needle probes during a slow backwards drive, which logically can only be started after a deep insertion of the needle into the tissue, leads to pO_2 values which are taken from injured tissue. The O_2 consumption of muscle fibres damaged at the sarcolemma, is most probably changed; moreover the local O_2 delivery to the tissue around a punctured canal is most probably changed by disturbances of microcirculation and capillary function. The histological findings presented here were obtained after a contact time of probe and living tissue of only 15 – 120 sec; tissue pO_2 measurements obtained by withdrawal of a hypodermic needle pO_2 probe, take at least a few minutes. Even within a time span of only 120 sec, we observed an aggravation of tissue damage near the punctured canal. We can therefore assume, that a variety of artifacts influence the pO_2 readings obtained by withrawal technique of hypodermic needles; on the one hand, artifacts may lead to an increase of the pO_2 reading (extravasation of erythrocytes, reduction of O_2 uptake of damaged muscle fibres, possibly increase of capillary flow within the outer tissue zone); yet on the other hand, artifacts may decrease the pO_2 reading (compression of tissue). In comparison to pO_2 profiles obtained by forwardly driven microneedle probes (Kunze 1969) or fast responding KIMOC® probes, muscle pO_2 profiles obtained by withdrawal of hypodermic needle probes of a small pO_2 catchment field radius (Beerthuizen et al. 1986; van der Kleij and de Koning 1981; van der Kleij et al. 1983; van der Kleij et al. 1984; de Koning and van der Kleij 1980) show pO_2 gradients that are levelled out; consequently in pO_2 histograms from those profiles, high and low values are reduced in frequency. This underestimation could be partly explained by a reduction of O_2 consumption within a layer of damaged tissue between the withdrawn hypodermic needle and the perfused O_2 consuming tissue (Fleckenstein et al., this book)

The histological findings in the punctured canal, of tissue injury and fast development of secondary tissue damage, give more reason to claim that local muscle pO_2 measurements with needle probes of high spacial resolution should be performed as fast as technically possible after the contact between the probe tip and the "virgin" tissue. The needles should be driven forward.

At the first glance, the results presented here seem to exclude the possibility of reliable measurements of mean tissue pO_2 with implanted catheters (e.g. performed by Brantigan et al. 1974; Furuse et al. 1973; Jussila 1980; Niinikoski and Halkola 1977); these types of catheters integrate the local pO_2 distribution within microcirculation over comparably long distances of 0.5 to 2 cm. However, if the pO_2 catchment field from which tissue pO_2 values are taken, reasonably exceeds the zone of compressed tissue, or if the O_2 consumption of muscle fibres adjacent to the probes is markedly reduced in course of implantation time or absent, then the restrictions of pO_2 measurement with "thick" probes are not valid in any respect. From own measurements in skeletal muscle and myocardium using implanted pO_2 catheter probes of comparably high pO_2 catchment radius made from soft plastic tubes (Eberhard et al. 1979) we got the impression that miniaturisation, weakness and flexibility of the catheter plays an important role in order to obtain reliable mean tissue pO_2 readings. In comparison to steel needles, there is possibly less muscle tissue compression if a soft catheter lies snaky, and adapted in the cross-sectional form, between the muscle bundles. It should be seriously kept in mind that mean tissue pO_2 measurements that are integrating over some milimeters or centimeters do not deliver any information about the tissue pO_2 distribution within microcirculation.

In this paper, tissue injury was discussed regarding problems of pO_2 measurement of high spacial resolution within microcirculation. Spoken in terms of clinical medicine, the muscular injury exerted by hypodermic needle probes ($\varnothing$ 350 μm) was rather small. In only one out of 30 punctures, examined by serial sections in the light microscope, an arterial resistance vessel was punctured.

References

1. Baumgärtl H, Lübbers DW (1983) Microcoaxial needle sensor for polarographic measurement of local O_2 pressure in the cellular range of living tissue. Its construction and properties. In: Gnaiger and Forstner (eds) Polographic Oxygen Sensors. Springer, Berlin, 37-65

2. Beerthuizen GIJM, Goris RJA, Kimmich HP, Kleij van der AJ, Kreuzer F (1986) Normoxia and hypoxia in patients with severe burns. In: Ehrly AM, Hauss J, Huch R (eds) Clinical Oxygen Pressure Measurement. Springer, Heidelberg, 76-78

3. Brantigan JW, Ziegler EC, Hynes KM, Miyazawa TY, Smith M (1974) Tissue gases during hypovolemic shock. J Appl Physiol 37:117

4. Eberhard P, Fehlmann W, Mindt W (1979) An electrochemical sensor for continuous intravascular oxygen monitoring. Bio- telemetary and Patient Monitoring 6:16

5. Ehrly AM (1981) Messungen des Gewebesauerstoffdruckes im ischämischen Muskelgewebe von Patienten mit arteriellen Verschlußkrankheiten mittels Mikro-Platin-Stichelektroden. In: Ehrly AM (ed) Messung des Gewebesauerstoffdruckes bei Patienten. Witzstrok, Baden-Baden, 36-45

6. Fleckenstein W. (1982) In vivo measurements of pO_2 histograms using a hypodermic needle electrode system. Pflüg Arch 392 R:2098

7. Fleckenstein W, Weiss C, Heinrich R, Schomerus H, Kersting T (1984) A New method for the bed-side recording of tissue pO_2 histograms. Verh Dtsch Ges Inn Med 90:439

8. Fleckenstein W (1985) Ein neues Gewebe pO_2 Meßverfahren zum Nachweis von Mikrozirkulationsstörungen. Med Diss, Med. Univ. Lübeck

9. Fleckenstein W, Weiss C (1984) A comparison of pO_2 histograms from rabbit hind limb muscles obtained by simultaneous measurements with hypodermic needle electrodes and with surface electrodes. Adv Exp Med Biol 169:447

10. Fleckenstein W (1987) Die Entwicklung der Feinnadel-Gewebe- pO_2-Histographie zum klinisch eingesetzten Diagnoseverfahren. In: Präsident der FU Berlin (ed) 2. Forum Medizintechnik. Verlag Forschungsvermittlung, Berlin, 92-105

11. Fleckenstein W, Schäffler, Heinrich R, Petersen, Günderoth-Palmowski, Nollert (this book) On the differences between muscles pO_2 measurements obtained with hypodermic needle probes and with multiwire surface probes.

12. Furuse A, Brawley RK, Struve E, Gott VC (1973) Skeletal muscle gas tension: Indicator of cardiac output and peripheral tissue perfusion. Surgery 74:214

13. Gaehtgens P (1981) Mikrorheologie des Blutes in Kapillaren. Arzneim Forsch, Drug Res 31:1995

14. Jussila E, Niinikoski J, Vänttinen E (1980) Intraoperative recording of tissue gas tension in calf muscles of patients with peripheral arterial disease. J Surg Res 29:533

15. Kleij van der AJ, Koning de J (1981) Tissue oxygen electrode for routine clinical application. In: Kimmich HP (ed) Monitoring of Vital Parameters during Extracorporeal Circulation. Karger, Basel, p 95-100

16. Kleij van der AJ, Koning de J, Beerthuizen GIJM, Goris RJA, Kreuzer FJA, Kimmich HP (1983) Early detection of hemorrhagic hypovolemia by muscle pO_2 assessment. Surgery 93:518

17. Kleij van der AJ, Kimmich HP, Goris RJA, Kreuzer F, Koning de J, Beerthuizen GIJM (1984) Micro, surface, and needle oxygen electrodes: Comparison of physiological relevance and clinical acceptance. Adv Exp Med Biol 169:869

18. Koning de J, Kleij van der AJ (1980) An electrode for clinical pO_2 monitoring. Arzneim Forsch, Drug Res 30:2215

19. Kunze K (1966) Die lokale, kontinuierliche Sauerstoffdruckmessung in der menschlichen Muskulatur. Pflüg Arch. 292:151

20. Kunze K (1969) Das Sauerstoffdruckfeld im normalen und pathologisch veränderten Muskel. Springer, Berlin

21. Lübbers DW (1981) Grundlagen und Bedeutung der lokalen Sauerstoffdruckmessung und des pO_2-Histogramms für die Beurteilung der Sauerstoffversorgung der Organe und des Organismus. In: Ehrly AM (ed) Messung des Gewebesauerstoffdruckes bei Patienten. Witzstrock, Baden- Baden, p 11-22

22. Meuer HJ (this book) Local oxygen consumption of blood perfused skeletal muscle determined with oxygen microelectrodes under stop-flow conditions.
23. Niinikoski J, Halkola L (1977) Skeletal muscle pO_2: Indicator of peripheral tissue perfusion in haemorrhagic shock. Adv Exp Med Biol 94:585
24. Schneiderman G, Goldstick ThK (1978) Oxygen electrode design criteria and performance characteristics: Recessed cathode. J Appl Physiol 45:145
25. Weiss C, Fleckenstein W (1986) Local tissue pO_2 measurements with "thick" needle probes. Funktionsanalyse Biol Syst 15:155
26. Whalen WJ, Riley J, Nair P (1967) A microelectrode for measuring intracellular pO_2. J Appl Physiol 23:798
27. Whalen WJ, Spande JI (1980) A hypodermic needle pO_2 electrode. J Appl Physiol 48:186

Measurement of the Intramuscular Oxygen Partial Pressure in the Tibialis Anterior Muscle of Patients with Stage I-III Hypertension According to the WHO

W. Kolepke, F. Jung, H. Kiesewetter, C. Blum, W. Vogel, R. Bach, D. Jesinghaus, H. Schieffer, E. Wenzel, G.A. Jutzler

Introduction

In plethysmographic studies early changes in the peripheral vasodilator reserve of patients suffering from hypertension [3, 25] could be demonstrated. Furthermore, we succeeded in showing – by intravital microscopy – that there is a significant reduction in the perfusion of cutaneous capillaries as well as a loss of the vasomotor reserve in patients with longstanding hypertension [11, 12]. It is supposed that in such patients the intramuscular oxygen pressure is also affected. For this reason local oxygen partial pressure histograms in the tibialis anterior muscle of patients with hypertension in different WHO stages were determined.

Patients

Up to now n = 85 patients with arterial hypertension have been examined. Some clinical and demographic data on the entire group of patients and the subgroups in the WHO stages I, II and III are given in Table 1.

Table 1. Clinical and demographic data of patients

	Entire group	WHO I	WHO II	WHO III
n	85	17	54	14
Sex (m/f)	60/25	10/7	42/12	8/6
Age (yrs)	59.2 ± 10.4	57.5 ± 8.8	59.1 ± 9.9	57.7 ± 10.4
Height (cm)	171 ± 8.8	172 ± 8.2	170 ± 9.3	172 ± 7
Weight (kg)	78.0 ± 12.5	79.3 ± 15.4	78 ± 9.7	82.6 ± 22
Blood pressure (mmHg)				
systolic	143 ± 21	143 ± 25	143 ± 19	147 ± 18
diastolic	83 ± 16	88 ± 16	82 ± 15	87 ± 16
Heart rate p.m.	73 ± 10	76 ± 7	73 ± 11	71 ± 12
Duration of treatment (yrs)	12.2 ± 8.5	7.1 ± 6.4	12.2 ± 7.9	19.0 ± 12.9

Clinical Oxygen Pressure Measurement II
A.M. Ehrly et al. (Eds.)
© Blackwell Ueberreuter Wissenschaft Berlin 1990

Except for the duration of treatment the values indicated in Table 1 are comparable for the 3 subgroups.

The classification into WHO-stages was made according to the concomitant diseases [8]. Stage I of hypertension is marked by the non-existence of objective organic lesions; stage II by the presence of the following lesions: hypertrophy relating to the left ventricle, focal or generalized restriction of the retinal arteries, proteinuria or slightly increased serum creatinine; stage III by temporary decompensated insufficiency of the left heart, cerebral hemorrhage, hypertensive encephalopathy, retinal hemorrhage or exudate production with or without oedema of the optic disc.

Additionally, patients who had had a myocardial or cerebral infarction or suffering from an angiographically documented coronary heart disease or a peripheral arterial occlusive disease in at least stage II were included in stage III (WHO). The important concomitant diseases are shown in Table 2.

Table 2. Concomitant diseases

	Entire group	WHO I	WHO II	WHO III
n	85	17	54	14
Increased lipid values[1]	66	13	43	10
Diabetes mellitus	26	2	16	8
Rheumatic disease	13	2	8	3
Coronary heart disease	31	5	21	5
Nephropathy	18	0	14	4
Hyperuricaemia[2]	18	0	13	5

[1] Cholesterol over 220 mg/dl or triglyceride concentration greater than 200 mg/dl or HDL-cholesterol below 35 mg/dl for females and 45 mg/dl for males
[2] Uric acid greater than 7.5 mg/dl

The concomitant diseases between stage I and stages II and III increase significantly; but between stages II and III there are hardly any differences. All patients had received an antihypertensive treatment using drugs containing the following active substances (Table 3).

Table 3. Antihypertensive therapy

	Entire group	WHO I	WHO II	WHO III
n	85	17	54	14
Selective beta blockers	44	11	23	10
Diuretics	44	6	24	14
Calcium antagonists	44	9	27	8
ACE-inhibitor (Enalapril)	17	4	10	3
Alpha receptor antagonists	5	1	3	1

Under this therapy n=17 of the 85 patients were within the physiologic blood pressure range (below 140/90 mmHg) and n=34 patients within the borderline range (equal to or greater than 140/90 mmHg but below 160/95 mmHg). 34 patients had a blood pressure of at least 160/95 mmHg. The concomitant medication is presented in Table 4.

Table 4. Concomitant medication

	Entire group	WHO I	WHO II	WHO III
n	85	17	54	14
Lipid-lowering agent	9	3	5	1
Antidiabetics:				
– Sulphonyl urea	12	1	7	4
– Insulin	4	0	2	2
Analgetics	2	0	1	1
Coronary stimulant	53	8	33	12
Uricostatics	11	2	5	4
Vaso-active substances	19	1	13	5
Thrombocyte aggregation inhibitors	20	6	11	3

Test method

Intramuscular oxygen histograms were measured with the "Makroelektrode Typ: pO_2-Histograph KIMOC (Eppendorf Gerätebau GmbH, Hamburg)" according to the method developed by Fleckenstein et al. [5]. As the implementation of the measurement has not yet been standardized it is detailed in the following.

Prior to the examination patients were adapted to room temperature (waiting room kept at about 22° Celsius), the waiting period before measurement being about one hour. The skin surface temperature was controlled before measurement, the latter not being carried out until skin temperature exceeded 27° Celsius.

The pO_2 measurements were made in the tibialis anterior muscle. After preparation of the measuring point and a subcutaneous local anaesthesia a disposable puncture cloth was placed on the site of insertion of the needle. The puncture was effected lateral to the tibia edge so as to achieve the greatest muscular cross section possible. Then, an access for the pO_2 probe was made in cranial direction by means of an Abbocath®-vascular catheter at an angle of about 30° to the longitudinal axis of the muscle fibre. The measurement of the pO_2 values was only started after a period of rest of 15 mins. pO_2 values were taken account of so as to ensure that the measurement was only started in the muscular tissue.

The automatic, microprocessor-controlled probe advance was done according to the "Pilgerschrittverfahren" with a forward step of 1.0 mm and a backward step of 0.3 mm resulting in a real step of 0.7 mm and with a time interval between measurements of 1.4 s. In all 21 measurements per measuring cycle were done, producing a channel length of 1.47 cm, after which the probe returned to its starting position. After each cycle the probe was rotated round its own axis by 120°. Then a new tissue area was chosen for measurement, the probe being aimed in a slightly different direction and at a slightly different angle, so as to be able to cover as large a muscular area as possible. In all, 200 single values were recorded and thus a histogram of the oxygen pressure values drawn up.

Statistics

In order to compare the relative frequency (cathectic numbers of the categories of the oxygen partial pressure histogram) the Kolmogoroff-Smirnow test was applied [16].
Differences below the 5 % level were considered to be significant, and below the 10 % to be according to tendency.

Results

The oxygen partial pressure line histograms of hypertensive patients in comparison with a group of apparently healthy subjects is illustrated in Fig. 1.
The histogram of hypertensive patients shows a non-Gaussian distribution (Kolmogoroff-Smirnow test). The median value is 19.6 mmHg, i.e. 22.2 % lower than the median of a control group of same age of 42 healthy subjects (25.1 mmHg). These healthy subjects had been selected from an original group of 72 healthy subjects [10] matched according to age and sex.
The mean histograms of the two groups present differences which are only according to tendency ($p < 0.08$). Fig. 1 shows clearly that oxygen partial pressure values just under 30 mmHg are more frequent in hypertensive patients; values over 30 mmHg, however, are more frequent in healthy subjects.
Table 5 shows the results of one-stage classifications according to different drugs.
Significant differences were not observable. It is, however, striking that patients having received calcium antagonists, beta blockers, nitrates or ACE-inhibitors presented higher pO_2 values than patients without these drugs. Glycosides did not influence the pO_2 values whereas patients treated with diuretics had lower pO_2 values than those without diuretics. Figure 2 shows the mean oxygen partial pressure histograms of patients with hypertension stages I, II and III.

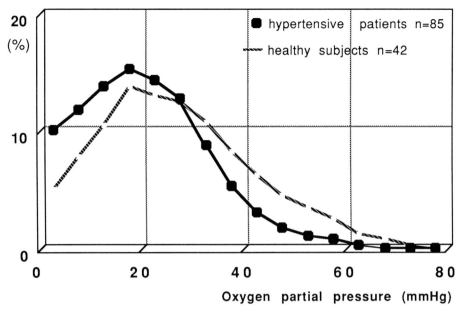

Fig. 1. Pool oxygen partial pressure line histogram of patients with arterial hypertension and healthy subjects

Table 5. Medication and mean intramuscular pO2 levels [+ = with, − = without]

		n	WHO I	WHO II	WHO III	mean pO_2
Nitrates	+	35	5	24	6	22.3 ± 7.2
	−	50	12	30	8	19.8 ± 7.6
Glycosides	+	18	3	9	6	20.0 ± 5.9
	−	67	14	45	8	20.5 ± 7.5
Diuretics	+	44	6	24	14	18.8 ± 7.4
	−	41	11	30	0	22.4 ± 7.4
Ca-Antag.	+	44	9	27	8	22.2 ± 6.2
	−	41	8	27	6	18.7 ± 7.6
Beta-Bl.	+	44	11	23	10	21.9 ± 7.2
	−	41	6	31	4	19.9 ± 7.7
ACE-Inh.	+	17	4	10	3	21.8 ± 8.1
	−	68	13	44	11	20.5 ± 7.3

Compared to healthy adults, patients in stage I have a slight shift to the right of the oxygen partial pressure histogram with a median oxygen pressure of 27.2 mmHg.

The group of patients in stage II, however, already presents a shift to the left compared to healthy adults, the median oxygen pressure being 19.4 mmHg. This shift to the left is only according to tendency, due to the low case numbers (p<0.09).

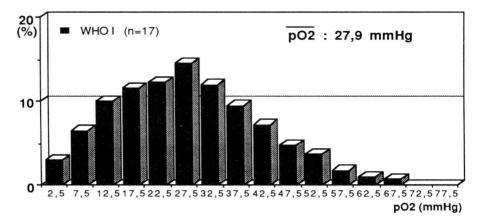

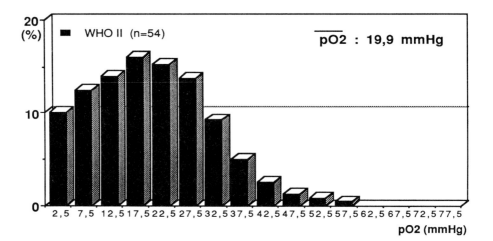

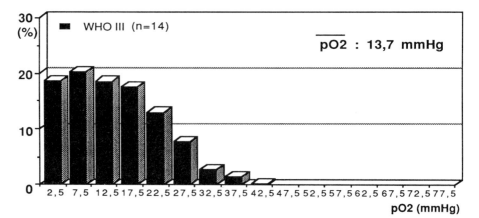

Fig. 2. Pool oxygen partial pressure histograms of patients with stage I – III hypertension according to the WHO

As for the patients in stage III a marked shift to the left, towards small oxygen partial pressure values, can be observed. The median oxygen pressure is 12.9 mHg. The pool histogram of this group differs significantly ($p<0.02$) from the mean histogram of healthy subjects.
The shift to the left of the mean histogram is according to tendency ($p<0.08$) for patients in stage II, but significant for patients in stage III ($p<0.01$), as compared to those of stage I. This shows that the extent of organic lesions corresponds to a significant reduction in the intramuscular oxygen supply.

Discussion

Compared to healthy subjects of same age, patients with arterial hypertension show a shift to the left of the intramuscular oxygen pressure histogram which is according to tendency, with markedly higher cathectic numbers in the oxygen categories below 30 mmHg and with the greatest differences in the smallest oxygen categories ($0 - 5$ mmHg).
According to Lübbers [18,19] a restricted pulmonary function, a shift to the left of the O_2-dissociation curve, an increase in O_2- oxygen consumption, a reduction in hematocrit, a decrease in capillary erythrocyte velocity as well as in capillary radius and number of capillaries (as enlargement of Krogh's cylinder) are to be considered as causes for the lower oxygen level. According to Kiesewetter et al. [15] a deterioration of blood fluidity is also a possible cause. Pulmonary function, arterial pO_2 as well as the acid-base balance of the hypertensive patients examined were within the normal range. Thanks to intravitalmicroscopical studies it is, however, known that the capillary erythrocyte velocity is significantly reduced in hypertensive patients compared to healthy subjects [11]. Besides dynamic changes there are also morphological alterations in the microcirculation influencing the oxygen pressure field in a negative way. Thus, Henrich and co-workers [9] were able to demonstrate that there is a significant reduction in the capillary density in patients with essential hypertension leading to an enlargement of the radius of Krogh's cylinder and to an extension of the diffusion distances and to reduced oxygen partial pressure values in the outer region of the cylinder. Besides, this is supported by the fact that the capillary radius in hypertenisve patients is probably smaller than in healthy subjects (this can only be concluded indirectly from the smaller erythrocyte column diameters of hypertensive patients compared to healthy persons [12]). In addition to these structural geometrical vascular changes the vessel content and the fluidity of blood is also altered. Thus a pathologic increase in plasma viscosity and erythrocyte aggregation could be demonstrated in hypertensive patients [2, 11]. Especially the increase in plasma viscosity represents an important determinant of the capillary perfusion velocity [7, 22] influencing the oxygen supply of the tissue directly [15].

The interindividual variation in the mean oxygen partial pressure of 34.8% for hypertensives is comparatively high. Some of the patients examined were supplied very well, but others very badly. For this inhomogeneous distribution several influencing factors may be accountable. By means of single-stage classifications the blood pressure (systolic and diastolic) as well as the antihypertensive therapy (classification according to drugs, see table 5) could be excluded as causes. It is striking that the patients under diuretic treatment showed lower pO_2 values than those without such treatment, whereas the opposite could be observed for all the other drugs we used. This agrees well with examinations of the capillary flow, where a restricted circulation combined with an increased plasma viscosity were observed [11].

Classification of the patients according to objective organic lesions following the WHO classification shows a clear dependence of the intramuscular oxygen supply on the WHO stage. The patients in stage I (n=17 patients without organic lesions and a mean duration of the disease of 7.1 yrs) even displayed, compared to healthy subjects, a sum histogram slightly shifted to the right with higher oxygen partial pressure values. This is quite conceivable, as in the initial stage of essential hypertension an increased cardiac output is frequent (so-called "minute volume hypertension") [24], which presumably accounts for an increased peripheral circulation. In plethysmographic examinations on the upper limb a similar result was found. Takeshita and Mark were able show that patients with borderline hypertension have yet no restriction in the vasodilator capacity [25].

With increasing duration of the disease, severe atherosclerotic vascular changes develop in the arterial periphery of hypertensive patients [4, 17, 23]. Due to chronic increase in blood pressure in combination with mechanical stress on the vessel wall a hypertrophy of the muscular vessel wall and, later on, atherosclerotic lesions appear which can lead to stenoses especially in the arteries with a small lumen [23] up to the precapillary resistance vessels [17]. Functionally, this atherosclerosis results in a restriction of the arterial or arteriolar ability to dilate, and thus to a reduction in the regulatory functional reserve [11]. It is likely that patients in stage II, but especially those in stage III with a mean duration of treatment of 19.0 years, present a considerably advanced sclerosis of the vessels – particularly in the precapillary system. Because of the simultaneous restriction in blood fluidity, there is a shift to the left of the oxygen partial histograms [12]. The patients in stage II have a median intramuscular oxygen partial pressure of 19.4 mmHg, and those in stage III present a value of 12.9 mmHg.

The restriction in capillary circulation combined with structural vascular changes in the macro- and microcirculation produces a significant reduction in the intramuscular oxygen supply in patients who have been suffering from hypertension for many years. The extent of the intramuscular oxygen deficit mainly correlates with the degree of atherosclerotic changes.

References

1. Block LH (1987) Hochdruck und Arteriosklerose. Münch Med Wschr 129:879
2. Chien S (1977) Blood rheology in hypertension and in cardiovascular diseases. Cardiovasc Med 2:3356
3. Conway J (1963) A vascular abnormity in hypertension. A study of blood flow in the forearm. Circulation 27:520
4. Dustan H (1974) Atherosclerosis complicating chronic hypertension. Circulation 50:871
5. Fleckenstein W, Heinrich R, Kersting Th, Schomerus H, Weiss Ch (1984) A new method for the bed-side recording of tissue pO_2 histograms. Verh Dtsch Ges Inn Med 90:439
6. Folkow B (1982) Physiological aspects of primary hypertension. Physiol Rev 62:347
7. Gaehtgens P (1977) Hemodynamic of the microcirculation. Physical characteristics of blood flow in the microvascular. In: Meessen H (ed) Handbuch der allgemeinen Pathologie III/7, Springer, Berlin, p 231
8. Ganten D, Ritz E (1985) Lehrbuch der Hypertonie. Schattauer, Stuttgart, p 4
9. Henrich HA, Romen W, Heimgärtner W, Hartung E, Bäumer F (1988) Capillary rarefaction characteristic of the skeletal muscle of hypertensive patients. Klin. Wochenschr. 66:54
10. Jung F, Bock M, Kolepke W, Heinrich R, Kiesewetter H, Wenzel E (1988) Intramuskulärer Sauerstoffpartialdruck im M. tibialis anterior bei anscheinend gesunden Probanden. To be published
11. Jung F, Spitzer S, Blum C, Feldman M, Konze R, Gilles M, Nüttgens HP, Kiesewetter H, Wenzel E, Jutzler GA (1987) Mikrozirkulatorische und hämorheologische Veränderungen bei Patienten mit arteriellem Bluthochdruck. In: Strauer BE, Ehrly AM, Leschke M (eds) Fortschritte in der kardiovaskulären Hämorheologie. Münch. Wiss. Publikationen, p 45
12. Jung F, Spitzer S, Kiesewetter H, Feldmann M, Kotitschke G, Blum C, Jutzler GA (1986) Comparative investigations of the microcirculation in patients with hypertension and healthy adults. Klin Wochenschr 64:956
13. Jung F, Berthold R, Wappler M, Konze R, Kiesewetter H, Wenzel E (1987) Referenzbereich der reaktiven Hyperämie anscheinend gesunder Probanden im Alter zwischen 6 und 65 Jahren. VASA Suppl 20:126
14. Jung F, Kiesewetter H, Roggenkamp HG, Nüttgens HP, Ringelstein EB, Gerhards M, Kotitschke G, Wenzel E, Zeller H (1986) Bestimmung der Referenzbereiche rheologischer Parameter: Studie an 653 zufällig ausgewählten Probanden im Kreis Aachen. Klin Wochenschr 64:375
15. Kiesewetter H, Jung F, Roggenkamp HG (1984) Einfluß der Fließfähigkeit des Blutes auf die Versorgung des Gewebes. In: Heilmann L, Kieswetter H, Ernst E (eds) Klinische Rheologie und Beta-1-Blockade. Zuckschwerdt, München, p 11
16. Kreyszig E (1979) Statistische Methoden und ihre Anwendung. Vandenhoeck & Ruprecht, Göttingen
17. Liebegott G (1976) Morphologie der hypertonischen Angiopathie. In: Zeitler E (ed) Hypertonie – Risikofaktor in der Angiologie. Witzstrock, Baden-Baden, p 15
18. Lübbers DW (1977) Quantitative measurement and description of oxygen supply to the tissue. In: Jöbsis FF (ed) Oxygen and physiological function. Professional Information Library, Dallas p 254
19. Lübbers DW (1977) Die Bedeutung des lokalen Gewebesauerstoffdruckes und des pO_2-Histogramms für die Beurteilung der Sauerstoffversorgung eines Organes. Prakt Anästh 12:184
20. Ross R, Glomset JA (1976) The pathogenesis of atherosclerosis. N Engl J Med 295:420
21. Sachs L (1984) Angewandte Statistik. Springer, Berlin
22. Schmid-Schönbein H (1982) Physiologie und Pathophysiologie der Mikrozirkulation aus rheologischer Sicht. Internist 23:359
23. Schwartz SM (1985) Hypertension as a vascular response to injury. In Folkow B, Nordlander M, Strauer BE, Wikstrand J (eds) Hypertension. Pathophysiology and clinical implications of structural changes. AB Hässle, Mölndal, p 74

24. Sivertsson R (1970) The hemodynamic importance of structural vascular changes in essential hypertension. Acta Physiol Scand Suppl 343
25. Takeshita A, Mark AL (1980) Decreased vasodilator capacity of forearm resistance vessels in borderline hypertension. Hypertension 2:610

Relationship between Muscle Tissue Oxygen Tension and Diabetes Duration in Insulin-Dependent Diabetic Patients: Evaluation with a New Polarographic Technique

K. Krönert, W. Grauer, M. Günderoth-Palmowski, A. Schuler, C. Zimmermann, R. Heinrich, D. Luft, M. Eggstein

Summary

The objective of the study was to evaluate 1. whether muscle tissue oxygen tension is changed in recently diagnosed insulin- dependent diabetic patients and 2. whether muscle tissue oxygen tension is related to the duration of the disease.

Muscle tissue oxygen tensions were measured with a new polarographic technique in seven recently diagnosed insulin- dependent diabetic patients (group I), in six diabetic patients with a longer duration of the disease (group II) but without obvious diabetic microangiopathy, and in six healthy subjects (group III).

The groups were matched for sex and age. In addition to parameters reflecting peripheral nerve function (sensory and motor nerve conduction velocities, electromyogram), four cardiovascular reflex tests were performed (E/I ratio, 30/15 ratio, Valsalva ratio, sustained handgrip test). Muscle tissue oxygen tension was analyzed while breathing ambient air and oxygen enriched air for a period of 30 minutes.

Hemodynamic and rheological data as well as automatic nerve function tests did not significantly differ between the three groups. Long-term diabetic subjects had significantly lower nerve conduction velocities than healthy subjects.

While breathing ambient air, muscle tissue oxygen tension was significantly higher in both diabetic groups compared with the controls. After inhalation of oxygen enriched air, capillary pO_2 significantly increased in all subjects studied. In contrary to the controls who significantly augmented muscle tissue pO_2 by breathing oxygen enriched air, the short-term diabetic patients did not change muscle oxygenation and the long-term diabetics even decreased muscle tissue oxygen tension. Although it is difficult to explain these results, they do not support the assumption that local hypoxia is one of the leading causes for the hemodynamic changes observed in early phases of diabetes mellitus.

Pathogenesis and development of diabetic microangiopathy are still unknown. Furthermore, the relationship between hyperglycemia and the small vessel disease is obscure and has to be elucidated. In early stages of

Clinical Oxygen Pressure Measurement II
A.M. Ehrly et al. (Eds.)
© Blackwell Ueberreuter Wissenschaft Berlin 1990

diabetes mellitus, a generalized microvascular dilatation has been documented for the retina and for the kidneys [1, 2, 3]. These hemodynamic changes in the microcirculation seem to be causally related to the subsequent development of diabetic microangiopathy [4]. The mechanism initiating the alterations in microcirculation is also unknown. Several hypotheses concerning the development of vasodilatation have been postulated. The most popular one suggests a general tissue hypoxia leading to the hemodynamic changes in the microcirculation because microvessels are highly sensitive to variations in oxygen tension [5, 6]. Until now, it was difficult to determine tissue oxygen tension. In 1984, Fleckenstein et al. [7] presented a new method for the bedside recording of tissue oxygen tension. This technique uses thin steal coated polarographic needle probes for the measurement of tissue oxygen tension.

The following investigation deals with muscle tissue oxygenation of insulin-dependent diabetes of varying duration. The specific questions asked were:

1. Is muscle tissue oxygen tension altered in recently diagnosed insulin-dependent diabetic patients?
2. Does muscle tissue oxygen tension differ between recently diagnosed diabetic patients and diabetes with a longer duration?

Subjects and Methods

The study protocol was approved by the local ethical committee. Seven recently diagnosed insulin-dependent diabetic patients (group I) and six diabetic patients with a diabetic history of 11 ± 3 years ($\bar{x} \pm SD$) (group II) participated after written consent. Both groups were matched for sex and age. Group II diabetic patients had no signs of diabetic microangiopathy documented by fundoscopy and Albustix® control of the urine.

Both groups received intensive conventional therapy consisting of two injections of NPH insulin in the morning, before breakfast, and in the evening, at 10 pm, and variable amounts of regular insulin before each main meal. Mean blood glucose was acceptable, at least during the last ten days before the beginning of the study. However, concentrations of glycohemoglobin were variable. Patients with other diseases apart from diabetes mellitus as well as those taking drugs known to influence microcirculation were excluded.

Six healthy subjects (group III) matched for sex and age served as controls.

Clinical data of the individual subjects studied are summarized in Table 1. In addition to detailed clinical and neurological examinations, electromyogram of the left anterior tibial muscle, motor (right median nerve, left tibial nerve), and sensory nerve (right median nerve, left sural nerve) conduction velocities were obtained with standard methods. During the measurement, skin temperature was kept constant at 34°C. Four different cardiovascular reflex tests (heart rate variation during deep

Table 1. Clinical data of the 3 groups studied

Group	Age (yr)	Sex	BMI (kg/m²)	diab.duration (mths)	MBG (mg/dl)	HbA₁ (%)
I 1	21	m	22.5	12	86 ± 25	8.8
2	24	f	22.5	2	210 ± 49	9.0
3	21	m	21.9	1	105 ± 41	12.3
4	22	f	17.2	1	138 ± 45	13.4
5	42	m	20.5	11	125 ± 30	8.0
6	24	m	24.1	1.5	115 ± 34	11.3
7	36	m	22.5	1.5	96 ± 38	14.7
II 1	40	m	26.0	168	145 ± 41	10.1
2	19	f	25.4	72	118 ± 41	12.1
3	20	m	23.3	84	126 ± 19	8.5
4	21	f	18.2	60	136 ± 43	8.3
5	21	m	22.8	156	145 ± 60	7.1
6	28	m	27.0	252	153 ± 23	10.6
III 1	26	m	22.5	–	90 ± 6	5.9
2	25	m	22.8	–	82 ± 3	5.0
3	26	m	26.3	–	87 ± 6	5.4
4	36	f	18.3	–	100 ± 2	5.6
5	26	m	21.6	–	93 ± 6	5.7
6	22	f	17.5	–	108 ± 3	5.5

breathing – E/I ratio, heart rate variation while lying and standing – 30/15 ratio, heart rate variation during the Valsalva manoeuvre – Valsalva ratio, and the sustained hand griptest – 30 % of maximal voluntary contraction) were performed twice in succession in order to evaluate cardiac autonomic nerve function. The mean of the two measurements was calculated.

Blood samples were collected to make blood cell counts and to determine hematocrit and total serum protein concentration.

Oxygen tensions of the right anterior tibial muscle were analyzed by a steal coated polarographic needle probe. The method has been described in detail elsewhere [7]. Each examination provided 200 individual tissue pO₂ values which finally combined to establish a pO₂ histogram (KIMOC 250, Gewebe pO₂- Histograph, Ges. für Med. Sondentechnik mbH, Kiel-Mielkendorf, FRG).

Fig. 1 demonstrates the study design. The examinations began at 9 am, after the usual breakfast. Control subjects were allowed to eat ad lib, the diabetic patients had their usual diet. Tea, coffee, and nicotine were not allowed. Measurements were performed at rest, while comfortably lying on a bed. The room was air- conditioned at a temperature of 20 – 23° C.

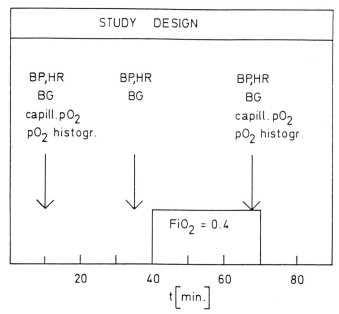

Fig. 1. Study design: Measurements of muscle tissue pO_2 were performed at rest while breathing ambient air and after inhalation of oxygen enriched air (40 %) for a period of 30 minutes. **BP** = blood pressure; **HR** = heart rate; **BG** = blood glucose capill.; pO_2 = capillary pO_2; **pO_2 histogr.** histogram of muscle tissue pO_2; **FiO_2** = fraction of inspired oxygen

Subjects were wearing underwear and were covered with a blanket according to their subjective feeling of thermal comfort. After local anesthesia, a teflon cannula (Abbocath, 18 g, Criticon TM, GmbH, Norderstedt, FRG) which served as a guide-way for the needle probe was inserted into the skin above the right anterior tibial muscle. Muscle tissue pO_2 values were measured while breathing 1. ambient air, and 2. oxygen enriched air with an oxygen concentration of about 40 % for a period of 30 minutes (Bard Inspiron, Accurox Mask, Bard Limited, Pennywell Industrial Estate, Sunderland, England).

Simultaneously, heart rates, blood pressures, and blood glucose concentrations, pO_2, pCO_2, and pH were determined in arterialized capillary blood drawn from the hyperemic ear lobe (Forapin Salbe, Mack, Illertissen, FRG).

Statistical Methods

Means ($\overline{x}$), and standard deviations (SD) were calculated with standard methods. The values of the different groups were compared using the U test of Wilcoxon, Mann, and Whitney. The t-test was used for paired and normally distributed measurements. $p < 0.05$ was considered significant (8).

Results

Blood cell counts, hematocrits, and total serum protein concentrations did not significantly differ between the three groups studied. Nor did blood pressures and heart rates (Table 2).

Table 2. Laboratory and hemodynamic data ($\bar{x} \pm$ SD) of the 3 groups studied (BP = blood pressure)

	Group I (n = 7)	Group II (n = 6)	Group III (n = 6)
leucocytes (ul⁻¹)	6600 ± 1700	6700 ± 2200	6400 ± 1200
hemoglobin (g/dl)	14.4 ± 2.0	14.8 ± 1.4	14.4 ± 0.8
hematocrit (%)	43.5 ± 5.2	44.6 ± 4.3	44.7 ± 2.6
thrombocytes (ul⁻¹)	284000 ± 49000	258000 ± 94000	261000 ± 59000
total serum protein (g/dl)	7.0 ± 0.8	7.2 ± 0.8	7.4 ± 0.3
syst. BP (mmHg)	114.8 ± 8.3	112.5 ± 10.8	112.8 ± 9.0
diast. BP (mmHg)	81.7 ± 9.8	76.7 ± 8.2	74.5 ± 9.4
heart rate (min⁻¹)	70.9 ± 6.3	69.3 ± 7.4	67.3 ± 12.1

During the examination period, mean blood glucose concentrations of group II subjects were significantly higher than those of the controls. However, mean blood glucose concentrations of group I diabetics and control subjects did not significantly differ. At least during the period of examination, diabetic patients did not suffer from severe insulin deficiency, as indicated by mean blood glucose concentrations (Fig. 2).
Variables of the peripheral nervous system and the results of the cardiovascular reflex tests are listed in Table 3. In group II diabetic patients, nerve conduction velocities were significantly reduced in comparison with the control subjects ($p < 0,01$, $p < 0,025$, respectively). Nerve conduction velocities of groups I and III did not significantly differ, nor did the results of the cardiovascular reflex tests of all subjects studied.
Mean **capillary** pO₂ values of all subjects were not significantly different, although at all time points they were significantly higher in the controls. In all subjects, both controls and diabetics, capillary pO₂ significantly increased while breathing oxygen enriched air for a period of 30 minutes ($p < 0,05$) (Fig. 3).
However, while breathing ambient air, both diabetic groups exhibited significantly elevated **muscle** pO₂ values compared with the control subjects ($p < 0,025$, $p < 0,005$, respectively).

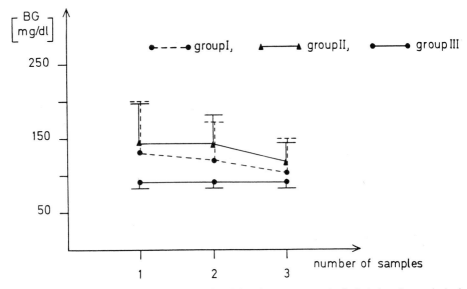

Fig. 2. Blood glucose concentrations (BG) of the three groups studied during the period of examination ($\overline{x} \pm$ SD)

Table 3. Variables of the peripheral and automatic nervous system ($\overline{x} \pm$ SD). MNCV = motor nerve conduction velocity; SNCV = sensory nerve conduction velocity; SHG = sustained hand grip test.

	group I (n = 7)	group II (n = 6)	group III (n = 6)
MNCV – tibial nerve (m/s)	42.9 ± 8.2	37.9 ± 2.2[+]	46.0 ± 3.3
MNCV – median nerve (m/s)	55.9 ± 8.0	–	64.3 ± 6.4
SNCV -median nerve (m/s)	51.3 ± 7.6	–	52.7 ± 3.9
SNCV – sural nerve (m/s)	50.0 ± 10.7	42.8 ± 4.4[++]	52.5 ± 4.5
E/I ratio	1.29 ± 0.11	1.20 ± 0.10	1.33 ± 0.06
30/15 ratio	1.18 ± 0.19	1.17 ± 0.14	1.24 ± 0.06
Valsalva ratio	1.51 ± 0.22	1.34 ± 0.22	1.55 ± 0.26
SHG (mmHg)	28.6 ± 10.7	22.5 ± 4.2	30.0 ± 8.8

[+]$p < 0.01$ [++]$p < 0.025$

After inhalation of oxygen enriched air, muscle tissue oxygen tensions significantly increased in the control subjects ($p<0,05$). Despite an equal increase in capillary pO_2, muscle tissue oxygen tensions remained unchanged in group I diabetics and even significantly declined ($p<0,005$) in group II diabetics while breathing oxygen enriched air (Fig. 3).

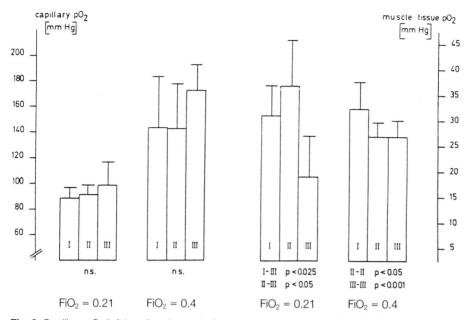

Fig. 3. Capillary pO$_2$ (left hand) and muscle tissue oxygen tension (right hand) of the three groups studied while breathing ambient air and oxygen enriched air (40 %). Values are expressed as means ± SD

Table 4. Muscle tissue oxygen tension (pO$_2$) while breathing **a)** ambient air (21 %) and **b)** oxygen enriched air (40 %) ($\bar{x}$ ± SD).

	Muscle tissue pO$_2$ (21 %) (mmHg)	Muscle tissue pO$_2$ (40 %) (mmHg)
group I (n = 7)	31.0 ± 5.9	32.5 ± 4.8
group II (n = 6)	37.2 ± 9.0	26.7 ± 1.6
group III (n = 6)	19.2 ± 8.2	26.7 ± 2.9

$^+$p < 0.025 $^{++}$p < 0.005

Although recently diagnosed insulin-dependent diabetic patients did not augment muscle tissue pO$_2$ by inhalation of oxygen enriched air, their muscle tissue oxygen tensions were still markedly elevated in comparison with the control subjects (p<0,025) (Table 4).

Pooled pO$_2$ histograms differed considerably between the three groups studied (Fig. 4): in contrast to the control subjects, the pO$_2$ histograms of all diabetic patients were shifted towards higher pO$_2$ concentrations without a definite peak. After breathing oxygen-enriched air, the pO$_2$ values of the diabetic patients displayed abnormal distributions, forming two separate bell-shaped peaks.

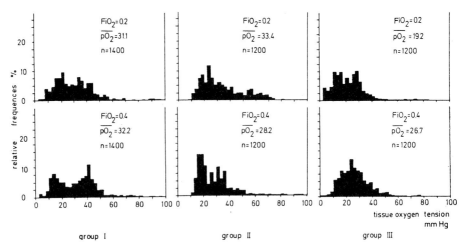

Fig. 4. Pooled pO$_2$ histograms of the three groups studied while breathing ambient air (upper pannel) and oxygen enriched air (lower pannel)

Discussion

The objective of this study was to evaluate 1. whether muscle tissue oxygen tension is altered in recently diagnosed insulin- dependent diabetic patients, and 2. whether tissue oxygen tension is related to the duration of the disease.

The results demonstrate clearly that muscle tissue oxygen tension is markedly elevated in recently diagnosed insulin- dependent diabetic patients and in long-term diabetes mellitus without obvious microangiopathy as well. After inhalation of oxygen enriched air, the diabetic groups react in different ways: while muscle tissue oxygen tension does not change in short-term diabetic patients, it significantly decreases in long-term diabetes mellitus.

Microangiopathy is the hallmark of diabetes mellitus. Although diabetic retinopathy was described more than 125 years ago and diabetic nephropathy was reported nearly 50 years ago, the mechanisms responsible for diabetic microvascular disease have not yet been resolved. Recent evidence suggests that hemodynamic changes in the microcirculation precede the development of microangiopathy. In early phases of insulin-dependent diabetes mellitus, renal and retinal vessels are dilated. Blood flow is elevated within these dilated capillaries [1, 2]. Vasodilatation has been shown to fluctuate with the state of metabolic control. Furthermore, blood flow is considerably elevated in muscular and cutaneous tissues of the forearm [9] as well as in abdominal adipose tissue of short-term insulin-dependent diabetic patients [10]. After initiation of insulin therapy, a significant decrease in capillary blood flow was observed (10).

Dilatation of the venous end of the capillaries of the toe nailfold has also been reported [11]. Studies performed in experimental diabetes likewise demonstrate a state of widespread hyperperfusion in the early phases of diabetes mellitus [12, 13].

These hemodynamic changes in the microcirculation, namely vasodilatation associated with elevated blood flow and with increased intracapillary pressure seem to cause increased permeability to macromolecules, capillary wall proliferation, consequent thickening of basement membranes, and luminal narrowing [14, 15].

The process mediating these early hemodynamic abnormalities is still unknown. Several mechanisms contributing to generalized vasodilatation have been discussed:

1. reduced plasma renin activity in insulin-dependent diabetes mellitus [16],
2. lower angiotensin receptor density in insulin-dependent diabetic patients [17],
3. reduced vascular reactivity to catecholamines in insulin- dependent diabetic patients [18],
4. chronic plasma volume expansion due to hyperglycemia [3],
5. increased production of vasodilatory substances like prostaglandin E [19],
6. local tissue hypoxia due to insulin.

The last hypothesis citing local tissue hypoxia due to insulin as one of the main causes for microvascular dilatation is a very popular hypothesis. Since microcirculation has been shown to be very sensitive to variations in oxygen tension [6, 20], microvascular dilatation is thought to be an autoregulatory response to relative tissue hypoxia providing a better tissue perfusion and improving tissue oxygen delivery. Ditzel and Standl [5] observed elevated concentrations of 2,3-diphospho-glycerate (DPG) in diabetic patients depending upon the state of metabolic control. They presumed that the increase in 2,3-DPG leading to a shift to the right of the oxyhemoglobin dissociation curve compensates tissue hypoxia [5]. Furthermore, total oxygen consumption is elevated in diabetes mellitus, which might aggravate local tissue hypoxia [21].

Our results contradict the common opinion concerning the pathogenesis of diabetic microangiopathy. Taking all the above mentioned facts into account, the interpretation of our results – highly elevated muscle tissue oxygen tension in diabetic patients with varying duration of the disease – is rather difficult.

Several mechanisms might be involved in augmenting tissue oxygen tension:

1. Tissue hyperperfusion. This assumption may be supported by previous studies which showed generalized vasodilatation and increased capillary blood flow in early phases of diabetes mellitus.
2. Increased oxygen diffusion capacity may also elevate tissue oxygen tension. Increased oxygen diffusion capacity might be the result of abnormal permeability of capillary basement membranes not only to plasma proteins but also to oxygen [22].

3. Moreover, increased tissue oxygen tension may be due to an abnormal regulation of microcirculation leading to an altered distribution of blood within the capillary network.

The last two hypotheses need further evaluation.

Capillary hyperperfusion has been shown to depend on the state of metabolic control and to normalize after initiating an adequate insulin therapy [10]. In our diabetic patients, who had received an adequate therapy, insulin application did not reverse the hemodynamic changes we observed. Mean blood glucose concentrations of both diabetic groups reflected rather good metabolic control. However concentrations of glycated hemoglobin varied considerably.

In contrast to the control subjects, newly diagnosed insulin- dependent diabetic patients did not augment muscle tissue oxygen tension while breathing oxygen enriched air. In patients with a longer diabetic history, muscle tissue oxygen tension even declined after a period of increased oxygen supply. These different reactions may point either to an abnormal regulation of microcirculation or to varying reactivities of the small vessels to increased capillary pO_2. Data providing a more detailed or exact explanation of this phenomenon are not available.

In conclusion, 1. we found markedly elevated muscle tissue oxygen tensions in recently diagnosed insulin-dependent diabetes mellitus and in diabetic patients with a longer duration of the disease but without obvious microangiopathy. 2. These elevated muscle tissue oxygen tensions could not further be augmented by inhalation of oxygen enriched air in short-term diabetic patients and even significantly decreased in diabetes of longer duration. Our results do not support the assumption that hypoxia is a leading cause of the hemodynamic changes particularly in the early phases of diabetes mellitus.

Acknowledgements. This study was supported by grant HE 1293-1/2 of the DFG (Deutsche Forschungsgemeinschaft).

References

1. Kohner EM, Hamilton AM, Saunders SJ, Suttcliffe BA, Bulpitt CJ (1975) The retinal blood flow in diabetes. Diabetologia 11:27
2. Hostetter TH, Troy JL, Brenner BM Glomerular hemodynamics in experimental diabetes mellitus. Kidney Int 19:410
3. Brocher-Mortensen J (1973) Glomerular filtration rate and extracellular fluid volumes during normoglycemia and moderate hyperglycemia in diabetes. Scand J Clin Lab Invest 32:311
4. Zatz R, Brenner BM (1986) Pathogenesis of diabetic microangiopathy. A hemodynamic view. Am J Med 80:443
5. Ditzel J, Standl E (1975) The problem of tissue oxygenation in diabetes mellitus. I. Its relation to early functional changes in the microcirculation of diabetic subjects. Acta Med Scand, Suppl 578:49
6. Hansen M, Madsen J (1973) Estimation of relative changes in testing muscle blood flow by ^{133}Xe washout: The effect of oxygen. Scand J Clin Lab Invest 31:133

7. Fleckenstein W, Weiss Ch, Heinrich R, Schomerus H, Kersting Th (1984) A new method for the bed-side recording of tissue pO$_2$ histograms. Verh Dtsch Ges Inn Med 90:439
8. Sachs L (1987) Angewandte Statistik. Springer, Berlin
9. Christensen NJ (1970) A reversible vascular abnormality associated with diabetic ketosis. Clin Sci 39:539
10. Gundersen HJG (1974) Peripheral blood flow and metabolic control in juvenile diabetes. Diabetologia 10:225
11. Landau J, Davis E (1960) The small blood vessels of the conjunctiva and nailbed in diabetes mellitus. Lancet ii:731
12. Bohlen HG, Hankins KD (1982) Early arteriolar and capillary changes in streptozotocin-induced diabetic rats and intraperitoneal hyperglycemic rats. Diabetologia 22:344
13. McCuskey PA, McCusky RS (1984) In vivo and electron microscopic study of the development of cerebral diabetic microangiopathy. Microcirc Endothel Lymphat 1:221
14. Parving H-H, Noer I, Deckert T (1976) The effect of metabolic regulation on microvascular permeability to small and large molecules in short-term juvenile diabetes. Diabetologia 12:161
15. O'Hare JA, Ferris JB, Twomey B, O'Sullivan DJ (1983) Poor metabolic control, hypertension and microangiopathy independently increase the transcapillary escape rate of albumin in diabetes. Diabetologia 25:260
16. Christlieb AR, Kaldany A, D'Elia JA (1976) Plasma renin activity and hypertension in diabetes mellitus. Diabetes 25:969
17. Ballermann BJ, Skoredei KL, Brenner BM (1984) Reduced glomerular angiotensin-II-receptor density in early untreated diabetes mellitus in the rat. Am J Physiol 247:F110
18. Christlieb AR, Janka H-U, Kraus B (1976) Vascular reactivity to angiotensin II and to norepinephrine in diabetic subjects. Diabetes 25:268
19. Halushka PV, Lurie D, Colwell JA (1977) Increased synthesis of prostaglandin-E-like material by platelets from patients with diabetes mellitus. N Engl J Med 297:1306
20. Ross JM, Fairchild HM, Weldy S, Guyton AC (1962) Autoregulation of blood flow by oxygen lack. Am J Physiol 202:21
21. Horstmann P: The oxygen consumption in diabetes mellitus. Acta Med Scand 139:326
22. Leinonen H, Matikainen E, Juntunen J (1982) Permeability and morphology of skeletal muscle capillaries in type I (insulin- dependent) diabetes mellitus. Diabetologia 22:158

Intramuscular Oxygen Pressure in Patients with Chronic Occlusive Arterial Disease

K. Grossmann

Introduction

The extent of collateral blood flow in claudicants is not correlated to the stage of the occlusive arterial disease. To get more detailed information on the kinetics of the pathophysiological processes in intermittent claudication, direct measurements at the cellular level of the muscle tissue are required [4].

In the present investigation we used micro-gold-electrodes in order to gather relative data on intramuscular oxygen pressure. The measuring procedure was constructed so that each measurement could be carried out over an extended period of time [1, 2]. Earlier results have shown that for this kind of investigation the best localization of the electrodes is the tibialis anterior muscle [7].

We directed our attention to the following three questions:

1. Using this polarographic method, which parameter allows for reproducibility and for differentiation between healthy volunteers and patients with occlusive arterial disease?
2. What is the correlation between intramuscular oxygen pressure (pO_2) values and blood flow values when an ischemic reaction is created?
3. What is the influence of drug therapy on the intramuscular pO_2 levels?

Subjects and methods

Measurements were performed in the tibialis anterior muscle in recumbent human subjects with legs fixed. After local anesthesia of the skin, a plastic injection needle was introduced into the muscle to a depth of 15 mm and then cut 2 mm above the surface of the skin. The pO_2 electrode was then introduced 20 mm into the muscle tissue. The electrodes had a tip diameter of 4 μm and were covered with polystyrole [2, 7]. Recording of pO_2 in the muscle tissue was started with an ischemic time interval and was continued for a certain period of time [5, 7].

Clinical Oxygen Pressure Measurement II
A.M. Ehrly et al. (Eds.)
© Blackwell Ueberreuter Wissenschaft Berlin 1990

In 59 single tests carried out on 20 healthy volunteers we explored the reaction of the pO_2 level following various ischemic times. We were able to show that the reaction of the pO_2 level after after 1 minute ischemia was not reproducible, whereas the ischemic reaction after 3 and 5 minutes displayed comparable courses [7]. For comparison between pO_2 measurements we studied the pO_2 recovery time in each record, i.e. the time interval between the end of ischemia and the point at which the pO_2 curve rejoins the original level [7].

Next we investigated 27 patients (mean age 55.1 years) with chronic occlusive arterial disease, as ascertained by an intensive angiological diagnosis. The arterial occlusions were found in the arteries of the pelvis and/or the upper part of the thigh. All patients in this group suffered from severe intermittent claudication stage II according to Fontaine and had pain-free walking distances of less than 200 m (group B).

27 healthy subjects as ascertained by angiological diagnosis (mean age 29.9 years) were used as controls (group A).

In both groups pO_2 levels were measured before, during and after a 3 minute ischemia. Synchronously we registered the arterial blood flow in the same calf segment using venous occlusion plethysmography (pneumatic system) [6].

The data represent the arithmetic means and the standard derivation (Table 1). In the upper part we can see the blood flow values of groups A and B. The lower part shows the pO_2 recovery times for both groups. The difference between them was significant.

Table 1. Correlation between pO_2 recovery time and circulatory parameters in healthy subjects (group A, n=27), and patients with chronic occlusive arterial disease (group B, n=27).

	group A	group B
blood flow (ml/min./100 ml tissue)		
first flow	18.4 ± 5.9	5.9 ± 3.8
peak flow	19.6 ± 10.7	10.0 ± 4.9
time values (s)		
peak flow time	1.8	30.6 ± 13.5
whole hyperemic time	52.4 ± 9.6	79.3 ± 29.7
pO_2-recovery time	60.2 ± 21.5	125.3 ± 33.0

It is noteworthy that pO_2 recovery times in the patients were longer in relation to the whole hyperemic blood flow time. The results obtained in this study support the theory of Ehrly and Schroeder according to which microcirculatory blood flow in ischemic tissue is inhomogenously distributed [4].

In a further study we registered intramuscular pO_2 during intraarterial drug application. In 45 patients with chronic occlusive arterial disease

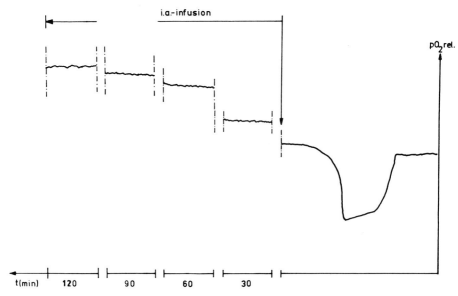

Fig. 1. Intramuscular oxygen pressure level in a 53 year old man with an occlusion of the A. femoralis superficialis during intraarterial infusion therapy

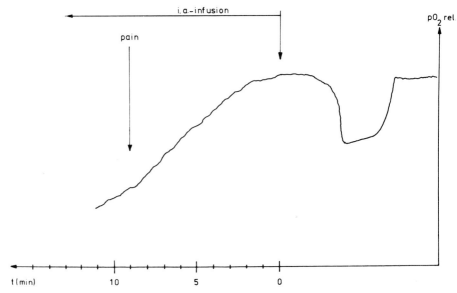

Fig. 2. Original pO_2 registration during intraarterial infusion with 1.0 g hydroxymethylpyridin: pO_2 level falls and later pains reappear

stage III according to Fontaine we applied an intraarterial infusion consisting of 500 mg pentoxifylline in 500 ml low molecular dextran over a period of 2 hours.

The intraartieral drug application was performed by means of a catheter introduced according to the Seldinger method [8]. The catheter tip was shifted right into the region of the arterial occlusion.

The pO_2 levels recorded varied greatly. Fig. 1 shows stepwise increases of pO_2 level during drug application. When vasoacitve (dilatory) drugs are applied, the steal phenomenon can be observed (Fig. 2): the pO_2 level fell, and later patients complained of pains in foot and calf.

The results indicate that measurements of muscle tissue pO_2 with micro-gold-electrodes seem to be an objective method for the investigation of oxygen supply to ischemic muscles, and that the results correlate both with ischemic reactions and with therapeutic procedures.

The disadvantage was that these measurements indicated relative changes only. In the coming period we want to continue our investigations using a quantitative pO_2 measuring system.

Summary

The investigation reports the results of intramuscular measurements of oxygen pressure carried out in the tibialis anterior muscle.

In a first study we compared the intramuscular oxygen pressure with the findings of venous occlusion plethysmography. The pO_2 recovery time after 3 minutes ischemia was found to be a reproducible parameter. Yielding 60 secs. in healthy subjects (n=27) and 126 secs. in patients with disturbances of arterial circulation (n=27), it allowed for a reliable distinction between the two groups.

In a second study we registered the pO_2 level during intraarterial drug therapy. In 45 patients with arteriosclerotic occlusive arterial disease stage III according to Fontaine the intramuscular oxygen pressure proved to be a very sensitive parameter to the treatment. The steal phenomenon in muscle circulation was revealed at an early stage. The disadvantage was that these measurements indicated relative changes only.

References

1. Ardenne Mv (1976) In vivo-Gewinnung von Richtwerten über O_2- Mangelzustände und Therapiewirkungen in erkrankten Körpergeweben durch pO_2-Messung mit Mikroelektroden. Z Med Lab Technik 17:116
2. Böhme G, Kaltofen S, Petzold D (1981) Entwicklung polarographischer Meßsysteme zur transkutanen, extrakorporalen und Gewebe-pO_2-Bestimmung. Dtsch Gesundh Wesen 36:675
3. Doermer C, Schroeder W (1975) Blood flow and tissue pO_2 in trained and untrained gastrognemius muscle of the anesthetized Guinea pig. Europ J Appl Physiol 34:33
4. Ehrly AM, Schroeder W (1977) Oxygen pressure in ischemic muscle tissue of patients with chronic occlusive arterial disease. Angiology 28:101

5. Ehrly AM (1981) Messung des Gewebesauerstoffdruckes bei Patienten. G. Witzstrock, Baden-Baden
6. Grossmann K (1979) Venenverschlußplethysmographie. In: Thiele P. Diagnostikfibel arterieller Durchblutungsstörungen. G. Fischer, Jena
7. Grossmann K, Weiss D, Petzold D, Kaltofen S (1986) Die Registrierung des intramuskulären Sauerstoffpartialdruckes bei gesunden Probanden und bei Patienten mit einer arteriellen Verschlusskrankheit. Z Klin Med 41:453
8. Grossmann K, Knischka A (1987) Die intraarterielle Therapie bei arterieller Verschlußkrankheit der Extremitäten. Z Ärztl Fortbild 81:879
9. Hlavova A, Linhardt J, Prerovsky I, Ganz V, Fronek A (1966) Leg oxygen consumption at rest and during exercise in normal subjects and in patients with femoral artery occlusion. Clin Sci 30:377
10. Jussila E, Ninikoski J, Inberg MV (1979) Tissue gas tensions in the calf muscles of patients with lower limb arterial ischemia. Scand J Thor Cardiovasc Surg 13:77
11. Kessler M, Lübbers DW (1966) Aufbau und Anwendungsmöglichkeiten verschiedener pO_2-Elektroden. Pflügers Arch Ges Physiol 291:82
12. Thompson LP, Mohrman DE (1983) Blood flow and oxygen consumption in skeletal muscle during sympathetic stimulation. Amer J Physiol 245:66

Skeletal Muscle pO_2 Assessment, Hemodynamics and Oxygen-Related Parameters in Critically Jll Patients

G.I.J.M. Beerthuizen, R.J.A. Goris, F.J.A. Kreuzer

Introduction

The function of blood circulation is to deliver an adequate volume of oxygen at an adequate partial pressure to replace the oxygen used at the terminal oxidase of the respiratory chain in the mitochondria. This oxygen supply is vital, as 95 % of the energy generated by the body normally originates from aerobic pathways and the entire oxygen store of the body would support resting needs for maximally 5 minutes [1]. Therefore, inadequate tissue perfusion results in inadequate oxygen transport to the mitochondria.

However, direct measurement of tissue perfusion and/or oxygenation is still difficult. Until now only systemic parameters such as arterial blood pressure, central venous pressure, pulmonary arterial pressure and cardiac output have been monitored. In critically ill patients, these parameters are meticulously controlled, but the therapeutic interventions may themselves actually impair tissue perfusion and tissue oxygenation.

Measurement of skeletal muscl pO_2 may provide an index of peripheral tissue oxygenation [2, 3]. Skeletal muscle pO_2 depends on the balance between rate of oxygen delivery to the tissue and rate of oxygen consumption by the tissue [4]. Each of these in turn depend upon a complex series of interrelated factors. In critically ill patients, one or more of these factors may be influenced by the treatment instituted. These alterations might lead to an increase or decrease in skeletal muscle pO_2. We studied the relationship between skeletal muscle pO_2, hemodynamics and oxygen-related parameters in critically ill patients.

Patients and methods

In 6 critically ill patients a Swan-Ganz catheter (Gould Swan-Ganz catheter, Siemens monitor) allowing for extensive monitoring was inserted for treatment at the time of entry into the study. Systolic arterial blood pressure, mean arterial blood pressure, heart rate, central venous pressure, pulmonary arterial pressure and pulmonary arterial wedge pressure were

Clinical Oxygen Pressure Measurement II
A.M. Ehrly et al. (Eds.)
© Blackwell Ueberreuter Wissenschaft Berlin 1990

determined. Cardiac output was obtained using the thermodilution method with the aid of a cardiac output computer (Edwards cardiac output computer). Arterial and mixed venous blood gases (ABL-3, Radiometer), arterial and mixed venous oxygen saturation (Oximeter, Instrumentation Laboratories) as well as hemoglobin and hematocrit were determined. Skeletal muscle pO_2 was measured in the quadriceps femoris muscle using a polarographic needle electrode. The electrode was calibrated before the measurement and positioned in the vastus lateralis of the quadriceps femoris muscle approximately 3 to 4 cm deep using a 20-gauge needle as a guiding canula. The electrode was withdrawn stepwise, and after each step of 200 μm a pO_2 value was measured. In this way 100 pO_2 values from 100 different places in the skeletal muscle were obtained. From these 100 pO_2 values the median was calculated, giving us the skeletal muscle pO_2 assessment. At the end of each such assessment, the electrode was withdrawn from the patient. One complete assessment takes 5 minutes. All measurements were performed at the start of the study and again after 2, 4, 6, 8 and 16 hours. Stroke volume, left and right ventricular stroke work index, systemic vascular resistance, pulmonary vascular resistance, arterial oxygen supply, arterio-venous oxygen difference, oxygen extraction ratio, oxygen consumption and p50 of the oxyhemoglobin dissociation curve were calculated. Correlation between skeletal muscle pO_2 and the other parameters was studied by calculating the Pearson correlation coefficient transformed according to Hotelling [5]. Differences were considered significant where $p < 0.05$.

Results

6 critically ill patients being treated for septic shock, multiple abdominal abscess, pulmonary edema, cardiac insufficiency, shock and multiple organ failure respectively were studied. All the patients were mechanically ventilated. Their ages ranged from 37 to 70 years. They displayed a wide variation in cardiac output, systemic vascular resistance, F_iO_2, arterial oxygen supply, arterio-venous oxygen difference, oxygen extraction, oxygen consumption, arterial pO_2, mixed venous pO_2 and skeletal muscle pO_2. Correlation between skeletal muscle pO_2 and the other parameters is presented in Table 1.

No significant correlations were found between skeletal muscle pO_2 and hemodynamic parameters in these patients. A significant within-patient correlation was found only between skeletal muscle pO_2 and arterial sO_2, mixed venous sO_2 and arterio-venous oxygen difference.

Discussion

Adequacy of tissue oxygenation cannot be predicted solely from measurement of arterial pO_2 since normal arterial values may be associated

Table 1. Correlation between skeletal muscle pO$_2$ and other variables (6 pts)

Parameter	Mean	
	Pearson coeff	p-value
Systolic arterial blood pressure	0.28	0.16
Heart rate	0.34	0.07
Central venous pressure	0.02	0.99
Mean arterial blood pressure	0.24	0.21
Cardiac output	0.01	0.96
Oxygen consumption	− 0.33	0.09
Arterial oxygen supply	0.08	0.68
Oxygen extraction ratio	− 0.36	0.06
Arterial pH	0.12	0.28
Arterial pO$_2$	− 0.07	0.73
Arterial sO$_2$	0.37	0.02
Mixed venous pH	0.16	0.42
Mixed venous pO$_2$	0.24	0.21
Mixed venous pCO$_2$	0.07	0.72
Mixed venous sO$_2$	0.46	0.02
Arterio-venous oxygen difference	− 0.41	0.03

with inadequate tissue oxygen supply [3]. Measurement of mixed venous pO$_2$ also does not reliably reflect adequacy of tissue perfusion since, in sepsis, mixed venous pO$_2$ may be elevated due to inadequate oxygen extraction in the microcirculation [6]. Monitoring pO$_2$ in the tissue may allow early detection of a disturbance in tissue oxygenation and may indicate how far the various compensatory mechanisms have been mobilized.

Skeletal muscle pO$_2$ depends upon the balance between rate of oxygen delivery to tissue and rate of oxygen consumption by tissue. Each of these in turn depend upon a complex series of interrelated factors. Oxygen delivery to muscle depends on blood flow to the muscle, which in turn depends on cardiac output and its distribution to different organs and on the oxygen content of the blood. This latter parameter depends on arterial pO$_2$, arterial sO$_2$ and hemoglobin concentration. Skeletal muscle oxygen tension is therefore not solely dependent upon the rate of oxygen consumption by the tissue. If oxygen delivery increases, but oxygen consumption increases even more, then tissue oxygen tension decreases.

Arterial sO$_2$, mixed venous sO$_2$ and arterio-venous oxygen difference are parameters which most closely reflect the balance between oxygen supply and oxygen consumption. These parameters were the only ones that correlated significantly with skeletal muscle pO$_2$. This underlines the value of skeletal muscle pO$_2$ assessment in determining the balance between oxygen supply and oxygen consumption in skeletal muscle tissue in critically ill patients. These findings are in agreement with previous results found in patients after extracorporeal circulation [7].

In conclusion, in critically ill patients skeletal muscle pO_2 assessment indicates the balance between oxygen supply and oxygen consumption in the muscle. If skeletal muscle pO_2 decreases in critically ill patients, measurement of hemodynamics, especially of oxygen-related parameters such as oxygen extraction, can reveal the cause of this decrease.

References

1. Kreuzer F, Cain SM (1985) Regulation of the peripheral vasculature and tissue oxygenation in health and disease. Crit Care Clin 1:453
2. Niinikoski J, Halkola L (1978) Skeletal muscle pO_2: Indicator of peripheral tissue perfusion in haemorrhagic shock. Adv Exp Med Biol 94:585
3. Kessler M, Hoper J, Krumme BA (1976) Monitoring of tissue perfusion and cellular function. Anesthesiology 45:184
4. Snyder JV, Carroll GC (1982) Tissue oxygenation: A physiologic approach to a clinical problem. Curr Probl Surg 19:650
5. Hotelling H (1953) New light on the correlation coefficient and its transforms. J R SS Series B, 15:193
6. Miller MJ (1982) Tissue oxygenation in clinical medicine: An historical review. Anesth Analg 61:527
7. Beerthuizen GIJM, Goris RJA, Bredel JJ, Mashhour YA, Kimmick HP, v.d. Kley AJ, Kreuzer F (1988) Muscle oxygen tension, hemodynamics, and oxygen transport after extracorporal circulation. Crit Care Med 16:748

Distribution of Oxygen Pressure in the Periphery and Centre of Malignant Head and Neck Tumors

W. Fleckenstein, J.R. Jungblut, M. Suckfüll

Introduction

In most cases, clinically observed malignant tumors have a volume of more than 2 cm³. Even in small tumors it can be expected that the convective and diffusive transport of O_2 and substrates is disturbed, at least in the centre of the tumor (Vaupel et al. 1981).

Microcirculation in malignoma cannot be physiologically regulated (Peterson 1982). Due to the chaotic growth of microvessels (Reinhold 1979), the flow rates of those capillaries and sinosoids arranged in parallel can differ extremely. Wide sinosoids can be fed by small microvessels. Hence, blood sludge within and microinfarction of tumor tissue easily occurs. The specific tissue perfusion decreases together with the growth of a malignoma because the vascular bed is compressed by the proliferating tumor cells (Vaupel and Müller-Klieser 1982; Endrich et al. 1982). Blood flow is further reduced due to bleeding in the tumor tissue and also because the vascular growth cannot sufficiently keep pace with the tumor cell growth (Vaupel 1977; Müller-Klieser and Vaupel 1982).

Diffusive transport rates in tumor tissue are reduced as the distance between the capillaries is increased during the tumor growth process (Vaupel and Müller-Klieser 1982). The O_2 diffusion coefficient of tissue probably remains unchanged during malignant transformation (Grote et al. 1977).

Disturbance of microcirculation in tumor tissue leads to regional or disseminated hypoxia, resulting in decreased cellular O_2 metabolism and pH value (Vaupel 1977; Vaupel et al. 1981). Cell proliferation in these tissue areas is then slowed down or stopped (Brammer et al. 1979; Rabes 1979). These areas can be resistant to therapy because here convective and diffusive transport of cytostatic agents is hindered. Moreover, cytostatics are less toxic on non-proliferating cells (Bhuyan 1979). Also, the cytotoxic effect of gamma radiation is comparatively low on hypoxic and non-proliferating tissue (Gray et al. 1953; Trott 1982). Hence, in most cases, at least some cell nests within the tumor are resistant to a monotherapy both by cytostatics and by irradiation.

By means of O_2 pressurized cabins, attempts were made to reduce the recurrence rate of malignant growth by increasing the arterial pO_2 value during irradiation; the intention behind this procedure was to elevate the

Clinical Oxygen Pressure Measurement II
A.M. Ehrly et al. (Eds.)
© Blackwell Ueberreuter Wissenschaft Berlin 1990

tissue pO_2 of the tumor. However, the outcome of these trials was not convincing. A weak point of this therapy concept may be that in tissue with a nonphysiological regulation of microflow, pO_2 can "paradoxically" be decreased as arterial pO_2 is increased (Fleckenstein et al. 1984; Fleckenstein 1985; Fleckenstein and Petersen, this book); and as shown in skin tumors, pO_2 of tumor tissue can remain at a constant level during arterial hyperoxia (Urbach and Noell 1958). Further pO_2 measurements are required in order to get more information about tumor tissue pO_2 regulation during hyperoxic treatment.

The application of hyperthermic therapy not in excess of 42°C results in an increase of blood flow, tissue pO_2 (Bicher et al. 1980; Vaupel et al. 1983; Otte 1984) and irradiation sensibility (Ben Hur 1972; Dewey et al. 1977). However, in spite of an increase in mean tumor blood flow and pO_2, it cannot be excluded that during such a therapy certain areas of the tumor remain ischemic and hypoxic.

After an initial phase of hyperemia, a hyperthermia of more than 30 minutes and in excess of 43°C leads to a stasis of flow within the tumor capillaries, which in turn leads to a cell-killing ischemia (reviewed by Otte 1984). Above 43°C, only a hyperthermia can be cytotoxic; especially the chronically hypoxic (Overgaad 1981; Teicher et al. 1981) and acidotic (Vaupel et al. 1983) tumor cells are less resistant to heat than sufficiently supplied tumor cells.

Applying inert-gas-clearance-techniques (Ingvar and Lassen 1962; Zierler 1965), no information about the regional inhomogeneity of tumor blood flow is obtainable because the spacial resolution of these methods is not sufficiently high. When using surface multiwire O_2 and H_2 pressure probes (Kessler and Grunewald 1969) under clinical conditions, pO_2 and flow values can be determined from the tumor tissue (Schultheiss et al. 1986). This surface method is not conclusive with regard to the biological environment of cells prevailing deep in the tumor. Applying pO_2 and pH_2 microneedle electrodes, pO_2 and flow values can be measured with high spacial resolution. Glass-sealed microneedles (Kunze, 1966; Stosseck et al. 1974; Bergsjo and Evans 1968; Badib and Webster 1969; Kolstad 1968; Urbach and Noell 1958) cannot be clinically applied because they are fragile and not commercially available. Mechanically stable hypodermic needle probes were used by Gatenby et al. (1985) and by Bergsjo and Evans (1969). These were implanted in a stationary manner at different sites within the tumor. On the one hand, by this method not enough single local pO_2 values could be obtained in order to get statistically significant tissue pO_2 distributions. On the other hand, when hypodermic needle sensors are applied in a stationary position, the biological significance of pO_2 measurements can be reasonably doubted. This is because the tissue pO_2 in the vicinity of the needle is markedly changed only seconds after the probe insertion (Schramm et al., this book). In particular, bleeding at the tip of the hypodermic needle probe may occur in tumor tissue with its highly fragile vasculature (see the high, almost arterial pO_2 values measured by Bergsjo and Evans (1969) in cervical cancer).

In tumor tissue, pO_2 values are correlated with blood flow rates (Bicher et al. 1980; Vaupel et al. 1983); however, one cannot assume that this correlation is linear because the specific O_2 uptake and specific flow rates are reduced as the tumor grows (Vaupel 1977). Ischemic tissue areas of a tumor can be detected by the hypoxic pO_2 values within these zones (Vaupel 1977; Vaupel et al. 1981). O_2 uptake by the tumor tissue can be qualitatively estimated from the slope of the pO_2 gradients caused by O_2 transport to O_2 metabolizing cells.

In order to obtain an insight into the microcirculatory O_2 supply in tumor tissue, in this study, pO_2 profiles from 7 patients with malignant head and neck tumors were recorded by stepwise driven hypodermic needle probes. This technique was shown to be suitable for clinical tissue pO_2 measurements of high spacial resolution (Fleckenstein 1985).

Patients and Methods

5 out of the 7 patients examined suffered from a squamous cell carcinoma of the oral mucosa. 1 patient was affected by an acinic cell carcinoma and 1 patient suffered from a metastasis of a squamous cell carcinoma situated retroauricarly (see details in Table 1). The parameters of the systemic O_2 transport in all patients were normal (mean values: mean blood pressure 96.3 ± 7.3 mm Hg; arterial pO_2 76.6 ± 7.0 mm Hg; arterial pCO_2 37.1 ± 6.5 mm Hg; blood HB-concentration 135.6 ± 18.9 g/l).

For tissue pO_2 measurement, polarographic hypodermic needle pO_2 probes were used (diameter 0.35 mm); these probes are flexible, unbreakable and sterilizable. The stepwise movements of the probes in the tissue (each 1.5 sec. a step of 0.8 mm is performed), and the calibration and calculation of pO_2 profiles and pO_2 histograms, were performed by a microcomputer (KIMOC® device, mfg. by GMS, Kiel-Mielkendorf, FRG).

Table 1. Patients and examined tumors

num-ber	age	sex	histological finding	localisation	projection (L * D, mm)	post. op. TNM classification
1	57	m	squamous cell carcinoma (1)	tongue	30 * 25	$T_4N_0M_x$
2	48	m	squamous cell carcinoma (1)	floor of mouth	45 * 20	$T_3N_1M_x$
3	84	m	spinocellular carcinoma	skin of head	40 * 40	$T_3N_0M_x$
4	61	m	metastasis of squ. c. carc. (1)	neck lymph node	60 * 45	$T_4N_3M_x$
5	52	m	squamous cell carcinoma (2)	tonsil	45 * 25	$T_4N_3M_x$
6	56	m	squamous cell carcinoma (1)	tongue	30 * 25	$T_3N_1M_x$
7	74	f	acinous cell carcinoma	parotideal gland	60 * 50	$T_4N_2M_1$

(1): cornifying
(2): not cornifying

Details about the method are reported elsewhere (Fleckenstein 1985; Fleckenstein 1987).

The size and the geometrical centre of tumors were macroscopically determined by palpation and in most cases by computer tomography. For the measurements, the probe was inserted step by step into the tumor tissue from the surface. The paths of the probe were directed parallel to the long axis of a tumor, yet slightly deviated in order to reach the centre point; the lengths of the long tumor axes lay between 30 and 60 mm (see Table 1). After the tumor centre was reached, the pO_2 probe was withdrawn and once again inserted at least 5 mm away from the last puncture point on the tumor surface. For each examination of tumor pO_2, the needle was inserted at least 3 times consecutively in order to obtain at least 3 pO_2 profiles. A risk of formation of metastases within punctured healthy tissue was avoided by puncturing only free-lying surfaces of tumor tissue.

Results

In Fig. 1, a typical pO_2 profile of the tumor tissue of each patient before therapy is shown. The zero point of the abscissa of each diagram represents the midpoint of each tumor. In the centre of most of the tumors, the mean pO_2 lay below 10 mm Hg. Numerical tumor pO_2 data from each of the patients are given in Table 2. Near the periphery of the tumors a tissue layer of only approx. 5 mm in thickness, with a steep pO_2 gradient, was observed. The thickness of this layer seemed to be independent of the tumor magnitude. On the other hand, the radius of the central area,

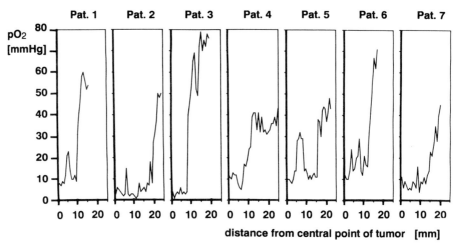

Fig. 1. Each diagram shows 1 typical pO_2 profile from each of the 7 patients. The zero point of each abscissa represents the centre of a tumor. The pO_2 needle probe was driven step by step (each step: 0.8 mm) through the tumor and stopped at each of the measuring sites for 1.5 sec for pO_2 measurements. Numbering of patients is the same as in Tab. 1

Table 2. Mean pO$_2$ values and pO$_2$ percentile quota of the tumor tissue pO$_2$ data. On the left side of the table, data from tissue within a radius of 1 cm around the macroscopically determined midpoints of the tumors; on the right side of the table, data measured from a distance of more than 1 cm from the tumor centres

patient number	pO$_2$ values in centre of tumor				pO$_2$ values in periphery of tumor			
	mean (mmHG)	percentile quota (mmHg): 10 %	50 %	90 %	mean (mmHG)	percentile quota (mmHg): 10 %	50 %	90 %
1	10.9	4.3	8.3	29.0	39.0	22.5	40.0	65.0
2	7.6	1.0	5.3	17.5	22.5	2.3	20.0	47.5
3	11.9	2.0	11.6	34.0	56.2	43.0	61.3	74.7
4	13.4	7.9	12.1	19.8	34.8	23.5	35.2	47.0
5	14.9	5.1	12.8	33.0	26.9	8.3	27.5	48.3
6	16.4	5.9	14.0	37.5	25.5	10.3	24.0	62.5
7	8.5	5.3	7.9	14.0	22.3	6.9	20.7	43.3
mean:	11.9	4.5	10.3	26.4	32.5	16.7	32.7	55.5
std. dev.:	3.2	2.3	3.2	9.2	12.2	14.1	14.6	11.9

which had low tissue pO$_2$, was approximately correlated to the magnitude of the tumor as a whole. In diagram 2c, a pO$_2$ histogram, pooling all pO$_2$ values (from all patients) taken from the tumor centres, is shown. The mean of all these pO$_2$ values, measured from a distance not exceeding 1 cm from tumor centres, lay at 11.9 mm Hg. The histogram shown in diagram 2d pools all pO$_2$ values (from all patients) taken within tumor tissue from a distance of more than 1 cm from the tumor midpoints. In these outer tumor areas, the mean pO$_2$ value lay at 32.5 mm Hg. The pO$_2$ histogram shown in diagram 2a was obtained from oral connective tissue and the pO$_2$ histogram shown in diagram 2b was from muscles of the floor of the mouth. Measurements from both of the latter histograms were taken from a healthy volunteer. In the normal oral tissues, pO$_2$ values below 5 mm Hg were virtually non-existent. In the tumor periphery, the tissue pO$_2$ values lay below those of normal connective or muscle tissues.

In each diagram of Fig. 2, three tumor pO$_2$ profiles, measured consecutively from the same patient, were superimposed. Profiles of diagram 3a were measured before irradiation therapy; tumor type was squamous cell carcinoma. The tumor was 60 mm in length and 45 mm in breadth, situated in a lymph node of the mandibular angle. Diagram 3b shows pO$_2$ profiles determined 14 days after the start of a series of irradiation doses to a sum of 32.5 Gy. Diagram 3c shows pO$_2$ profiles 28 days after start of therapy (total dosage by this time was 70 Gy).

Before irradiation (diag. 3a), pO$_2$ decreases from the surface to the centre of the tumor. pO$_2$ gradients are comparatively flat, so a low O$_2$-consumption of the tissue can be assumed. After an irradiation dosage of 32.5 Gy (diag 3b), a difference of pO$_2$ levels between the centre and the periphery of the tumor was absent. Mean pO$_2$ values lay at 10 mm Hg within almost

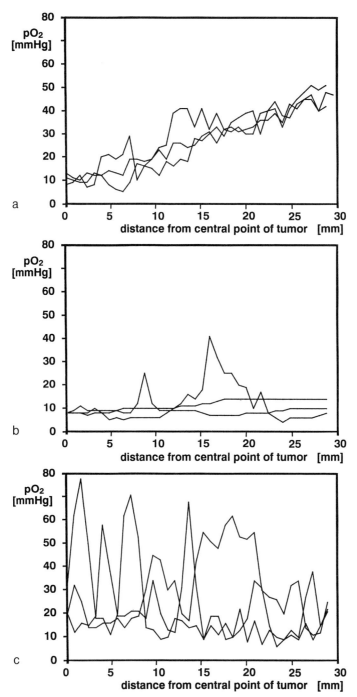

Fig. 2a–c. Each diagram shows 3 superimposed pO$_2$ profiles recorded during the same examination and in the same tumor (patient no. 4, metastasis of a squamous cell carcinoma): a) before gamma irradiation therapy; b) 14 days after start of irradiation therapy (32.5 Gy); c) 28 days after start of irradiation therapy (70 Gy)

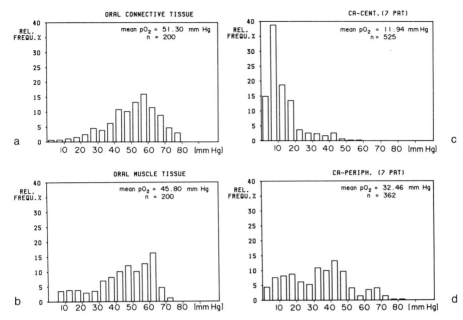

Fig. 3a–d. pO₂ histograms from different tissues: **a)** normal oral connective tissue of a healthy volunteer; **b)** muscles of the floor of the mouth measured from a healthy volunteer; **c)** pO₂ data from all patients were pooled in this histogram; data were obtained from central tumor tissue within a radius of 1 cm surrounding the macroscopically determined mid-points of the tumors; **d)** tumor tissue at a distance of more than 1 cm from the tumor centres; pO₂ data of all patients were pooled in this histogram

the entire tumor mass. Very few pO₂ gradients were present. From this data, it can be concluded that the O₂ uptake from the tissue as well as the perfusion of the tumor, were almost stopped. The very low frequency of pO₂ gradients, seen in diag. 3b, can be traced to discrete vital tissue. These areas could either be surviving tumor cell nests supplied with blood, or they could be cells which had freshly immigrated, being accompanied by spreading vessels, in the course of the organization of the irradiated tumor mass.

After irradiation with 70 Gy (diag 3c) in the centre and periphery of the tumor area, almost equal mean pO₂ levels were observed (mean pO₂ 24.9 mm Hg). The re-appearance of pO₂ gradient is a sign of recapture of oxidative metabolism of tissue. A histogram (not shown), of the pO₂ values of diag. 3c, compared with the pO₂ distribution of oral connective tissue (Fig. 3a), was shifted to the left.

Discussion

In all pO₂ profiles from the untreated tumors, a reduced O₂ supply to the centre areas as well as an inhomogeneity of tumor perfusion was evident.

In the histologically similar tumors (squamous cell carcinoma: Patients no. 1,2,4,5,6) the severity of central hypoxia was unequal. There is a chance that the recurrence-rate of malignant growth will be reduced if pO_2 data are taken into account when the individual patients' therapeutical program is decided upon. It remains to be examined to what extent the correlations between the parameters of microcirculation and the resistance to therapy – as in most cases observed in animal experiments – can be transferred to clinical conditions. Malignant tumors of the head and neck area are well suited to further development of new schemes of conservative therapy because they cannot often be radically extirpated, and because they can be locally heated to a temperature of over 43°C. With hypodermic needle probes, pO_2 profiles of head and neck tumors cannot only be externally measured, but can also be measured by oral access in the mouth and even deep in the throat (latter technique in narcosis, yet unpublished data). pO_2 measurements taken as the therapy progressed revealed significant changes in pO_2 profiles. pO_2 profiles enable one to draw conclusions about microcirculation and oxidative metabolism in the tumor area. These measurements can be repeated at will and inflict neither pain nor risk to the patient. With the method demonstrated in this study, information can be acquired regarding changes in microcirculation during the progress of repeatedly applied hyperthermia or irradiation.

Summary

The pO_2 supply of the tissue of malignant tumors of the head and neck area was estimated by pO_2 measurements of high spacial resolution. Fast responding hypodermic needle pO_2 probes ($\varnothing$ 350 µm) were stepwise driven forward in tumors of 7 patients. In all patients, varying degrees of tissue hypoxia were found in the tumor centre areas which were of variable widths. In the peripheral tumor zones, the tissue pO_2 values were lower than in the healthy tissue, although there was no hypoxia. In one patient, the examinations were repeated in the course of radiotherapy. Following an irradiation dose of 32.5 Gy, the pO_2 value was 10 mm Hg almost all over the tumor centre and periphery; obviously blood supply and O_2 consumption were interrupted within nearly the entire tumor tissue. After 70 Gy, high pO_2 gradients were observed and the mean pO_2 value elevated again, suggesting that the oxidative metabolism had been resumed.

References

1. Badib, A.O., Webster, J.H.: Changes in tumor oxygen tension during radiation therapy. Acta Radiol. Therap. Phys. Biol. 8, 247-257 (1969)
2. Ben Hur, E.: Thermally enhanced radiosensitivity of cultured chinese hamster cells. Nature 238, 209-211 (1972).

3. Bergsjo, P., Evans, J.C.: Tissue oxygen tension of cervix cancer. Comparison of effects of breathing a carbon dioxide mixture and pure oxygen. Acta Radiol. Ther. Phys. Biol. 7, 1-11 (1968)

4. Bergsjo, P., Evans, J.C.: Oxygen tension of cervical carcinoma during the early phase of external irradiation, 1. Measurements with a Clark micro electrode. Scand. J. Clin. Lab. Invest. Suppl. 106, 159-166 (1969)

5. Bhuyan, B.K.: Kinetics of cell kill by hyperthermia. Cancer Res. 39, 2277-2284 (1979)

6. Bicher, H.I., Hetzel, F.W., Sandha, T.S., Frinak, S., Vaupel, P., O'Hara, M.D., O'Brien, T.: Effects of hyperthermia on normal and tumor microenvironment. Radiology 137, 523-530 (1980)

7. Brammer, I., Zywietz, F., Jung, H.: Changes of histological and proliferative indices in the Walker carcinoma with tumor size and distance from blood vessel. Europ J. Cancer 15, 1329-1336 (1979)

8. Dewey, W., Thrall, D., Gilette, E.: Hyperthermia and radiation – A selective thermal effect on chronically hypoxic tumor cells in vivo. Int. J. Radiat. Oncol. Biol. Phys. 2, 99-103 (1977)

9. Endrich, B., Intaglietta, M., Messmer, K.: Besonderheiten der Mikrozirkulation in bösartigen Tumoren. 6. Jahrestagung der Gesellschaft für Mikrozirkulation, München, 26.-27.11.1982

10. Fleckenstein, W.: Ein neues Gewebe-pO₂-Meßverfahren zum Nachweis von Mikrozirkulationsstörungen. Med. Diss. Universität Lübeck (1985)

11. Fleckenstein, W, Heinrich, R., Huber, A., Grauer, W., Schomerus, H., Günderoth, M., Dölle, W., Weiss, Ch.: Muscle pO₂ distribution and pulmonary gas transfer conditions in patients with liver cirrhosis. In: Grote, J., Witzleb, E. (Hrsg.): Atemgaswechsel und O₂-Versorgung der Organe. Steiner, Wiesbaden, 125-129 (1984)

12. Fleckenstein, W.: Die Entwicklung der Feinnadel-Gewebe-pO₂- Histographie zum klinisch eingesetzten Diagnoseverfahren. In: Präsident der FU Berlin (Hsrg.): 2. Treffpunkt Medizintechnik, 92 (1987)

13. Fleckenstein W., Petersen, C.: On the effects of arterial hyperoxia on muscle oxygen supply of man and dog. This book

14. Gatenby, R.A. et al.: Oxygen tension in human tumors: In vivo mapping using CT-guided probes. Radiol. 156, 211-214 (1985)

15. Gray, L.H., Langer, A.D., Ebert, M., Hornsey, S., Scott, O.C.A.: The concentration of oxygen dissolved in tissues at the time of irradiation as a factor of radiotherapy. Br. J. Radiol. 26, 638- 648 (1953)

16. Grote, J., Süsskind, R., Vaupel, P.: Oxygen diffusivity in tumor tissue (Ds-carcinosarcoma) under temperature conditions within the range of 20-40°C. Pflügers Arch 372, 37-42 (1977)

17. Ingvar, D., Lassen, N.: Regional blood flow of the cerebral cortex determined by Krypton. Act Physiol. Scand. 54, 325-338 (1962)

18. Kessler, M, Grunewald W.: Possibilities of measuring oxygen pressurefields in tissue by multiwise platinum electrodes. Progr. Resp. Res. 3, 147-152 (1969)

19. Kolstad, P.: Intercapillary Distance, Oxygen tension and local recurrence in cervix cancer. Scand. J. clin. Lab. Invest. Suppl. 106, 145-157 (1968)

20. Kunze, K.: Die lokale, kontinuierliche Sauerstoffdruckmessung in der menschlichen Muskulatur. Pflügers Arch 292, 151 (1966)

21. Müller-Klieser, W., Vaupel, P.: Die Sauerstoffversorgung maligner Tumoren als kritischer Parameter der Therapie. 6. Jahrestagung der Gesellschaft für Mikrozirkulation, München, 26.-27.11. 1982

22. Otte, J.: Hyperthermie in der Behandlung maligner Tumoren – Biologische Grundlagen und Therapeutische Studien. Med. Habilschr., Lübeck 1984

23. Overgaad, J.: Effect of hyperthermia on the hypoxic fraction in an experimental mammary carcinoma in vivo. Br. J. Cancer 54, 245-249 (1981)

24. Peterson, H.I.: Tumor vessel innervation, influence of vasoactive drugs and control of tumor blood flow. 6. Jahrestagung der Gesellschaft für Mikrozirkulation, München, 26.-27.11. 1982

25. Rabes, B.: Proliferative Vorgänge während der Frühstadien der malignen Transformation. Verh. Dtsch. Ges. Pathol. 63, 18-39 (1979)
26. Reinhold, H.: In vivo observation of tumor blood flow. In: Peterson, H.I. (Hrsg.): Tumor blood circulation: Angiogenesis vascular morphology and blood flow in experimental and human tumors. CRC Press, Boca Raton, 115-128 (1979)
27. Schramm, U., Fleckenstein, W., Weber, C.: Morphological assessment of skeletal muscle injury caused by pO_2 measurements with hyperdermic needle probes. This book.
28. Schultheiß, R., Wüllenweber, R., Leninger-Follert, E.: Clinical results of local tissue pO_2 measurements on the surface of the brain during neurosurgical operations. In: Ehrly, A.M., Hauss, I., Huch, R. (Hrsg.): Clinical Oxygen Pressure Measurement. Springer, Berlin-Heidelberg-New-York-London-Paris-Tokyo 1986
29. Stosseck, K., Lübbers, D.W., Cottin, N.: Determination of local blood flow (microflow by electrochemically generated hydrogen, construction and application of the measuring probe). Pflügers Arch 348, 225-238 (1974)
30. Teicher, B.A., Kowal, C.D., Kennedy, K.A., Sartorelli, A.L.: Enhancement by hyperthermia of the in vitro cytotoxicity of mitomycin C toward hypoxic tumor cells. Cancer Res. 41, 1096-1099 (1981)
31. Trott, K.R.: Welche Konsequenzen ergeben sich aus den Besonderheiten der Tumormikrozirkulation für Strahlenbiologie und die klinische Onkologie? 6. Jahrestagung der Gesellschaft für Mikrozirkulation, München, 26.-27.11. 1982
32. Urbach, F., Noell, W.K.: Effects of oxygen breathing on tumor oxygen measured polarographically. J. Appl. Physiol. 13(1): 61-65 (1958)
33. Vaupel, P.: Atemgaswechsel und Glucosestoffwechsel von Implantationstumoren (DS-Carcinosarkom) in vivo. In: Thews, G. (Hrsg.): Funktionsanalyse biologischer Systeme I. Steiner, Wiesbaden, 1-138 (1974)
34. Vaupel, P.: Hypoxia in neoplastic tissue. Microvasc. Res. 13, 399- 408 (1977)
35. Vaupel, P.W., Frinak, S., Bicher, H.I.: Heterogenous, oxygen partial pressure and pH distribution in C_3H mouse mammary adenocarcinoma. Cancer Res. 41, 2008-2013 (1981)
36. Vaupel, P., Müller-Klieser, W.: Interstitieller Raum und Mikromilieu in malignen Tumoren. 6. Jahrestagung der Gesellschaft für Mikrozirkulation, München, 26.-27.11. 1982
37. Vaupel, P., Müller-Klieser, W., Otte, J., Manz, R., Kalinowski, P.: Blood flow, tissue oxygeneration and pH distribution in malignant tumors upon localized hyperthermia. Strahlentherapie 159, 73-81 (1983)
38. Zierler, K.: Equations for blood flow by external monitoring of radioisotopes. Circ. Res. 16, 309-321 (1965)

Optimal Hematocrit in Claudicants: Exercise-Induced Muscle pO$_2$ after Stepwise Isovolemic Hemodilution

H.-G. Höffkes, K. Saeger-Lorenz, A.M. Ehrly

Introduction

The flow properties of blood are among the factors which determine the microcirculatory blood flow. Hematocrit is the major determinant of whole blood viscosity.

If hematocrit values reach levels of over 50 % in patients with chronic arterial occlusive disease (hence leading to correspondingly high whole blood viscosity values), a reduction of packed cell volume is nowadays a standard therapy.

The question arises, however, to what extent a reduction in hematocrit values leading to a decrease in whole blood viscosity can be performed without interfering with the so-called systemic oxygen transport capacity. Clearly, a reduction in whole blood viscosity and a corresponding increase in blood flow in the microcirculation with a hematocrit value of 0 % won't allow for any oxygen transport whatsoever. But the question, to what extent the hematocrit should be lowered in patients with chronic arterial occlusive disease in order to improve tissue supply (optimal hematocrit) was and still is under debate, since objective measurements in patients in the course of a hemodilution therapy are very rare.

Former investigations on the optimal hematocrit value

During the last decade a number of theoretical calculations as well as animal experiments have been carried out in order to clarify the optimal hematocrit value.

Mathematical calculations were done by Castle and Jandl [1], Crowell et al. [2], Hint [3], Meiselman [4], Gordin and Ravin [5], Duvelleroy et al. [6], as well as Jan and Chien [7] and Ernst and Matrai [8].

Hint [3], Meiselman [4] and Duvelleroy [6] calculated an optimal hematocrit of about 30 %; Ernst and Matrai [8] of about 35 %; Castle and Jandl [1], Crowell [2], Gordin and Ravin [4], and Jan and Chien [7] values of about 40 %.

In-vitro experiments were performed by Stone et al. [9], Self et al. [10], Linderkamp [11] and Lingard [12].

Clinical Oxygen Pressure Measurement II
A.M. Ehrly et al. (Eds.)
© Blackwell Ueberreuter Wissenschaft Berlin 1990

Stone et al. investigated the influence of the erythrocytes' shape on blood viscosity. Red blood cells of camels and llamas are elliptical, in contrast to the disc-shaped biconcave red cells of other mammals. They deduced from these experiments an optimal hematocrit value for oxygen transport in humans of about 45 % [9].

Self et al. investigated the effect of hemodilution and hemoconcentration in patients with hemoglobinopathies. Using a Weisenberg Rheogoniometer they obtained the apparent whole blood viscosity of blood samples. From these experiments they deduced an optimal hematocrit for the arterial system of about 30 % and for the venous system of about 25 % [10]. Linderkamp performed in-vitro experiments measuring the blood flow

Table 1. Former investigations on the optimal hematocrit value

Optimal hematocrit (calculations)

Hint	(1968)	30 %
Meiselmann	(1971)	30 %
Duvelleroy	(1980)	30 %
Schmid-Schönbein	(1985	33 %
Ernst und Matrai	(1983)	35 %
Castle und Jandl	(1966)	40 %
Crowell	(1967)	40 %
Gordin and Ravin	(1979)	40 %
Jan und Chien	(1977)	40 %
Gaethgens and Marx	(1987)	42 %

Optimal hematocrit (in vitro studies)

Self	(1977)	30 %
Lingard	(1982)	35 %
Linderkamp	(1981)	40 %
Stone	(1968)	45 %
Linderkamp	(1981)	50 %

Optimal hematocrit (animal experiments)

Sunder-Plassmann and Messmer	(1971)	30 %
Richardson and Guyton	(1959)	40 %
Guyton and Richardson	(1961)	40 %
Erslev	(1966)	40 %
Smith and Crowell	(1963)	40 %
Crowell	(1959)	42 %
Murray	(1962)	45 %
Thorling and Erslev	(1968)	45 %
Smith and Crowell	(1967)	46 %
Gaethgens and Kreutz	(1979)	50–56 %

through glass tubes. From these experiments he deduced an optimal hematocrit value of 40 % for adults and of about 50 % for newborns [11]. Lingard investigated the influence of blood rheology and oxygen supply to tissue in a circulation model. From these experiments he deduced an optimal hematocrit value for the capillary bed of about 35 % [12].

Animal experiments were performed by Crowell [13], Smith and Crowell [18], Richardson and Guyton [14] and Guyton and Richardson [15], Murray et al [16, 19], Erslev [17], Thorling and Erslev [20], Sunder-Plassman and Messmer [21] as well as Gaetghens and Kreutz [22, 23] and Fan et al. [24].

Crowell et al. investigated the survival time of dogs following hemorrhagic shock as a function of hematocrit and found optimal results at values of about 42 % [13].

Richardson and Guyton investigated the influence of polycythemia and anemia on the cardiac output and other hemodynamic factors in healthy dogs. In these experiments the optimal hematocrit value was 40 % [14].

In addition to these experiments Guyton and Richardson investigated the influence of hematocrit on venous return in healthy dogs. In these experiments they found a negative correlation between hematocrit and venous blood flow, and deduced an optimal hematocrit of about 40 % [15].

Murray et al. investigated the influence of normovolemic hemodilution and hemoconcentration on the systemic oxygen transport in healthy adult dogs. The optimal hematocrit value in these experiments was found to be around 40 % [16].

Erslev investigated the influence of hematocrit variations in normovolemic healthy adult rabbits. In these experiments the optimal hematocrit value was found to be at about 40 % [17].

Smith and Crowell investigated the influence of the hematocrit value in healthy dogs, simulating an acute exposure to high altitude (40.000 and 50.000 ft). They found that under these acute conditions the optimal hematocrit is about 40 % [18], and that after altitude acclimatisation the optimal hematocrit shifts from 40 % to 46 % [19].

Murray et al. compared the influence of normovolemic and hypervolemic hemodilution on the optimal hematocrit value in healthy dogs and arrived at optimal values of about 40 % under normovolemic hemodilution and 38-40 % under hypervolemic hemodilution [20].

Thorling and Erslev performed experiments on mice and rats to determine the influence of the hematocrit value on the tissue oxygen tension in subcutaneous air pockets and the pneumoperitoneum. They found that under normovolemic conditions the optimal hematocrit is about 45 % and under hypervolemic conditions about 55 % [21].

Sunder-Plassmann and Messmer induced an acute preoperative isovolemic hemodilution in dogs. They showed that a decrease of hematocrit values to about 30 % does not impair systemic oxygen transport capacity [22]. It should be mentioned that these experiments do not simulate the condition of arterosclerotic disease in elderly patients.

Table 2. Isovolemic hemodilution in chronic arterial occlusive disease stage II according to Fontaine (clinical studies)

Author	n	Solution	Hematocrit ($\bar{x}$)	Success
Yates et. al. (1979)	10	Dextran 70	45 % -- > 35 %	impairment (n. s.)
Köhler et. al. (1981)	15	?	? % -- > 32 %	no change (n. s.)
Wolfe et. al. (1985)	17	Dextran 70	49 % -- > 33 %	impairment (n. s.)
Rudofsky et. al. (1981)	25	Albumin 4 %	?	improvement (sign.)
Gottstein et. al. (1971)	11	Dextran 40	46 % -- > 38 %	improvement (sign.)
Kiesewetter et. al. (1986)	15	HES 10 % (200/0.5)	49 % -- > 42 %	improvement (sign.)
	15	0.9 % NaCl	49 % -- > 42 %	improvement (sign.)
Kiesewetter et. al. (1987)	30	HES 10 % (200/0.5)	> 42 % -- > 40 %	improvement (sign.)
	30	Dextran 40	> 42 % -- > 40 %	improvement (sign.)
Ernst et. al. (1988)	25	HES 10 % (200/0.5)	48 % -- > 41 %	improvement (sign.)

Gaethgens and Kreutz investigated the influence of various hematocrit values in the isolated canine muscle and found optimal muscle tissue supply under exercise conditions at hematocrit values ranging from 50–56 % [23, 24].

Fan et al. induced isovolemic hemodilution and hemoconcentration in dogs. In particular they investigated the inflence of hematocrit on central organs such as brain, heart, etc. For the brain, liver and kidney they found an optimal hematocrit of about 57 %. The optimal hematocrit for the spleen was found to be about 44 %. Intestine and heart displayed no optimum but a plateau between 37 and 58 % [25].

Czer and Shoemaker investigated the optimal hematocrit value in critically ill patients. They found that a preoperative hematocrit value of about 33 % leads to a significantly higher survival ratio after surgery than other preoperative hematocrit values [26].

Jan et al. investigated the influence of blood transfusion on pO_2 in patients with sickle cell anemia and found a maximum pO_2 at a hematocrit of about 30 to 35 % [27].

In a great number of clinical studies in patients isovolemic as well as hypervolemic hemodilution was used to improve ischemic symptoms [28, 29, 30, 31, 32, 33]. In most of these studies the hematocrit values were decreased to around 40 % [28, 29, 30, 32, 33].

Table 3. Changes in whole blood viscosity, plasma viscosity, RBC aggregation and tcpO$_2$ during isovolemic hemodilution (IHD) (M ± SEM)

Rheological parameters	Before IHD	On 4th or 5th day	On 9th day
Hematocrit (%)	48.01 ± 1.88	39.00 ± 0.77	33.83 ± 0.85
Apparent blood viscosity (H$_2$O = 1)	5.32 ± 0.40	4.41 ± 0.40 $p < 0.0005$	3.90 ± 0.41 $p < 0.0025$
Plasma viscosity (H$_2$O =1)	1.74 ± 0.13	1.66 ± 0.16 $p < 0.01$	1.68 ± 0.03 $p < 0.01$
RBC aggregation (∢) α (degree))	36.50 ±8.80	25.50 ± 5.63 $p < 0.0005$	26.33 ± 3.40 $p < 0.0005$
tcpO$_2$ (Torr)	37.40 ±14.64	36.10 ± 17.07 n.s.	34.00 ± 30.74 n.s.

The above-mentioned disparities in the optimal hematocrit values are due to the difficulties of quantifying the efficacy of hemodilution therapy. This is easily explainable since the various patients and the experimental conditions differed very much.

In most of the above-mentioned studies objective parameters were missing. However, one objective parameter which proved to be especially useful is the muscle tissue oxygen pressure [34]

In earlier studies performing hypervolemic hemodilution Landgraf et al. [35] found that the reduction of hematocrit to about 40 % can indeed improve muscle tissue oxygen supply of claudicants at rest.

The aim of the present study was to verify the optimal hematocrit value for the oxygen supply in the lower limb muscles of patients with chronic arterial occlusive disease in the clinical stage II according to Fontaine (i.e. intermittent claudication).

Materials and Methods

In order to simulate the condition of intermittent claudication the present measurements were performed with a standardized pedal ergometric test according to Ehrly and Dehn [36].

Isovolemic hemodilution was achieved in the course of stepwise reduction of hematocrit by withdrawal of 500 ml blood and subsequent infusion of 500 ml hydroxyethylstarch solution ($\overline{MG}$: 200.000/0.5), Haes-steril® 10 %, Fresenius Company, Oberursel, Germany.

Stepwise isovolemic hemodilution was performed twice within 8-9 days in 10 patients (41-72 years old) suffering from intermittent claudication.

Muscle tissue pO₂ readings under exercise conditions were done using micro-pt-needle electrodes with a diameter of 2-4 micrometer shortly before and 3, 10, 20 and 30 minutes after a 4 minute pedal ergometric exercise at a work load of 5.7 ±0.2 Watt. Simultaneously some other hemodynamics and hemorrheological parameters were obtained.

The study design allowed us to obtain intraindividual data. For statistical analysis Wilcoxon-test and Student t-test were used.

Results

Figure 1 shows the muscle tissue pO₂ pattern given as medians from patients at different hematocrit values. The solid line demonstrates the reaction of tissue pO₂ after exercise before hemodilution at an average hematocrit value of 48.01 %. There is a stepwise increase in muscle tissue pO₂ values. We call this period "retarted reactive hyperoxia". The curve with the open circles represents the pattern after isovolemic hemodilu-

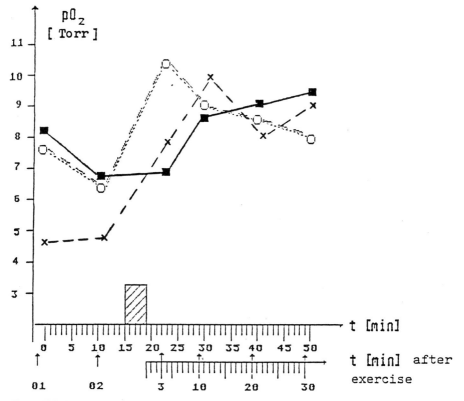

Fig. 1. This figure shows the muscle tissue pO₂ pattern in form of medians of patients at different hematocrit values. Solid line: average hematocrit of 48.01 %; open circle line: average hematocrit of 39 %; dotted line: average hematocrit of 33.83 %. pO₂ measurements at rest (01, 02) and after exercise (3, 10, 20, 30 minutes after exercise)

tion, when the average hematocrit value was now at 39.00 %. There is a sudden steep increase in tissue pO_2 3 minutes after the end of exercise followed by a subsequent reduction (normalization) of pO_2 values. The dotted line represents the tissue pO_2 pattern after repeated isovolemic hemodilution, when the average hematocrit was at 33.83 %. Again, there is a "retarded reactive hyperoxia" in muscle tissue pO_2, comparable to the situation before hemodilution, i.e. at high hematocrit values.

Figure 2 a–c shows a comparison of the pooled histograms of this group of patients at average hematocrit values of 48.01 %, 39 % and 33.83 %. It is obvious that the pO_2 behaviour after a moderate exercise is optimal at a level of 39 %, whereas at 48.01 % as well as at 33.83 % a shift to the left after the end of exercise can be seen. It should be noticed that pO_2 values at rest, i.e. before exercise, are comparable in the case of hematocrit values of 48.01 % and 39 %, whereas the tissue pO_2 at rest at a hematocrit value of 33.83 % is markedly lower.

In Table 3 some hemorrheological parameters are shown. As expected, there is a reduction in hematocrit, as well as apparent whole blood viscosity and plasma viscosity. There is however no statistically significant difference in transcutaneous pO_2 values, although arithmetic mean values do decrease after isovolemic hemodilution.

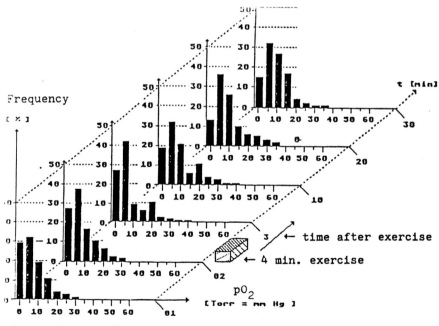

Fig. 2a   Hematocrit($\bar{x}$): 48.01%

Fig. 2a–c. Comparison of the pattern of pooled pO_2 histograms before (01, 02) and after standardized exercise test at different hematocrit values (arithmetic mean values: $\bar{x}$)

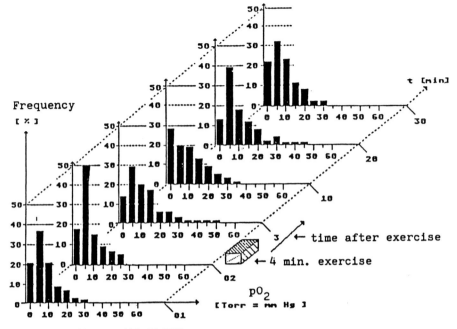

Fig. 2b   Hematocrit(x̄): 39.00%

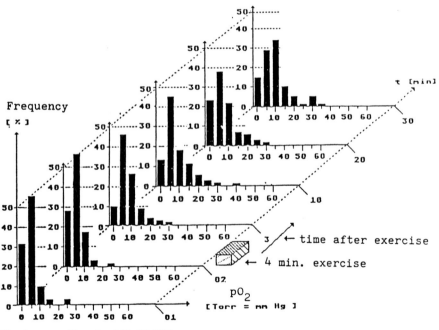

Fig. 2c   Hematocrit(x̄): 33.83%

Conclusion

A reduction of high hematocrit values in patients with intermittent claudication from 48.01 % to 39 % results in an improvement of tissue supply under exercise conditions.

Further reduction in hematocrit values then impairs tissue oxygen supply. This means that for this given disease at this stage the optimal hematocrit is about 40 %.

This result agrees well with earlier tissue pO_2 data from Landgraf and Ehrly [33] obtained during hypervolemic hemodilution at rest. The results presented here support those suggestions and data from animal experiments, in-vitro studies and theoretical studies which proposed an optimal hematocrit value of about 40 %.

However, the results of the present study only hold for this particular group of patients during **iso**volemic hemodilution. The optimal hematocrit value could differ in the case of different pathological conditions, e.g. shock, arterosclerosis, various stages and localizations of ischemic disease (brain, muscle, skin).

Hypervolemic hemodilution may lead to other optimal hematocrit values. Therefore further, more detailed studies are needed.

References

1. Castle WB, Jandl JH (1966) Blood viscosity and blood volume: Opposing influences upon oxygen transport in polycythemia. Seminars in Hematology 3:193
2. Crowell JW, Smith EE (1967) Determinant of the optimal hematocrit. J Appl Physiol 22:501
3. Hint H (1968) The pharmacology of Dextran and the physiological background for the clinical use of Rheomacrodex and Macrodex. Acta Anaesth Belg 19:119
4. Meiselman HJ (1972) In vivo viscometry: Effect of hemodilution. In: Hemodilution. Theoretical basis and clinical application. Int Symp Rottach-Egern 1971. Karger, Basel p 143
5. Gordin RJ, Ravin MB (1979) Rheology and anesthesiology. Anesth Analg 57:252
6. Duvelleroy MA, Duruble M, Martin JL, Gaudel Y, Teisseire B (1980) Hemodilution and oxygen. In: Stolz JF, Drouin P (eds) Hemorrheology and diseases. Doin p 615
7. Jan KM, Chien S (1977) Effect of hematocrit variations on coronary hemodynamics and oxygen utilization. Am J Physiol 233:106
8. Ernst E, Matrai A (1983) Zum Thema "optimaler Hämatokrit" – Rationale der Hämo-dilutionstherapie. Herz/Kreislauf 9:409
9. Stone HO, Thompson HK jr, Schmidt-Nielsen K (1968) Influence of erythrocytes on blood viscosity. Am J Physiol 214:913
10. Self F, McFuture LV, Zanger B (1977) Rheological evaluation of hemoglobin S and hemoglobin C hemoglobinopathies. J Lab Clin Med, Vol 89, 3:488
11. Linderkamp O, Meiselman HJ, Wu PYK, Miller FC (1981) Blood and plasma viscosity and optimal hematocrit in the normal newborn infant. Clin Hemorh 1:575
12. Lingard PS (1982) Blood rheology and oxygen supply to tissue. Clin Hemorh 2:13
13. Crowell JW, Ford RG, Lewis VM (1959) Oxygen transport in hemorrhagic shock as a function of hematocrit ratio. Am J Physiol 196:1033
14. Richardson TO, Guyton AC (1959) Effects of polycythemia and anemia on cardiac output and other circulatory factors. Am J Physiol 1976:1167

15. Guyton AC, Richardson TO (1961) Effect of hematocrit on venous return. Circ Res IX:157
16. Murray JF, Gold P, Johnson BL jr (1962) Systemic oxygen transport in induced normovolemic anemia and polycythemia. Am.J.Physiol. 203:720
17. Erslev AJ (1966) The erythropoietic effect of hematocrit variations in normovolaemic rabbits. Blood 27:629
18. Smith EE, Crowell JW (1963) Influence of hematocrit ratio on survival of unacclimatized dogs at simulated high altitude. Am J Physiol 205:1172
19. Smith EE, Crowell JW (1967) Role of an increased hematocrit in altitude acclimatization. Aerospace Medicine, January:39
20. Murray JF, Gold P, Johnson BC jr (1963) The circulatory effects of hematocrit variations in normovolaemic and hypervolaemic dogs. J Clin Inv 42:1150
21. Thorling EB, Erslev AJ (1968) The "tissue" tension of oxygen and its relation to hematocrit and erythropoesis. Blood 31:332
22. Sunder-Plassmann L, Klövekorn WP, Holper K, Hase U, Messmer K (1971) The physiological significance of acutely induced hemodilution. Proc 6th Eur Conf Microcirculation, Aalborg 1970. Karger, Basel, p 23
23. Gaetghens P, Kreutz F, Albrecht KH (1979) Optimal hematocrit for canine skeletal muscle during rythmic isotonic exercise. Eur J Appl Physiol Occup Physiol 41:27
24. Kreutz F (1979) Der optimale Hämatokrit für den arbeitenden Skelettmuskel. Dissertation, Köln
25. Fan FC, Chien RYZ, Schuessler GB, Chien SC (1980) Effects of hematocrit variations on regional hemodynamics and oxygen transport in the dog. Am J Physiol 238:H545
26. Czer LSC, Shoemaker WC (1978) Optimal hematocrit value in critically ill postoperative patients. Sur Gyn, and Obstr. 147:363
27. Jan K, Usani S, Smith JA (1982) Effects of transfusion on rheological properties of blood in sickle cell anemia. Transfusion 22:17
28. Bollinger A (1968) Wirkung von niedermolekularem Dextran auf Blutviskosität und Extremitätendurchblutung. Z Kreisl.-Forsch 57:456
29. Yates CJP, Andrews V, Berent A, Dormandy JA: Increase in leg blood flow by normovolaemic hemodilution in intermittent claudication. Lancet 11:166
30. Angelkort B, Kiesewetter H, Maurin N: Einfluß von Hämodilution und oraler Pentoxifyllinmedikation auf Muskeldurchblutung, Fließverhalten und Haemostase des Blutes bei chronischer arterieller Verschlußkrankheit. In: Breddin K (ed) Thrombose und Atherogenese. Witzrock, Baden-Baden, p 114
31. Rieger H (1982) Induzierte Blutverdünnung (Hämodilution) als neues Konzept in der Therapie peripherer Durchblutungsstörungen. Der Internist 23:375
32. Kiesewetter H (1984) Hämorrheologische Therapie für Patienten mit peripherer arterieller Verschlußkrankheit. In: Trübestein G (ed) Konservative Therapie arterieller Durchblutungsstörungen. Thieme, Stuttgart, p 213
33. Wolf JHN (1985) The effect of hemodilution upon patients with intermittent claudication. Surg Gynecol and Obs, p 160
34. Ehrly AM (1984) Überlegungen zur Quantifizierung von Wirkungen und Wirksamkeit einer medikamentösen Therapie der chronischen arteriellen Verschlußkrankheit. In: Trübestein G (ed) Konservative Therapie arterieller Durchblutungsstörungen. Thieme, Stuttgart, p 61
35. Landgraf H, Ehrly AM (1987) Verhalten Hämorrheologischer Parameter und des Gewebesauerstoffdruckes im Verlauf einer hypervolämischen Hämodilution bei Patienten mit arterieller Verschlusskrankheit. In: Heilmann L, Beez M (eds) Neuere klinische Aspekte zur Hämodilution. Schattauer, Stuttgart, p 115
36. Ehrly AM, Dehn R (1986) Verhalten des Muskelgewebesauerstoffpartialdruckes (pO$_2$) bei Gesunden und Patienten mit Claudicatio intermittens nach definierter fußergometrischer Belastung. Vasa Suppl 14 p 1

Effects of Hydroxyethylstarch (HES) on the Oxygen Tension in Skeletal Muscle of Critically Jll Patients

B. Steinberg, E. Kochs, H. Bause, J. Schulte am Esch

Introduction

In critically ill patients undergoing mechanical ventilation and parenteral feeding, hemodynamic functions are supported by infusion of blood substitutes (BS). Frequently those patients suffer from disorders in microcirculation. Hence, BS should not only be balanced in its contents, but should also foster an adequate microcirculation and cardiac output level [14]. Particularly, this applies to patients suffering from shock since shock of various origins can lead to tissue hypoxia. However, in the hyperdynamic stage of septic shock the cardiac output (CO) is increased. In most cases this leads to a CO-dependent increase in perfusion of the skeletal muscle [2]. It is unclear if endotoxines affect the smooth muscle of vessel directly; changes in circulation are attributed predominantly to mediators and their effects on endothelium, smooth muscle and blood components [6, 12]. In the hyperdynamic stage of septic shock with increased CO and organ perfusion [11], the peripheral microcirculation (of skin and muscle tissue) can be disturbed. These disorders correlate with the degree of endothelial cell damage and the extent of leucocyte sticking [9, 12].

In most clinical studies on hemodynamics of septic patients, systemic parameters are examined, e.g. oxygen content in arterial and mixed venous blood, mean arterial blood pressure (MAP), CO, central venous pressure (CVP), pulmonary arterial pressure (PAP) and lung capillary wedge pressure (PCWP). These parameters allow an estimation of myocardial function and the calculation of systemic and pulmonary vascular resistance values, as well as calculations of parameters regarding systemic oxygen transport. However, in septic patients, monitoring should include parameters rating the microcirculaton. The tissue oxygen pressure (pO_2) is a sensitive indicator of regional blood flow and its distribution within tissue [1, 3, 8]. Hence, we examined pO_2 distributions in the skeletal muscle of septic patients during infusion of Ringer's solution or of hydroxyethylstarch (HES). Two HES preparations of different mean molecular weights of 40000 and 270000 respectively, were tested.

Clinical Oxygen Pressure Measurement II
A. M. Ehrly et al. (Eds.)
© Blackwell Ueberreuter Wissenschaft Berlin 1990

Table 1. Parameters recorded simultaneously with tissue pO_2

Ventilation:	PEEP, FIO_2, frequency of ventilation
Blood:	pO_2, pCO_2, pH, S_aO_2, Bicarbonate, Hb
Hemodynamics:	ECG, heart rate, CVP, HCT

Patients and Methods

Between the 3rd and 9th day of postoperative intensive care, 30 hyper-dynamic septic patients aged between 19 and 72 years (on average 49 years) were examined. All patients were mechanically ventilated and got total parenteral nutrition.

Recorded parameters are shown in Table 1. All patients received Dopamine continuously i.v. in doses of up to 4 µg kg^{-1} min^{-1}. Noradrenaline was given intermittently in doses of 1.5 to 12 µg min^{-1} (average 3 µg min^{-1}). Sedation and analgesia were maintained by Fentanyl (0.2 to 0.6 µg h^{-1}) in combination with Midazolam (4.5 to 13.5 mg h^{-1}). Only those patients with stable respiratory and circulatory functions and who received constant medication throughout the period of observation, were included in the study.

Determination of oxygen partial pressure in tissue

A measuring device with sterilizable, polarographic hypodermic needle pO_2 probes of high spatial resolution (of about 3×10^{-6} µl) as well as a tissue pO_2 histography procedure, both developed by Fleckenstein [3, 4] and by GMS (KIMOC®, Ges. Med. Sondentechnik, Kiel-Mielkendorf, FRG), were used to determine pO_2 distributions in tissue. The process of measurement, the calibration of the probe as well as the calculation of pO_2 values and pO_2 histograms were controlled by a microprocessor device (pO_2 Histograph/KIMOC, Eppendorf Gerätebau, Hamburg, FRG). The histograms were calculated from 200 local pO_2 values determined within 6 min from a tissue volume of about 3 cm^3.

Procedure

The patients were subdivided into 3 groups, each group comprising 10 individuals, and received either 500 ml Ringer's solution or HES 40 (6%) solution (Onkohäs®, B. Braun, Melsungen, FRG) or HES 270 (6%) solution (B. Braun, Melsungen) respectively. After control data had been measured, the respective solutions were infused continuously within 60 min. Further measurements were taken 30, 60, 90, 120 and 150 min after the beginning of infusion. For statistical evaluations the Wilcoxon signed

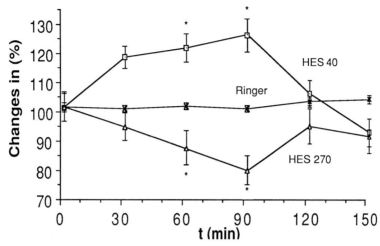

Fig. 1. Mean of change in medians of tissue pO_2 distributions; the relative data are referred to control values. Data obtained from 10 patients receiving HES 40 (square symbols), 10 patients receiving HES 270 (triangle symbols) and 10 patients receiving Ringer's solution (cross symbols). For each of the 6 measurements 200 local tissue pO_2 values were taken from all patients. Infusions were started after the first and ended after the 4th measurement (at t=90 min)

rank test was used. The zero hypothesis was rejected at a significance level of 5 %.

Results

Figur 1 shows the relative change in average tissue pO_2 which was induced by infusion of HES 40, HES 270 and Ringer's solution; in Figur 1 the median values of the individual patients' pO_2 distributions are averaged. In the patients receiving HES 40, 30 min after start of the infusion the average muscular pO_2 was significantly increased by about 20%, at decreased frequency of low tissue pO_2 values (s. Table 3). Surprisingly, in patients receiving HES 270, the average muscular pO_2 was reduced by 22%, and the 10% percentile of pO_2 distributions by 50% (s. Table 4). About 30 min after stop of the HES infusions of both preparations, the pO_2 distributions in tissue reattained the control levels. On the other hand, Ringer's solution had no effect on tissue pO_2 distributions. Significant changes in CVP, MAP, heart rate and arterio-venous difference in oxygen content (AVDO2) were not observed. In each of the 3 groups the infusions led to a slight decrease in hematocrit. Central venous oxygen saturation and arterial pO_2 were slightly increased. Tissue pO_2 data and parameters of systemic oxygen transport are summarized in Tables 2, 3 and 4; average values, standard errors (S$\bar{x}$) as well as the relative deviations from the control values are given.

Discussion

Infusion of HES 40 obviously leads to an increase in microcirculation and tissue oxygen offer. According to Halmagyi (1984) the infusion of 500 ml HES 40 has a volume effect of more than 86 % after 90 minutes and of

Table 2. Tissue pO_2 and systemic parameters in patients receiving Ringer's solution, infusion was started after the first and ended after the 4th measurement; arterial pO_2 (pO_2 art.); hematocrit (HCT); central venous oxygen saturation (SvO_2); mean arterial blood pressure (MAP); central venous pressure (CVP); heart rate (HR); arterio-venous oxygen content difference ($AvDO_2$); % = relative value with regard to control value; $S\overline{x}$ = standard error of mean

Ringer
n = 10

Time of measurement	0 min	30 min	60 min	90 min	120 min	150 min
Median of tissue pO_2 (mmHg)	23.7	23.6	23.8	23.6	24.1	24.3
%	100	99.0	100.4	99.6	101.7	102.5
$S\overline{x}$	1.7	1.3	1.3	1.1	1.1	1.4
10% percentile of tissue pO_2 (mmHg)	10.7	10.2	10.5	10.2	10.4	10.5
%	100	95.3	98.1	95.3	97.2	98.1
$S\overline{x}$	2.1	2.1	3	2.6	2.3	2.3
pO_2 art. (mmHg)	115.7	113.3	115.8	119.9	115	114.7
%	100	98.1	100.08	103.6	99.4	99.1
$S\overline{x}$	7.25	7.09	7.55	8.78	7.38	7.38
HCT (%)	34.8	33.3*	33.5*	34.1	34.4	34.5
%	100	95.7	96.3	98	98.5	99.1
$S\overline{x}$	0.92	0.63	0.52	0.82	0.78	0.4
SvO_2 (%)	76.6	77.4	77.4	77.5	77.2	77.1
%	100	101	101	101.2	100.8	100.7
$S\overline{x}$	2.12	2.35	2.55	2.07	1.69	1.95
MAP (mmHg)	76.2	77.9	78.4	78.5	76.8	78.6
%	100	102.2	102.9	103	100.8	103.1
$S\overline{x}$	4.68	3.85	3.99	3.92	3.47	3.98
CVP (mmHg)	6.9	6.7	6.9	7	6.8	7
%	100	97.1	100	101.4	98.6	101.4
$S\overline{x}$	0.77	0.81	0.8	0.7	0.63	0.7
HR (1/s)	84.8	84.8	84.9	85.1	84.6	85.3
%	100	100	100.1	100.4	99.8	100.6
$S\overline{x}$	5.5	5.5	5.8	5.5	5.2	4.5
$AvDO_2$ (ml/100ml)	3.6	3.5	3.3	3.3	3.5	3.4
%	100	97.2	91.7	91.7	97.2	94.4
$S\overline{x}$	0.3	0.4	0.3	0.3	0.4	0.4

more than 48 % even after 240 minutes. In general, it can be assumed that the effect of HES preparations of low molecular weights persists longer than 4 hours on intravascular volume [5]. However, in comparison with the duration of the volume effect, in patients receiving HES 40 the increase in tissue pO$_2$ was markedly shorter. Consequently a direct link between hemodilution and tissue pO$_2$ increase was not observed. The decrease in the muscular pO$_2$ after the infusion of HES 270 also cannot be

Table 3. Tissue pO$_2$ and systemic parameters in patients receiving HES 40, infusion was started after the first and ended after the 4th measurement; abbreviations see Tab. 2

HES-40
n = 10

Time of measurement	0 min	30 min	60 min	90 min	120 min	150 min
Median of tissue pO$_2$ (mmHg)	29	33.9	34.9*	36.1*	30.3	26.5
%	100	116.9	120.3	124.5	104.5	91.4
S$\bar{x}$	5	3.8	4.8	5.9	4.4	4.7
10% percentile of tissue pO$_2$ (mmHg)	14.4	16.7	18.8*	19.1*	13.8	10.7
%	100	114.4	123.9	125.5	97.1	66.5
S$\bar{x}$	3.8	2.8	4	5	3.3	2.9
pO$_2$ art. (mmHg)	116.2	115.8	117.1	127	127.4	128.4
%	100	99.6	100.78	109.2	109.6	110.4
S$\bar{x}$	13.1	13.1	13	12.8	12.7	12.4
HCT (%)	34.3	32.8*	32.4*	32.4*	32.3*	32.4*
%	100	95.4	94.1	94.1	93.8	94.1
S$\bar{x}$	1	0.8	0.9	0.7	0.8	0.7
SvO$_2$ (%)	73	73	74	75	75	74
%	100	100	101.4	102.7	102.7	101.4
S$\bar{x}$	2.6	2.5	2.1	2.1	2.2	2.2
MAP (mmHg)	74.7	78.3	76.9	77.3	75.3	75
%	100	104.8	103	103.5	100.8	100.4
S$\bar{x}$	5.1	5	4.5	4.7	5	5
CVP (mmHg)	6.4	6.4	6.3	6.9	6.8	6.7
%	100	100	98.4	107.8	106.3	104.7
S$\bar{x}$	0.9	0.9	0.9	0.8	0.9	0.8
HR (1/s)	89.3	90.3	88.7	87.9	89.2	89.4
%	100	101.1	99.3	98.4	99.9	100.1
S$\bar{x}$	6	4.9	5	5.1	5.2	5.3
AvDO$_2$ (ml/100 ml)	3.7	3.6	3.4	3.5	3.5	3.4
%	100	97.3	91.9	94.6	94.6	91.9
S$\bar{x}$	0.4	0.3	0.3	0.3	0.3	0.3

explained by hemodilution since the hemodilutant effect was nearly equal both in the cases of HES 40 and HES 270 infusions. The difference in tissue pO_2 effect of the compared HES preparations might be contributed to differences in the complex pharmacokinetics of HES particles of widely varying sizes. It can be assumed that the ratio of the intravascular to the perivascular concentration of HES molecules influences the microcirculation significantly. Consequently, results of tissue pO_2 measurements under HES infusion cannot be directly transferred from septic patients to

Table 4. Tissue pO_2 and systemic parameters in patients receiving HES 270, infusion was started after the first and ended after the 4th measurement; abbreviations see Tab. 2

HES-270
n = 10

Time of measurement	0 min	30 min	60 min	90 min	120 min	150 min
Median of tissue pO_2 (mmHg)	31	28.9	26.7	24.3	29	27.9
%	100	93.2	86.1	78.4	93.6	90
$S\bar{x}$	4.8	4.7	5.8	5	6.1	5.8
10% percentile of tissue pO_2 (mmHg)	15.3	11.7	11.3*	7.4*	8.9*	11*
%	100	76.5	73.9	48.4	58.2	71.9
$S\bar{x}$	3.8	2.9	3.3	2.8	2.8	3.2
pO_2 art. (mmHg)	115.8	114.9	117.6	120	115.8	114.9
%	100	99.2	101.6	103.6	100	99.2
$S\bar{x}$	7.4	7.8	13	8.8	7.6	7.4
HCT (%)	36.5	34.4*	33.6*	33.4*	33.5*	33.5*
%	100	94.3	92.1	91.5	91.8	91.8
$S\bar{x}$	1.3	1.3	1.6	1.3	1.3	1.3
SvO_2 (%)	75	74	75	76	73	73
%	100	98.7	100	101.3	97.3	97.3
$S\bar{x}$	2.1	2.1	2.2	2.1	2.6	2.5
MAP (mmHg)	76.9	75.8	80.8	80.8	80.8	76.6
%	100	98.6	105.1	105.1	105.1	99.6
$S\bar{x}$	3.1	2.2	3.8	3.3	3	3.1
CVP (mmHg)	6.8	7.1	8*	7.6	7.4	7.4
%	100	104.4	117.7	111.8	108.8	108.8
$S\bar{x}$	0.8	0.8	1.3	1.2	1.1	1.1
HR (1/s)	93.1	89.9	89.4	89.9	89.9	92.9
%	100	96.6	96	96.6	96.6	99.8
$S\bar{x}$	7.2	8	7.9	8.3	8.6	8.7
$AvDO_2$	3.7	3.7	3.5	3.4	3.6	3.8
%	100	100	94.6	91.9	97.3	102.7
$S\bar{x}$	0.3	0.3	0.3	0.4	0.3	0.3

non-septic ones with altered properties of capillary barrier. On the other hand, HES particles possibly influence the reactivity of septic shock mediators [7, 13], as well as the phagocytic activity of the reticulo-endothelial system.

Free circulating endotoxin can initiate numerous reactions, e.g. pyrogene reactions, stimulation of the immune and complement systems, coagulation, activation of monocytes and macrophages with the release of Interleukin. These reactions can induce a reduction in systemic vascular resistance, hypotension and arteriovenous functional shunting in microcirculation leading to insufficient tissue oxygen supply. This may result in local tissue acidosis and in tissue pO_2 distributions shifted to the left, reflecting an increase in frequency of hypoxic regions in tissue [10]. On the other hand, during hyperdynamic shock, tissue pO_2 also can be increased. In most of our patients, the mean tissue pO_2 levels and the frequencies of low pO_2 values lay within the normal ranges. Hence, infusion therapy and vasoactive drug administration were balanced in an appropriate manner. The method of determining the tissue pO_2 in skeletal muscle used in this study, allows early detection of changes in tissue oxygen supply and indirect monitoring of the microcirculation. The method provides diagnostic data and can be used for evaluation of new therapeutic measures. Yet, it remains unclear whether pO_2 distributions in peripheral tissue reflect the conditions of oxygen supply to parenchymatous organs.

Summary

Volume expansion for maintaining normal to hyperdynamic circulatory conditions in septic patients is part and parcel of a standard treatment concept and is supposed to favorably influence microcirculation. It was examined in 30 hyperdynamic septic patients whether the infusion of 500 ml hydroxyethylstarch (6%) with an average molecular weight of 40000 (HES 40) or 270000 (HES 270) changes the oxygen pressure distribution in the skeletal muscle; for comparison Ringer's solution was administered. A tissue pO_2 histography device equipped with a polarographic hypodermic pO_2 needle probe, was used to determine pO_2 distributions in the femoral quadriceps muscle. The patients received either 500 ml Ringer's solution or HES. After recording control values, the respective solutions were infused within 60 minutes. Measurements were taken 30, 60, 90, 120 and 150 minutes after the beginning of the infusion. In 10 patients receiving HES 40, the oxygen pressure in skeletal muscle was significantly increased. In contrast, infusion of HES 270 induced a significant reduction in muscular pO_2 in another 10 patients. No significant changes occurred in the Ringer group (10 patients). During infusions, no changes in the following parameters were noted: CVP, MAP, heart rate and AVDO2. The hematocrit showed a similar, significant drop in the three groups.

The differences in the effects of the compared HES preparations cannot primarily be attributed to a particular hemodilutant effect of HES 40, since in all groups hematocrit values were similarly reduced. The duration of HES effects on tissue pO_2 was markedly shorter than the hemodilution.

References

1. Ehrly AM, Schroeder W (1977) Oxygen pressure in ischemic muscle tissue of patients with chronic occlusive arterial diseases. Angiology 28: p 101
2. Finley RJ, Duff JH, Holliday RL, Jones D, Marchuk JB (1975) Capillary muscle blood flow in human sepsis. Surgery 78: p 87
3. Fleckenstein W (1985) Ein neues Gewebe pO_2 Meßverfahren zum Nachweis von Mikrozirkulationsstörungen. Med Diss Lübeck
4. Fleckenstein W (1987) Die Entwicklung der Feinnadel-Gewebe-pO_2-Histographie zum klinisch eingesetzten Diagnoseverfahren. In: Präsident der FU Berlin (ed), 2. Forum Medizintechnik. Forschungsvermittlung FU Berlin: p 92
5. Halmagyi M (1984) Zur Bewertung des kolloidalen Volumenersatzmittels 6% HÄS 40% 0,5. Anästhesist 33: p 73
6. Kohler P, Albrecht M, van Ackern K (1987) Kreislaufverhalten im septischen Schock. In: Schulte am Esch, J. (ed), Sepsis, experimentelle Befunde, klinische Erfahrungen, 3. Hamburger Anästhesiologisch/Intensivmedizinisches Symposium. Zuckschwerdt München, Bern, Wien: p 26
7. Kortilla K, Grohn P, Gordin A (1984) Effect of hydroxyethylstarch and dextran on plasma volume and blood hemostasis and coagulation. J Clin Pharmacol 24: p 273
8. Kunze K (1969) Das Sauerstoffdruckfeld im normalen und pathologisch veränderten Muskel. Schriftenreihe Neurologie. Springer Berlin, Heidelberg, New York.
9. Ley K, Gaehtgens P (1987) Mikrozirkulationsstörungen im Schock. In: Kilian J, Meßmer K, Ahnefeld FW (eds), Schock, Klinische Anästhesiologie und Intensivtherapie 33. Springer Berlin, Heidelberg, New York: p 19
10. Meßmer K, Sunder-Plassmann L (1975) Schock. In: Lindenschmidt TO (ed), Pathophysiologische Grundlagen der Chirurgie. Thieme Stuttgart: p 159
11. Meßmer K (1982) Pathophysiologie des septischen Patienten. In: Lawin P, Peter K, Hartenauer U (eds), Infektion – Sepsis -Peritonitis. Thieme Stuttgart: p 12
12. Neuhof H (1987) Humorale Veränderungen im Schock: Die pathogenetische Bedeutung der Mediatoren. In: Kilian J, Meßmer K, Ahnefeld FW (eds), Schock, Klinische Anästhesiologie und Intensivtherapie 33. Springer Berlin, Heidelberg, New York: p 37
13. Stump DC, Strauss RG, Henriksen RA (1985) Effects of hydroxyethylstarch on blood coagulation, particularly factor VIII. Transfusion 25: p 349
14. Sturm JA, Wisner DH (1985) Fluid resuscitation of hypovolemia. Intensive Care Med 11: p 127

The Polarographic Measurement of pO_2-Changes on the Human Cerebral Cortex caused by Pentoxifylline

R. Leuwer, R. Schultheiß, R. Wüllenweber

Introduction

During intracranial operations the character of the perifocal brain edema is of great importance for cerebral microcirculation and thus the prognosis of postoperative recovery. Relevant disturbances of tissue oxygenation may be monitored by measurement of tissue pO_2. The polarographic multiwire-surface-electrode developed by Kessler and Lübbers (1966) can be used for intraoperative measurement of cerebral oxygen supply (Leuwer 1988).

Cortical oxygen supply may be specifically influenced by the following factors:
– extent of brain edema in the region of interest
– extent of raised intracranial pressure by the tumor
– blood supply and oxygen consumption of the tumor itself (Assad et al. 1984, Gänshirt and Tönnis 1956)
– size of the bone defect caused by the trepanation and its influence on the relation between extent of brain edema and intracranial pressure (Reichardt 1905)
– age of the patients and extent of atherosclerosis

In this study, the effect of Pentoxifylline on cortical pO_2 distributions was examined. In a first group of patients cerebral microcirculation was disturbed by primary arterial vascular diseases of intracranial vessels and in another group by an increase in intracranial pressure and brain edema.

Patients and Methods

The first group of 8 patients with arterial vascular disease underwent extracranial-intracranial bypass-surgery; measurements were performed intraoperatively before inosculation.

The second group of 6 patients suffered from brain tumors, raised intracranial pressure and brain edema. The patients of this group differed

Clinical Oxygen Pressure Measurement II
A.M. Ehrly et al. (Eds.)
© Blackwell Ueberreuter Wissenschaft Berlin 1990

Table 1. Data of the patients suffering from intracranial tumors

Patient	Age	Sex	Tumor Histology	Localization	extent of edema
1	47	f	Glioblastoma	r. parietal	+
2	65	m	Metastasis (renal ca.)	r. temporoparietal	+++
3	38	f	Astrocytoma II	r. frontoparietal	++
4	37	f	Glioblastoma	l. parietooccipital	+++
5	33	f	Meningeoma	l. frontobasal	(+)
6	62	f	Glioblastoma	r. parietal	++++

+ = very little; ++ = little; +++ = marked; ++++ = very marked

clearly regarding age, extent of brain edema and the histology of their tumor (see Table 1). The evaluation of the edema in the region of pO_2 measurement was graded by CT-findings and the pathomorphology of the tissue.

Measurements of cortical pO_2 distributions were started immediately after the opening of the dura mater; 10 min after a subsequent infusion of 300 mg Pentoxifylline in 5% glucose solution was ended, the cortical pO_2 was measured once more under new steady-state conditions. Before and after the tissue pO_2 measurements, blood pressure, pulse rate, respiratory minute volume, inspiratory oxygen fraction and expiratory pCO_2 were recorded; from arterial samples blood gas values, acid/base status, oxygen saturation, hemoglobin concentration, hematocrit, Na^+ and K^+ were determined.

Results and Discussion

In 7 of the 8 Patients with primary arterial vascular disease, the injection of Pentoxifylline led to a relevant increase in mean cortical pO_2.

However, in one young female patient suffering from a Moya-Moya-Syndrome only a discrete shift of the histogram to the right was observed after the application of Pentoxifylline (see Fig.1); the broadly scattered oxygen distribution is not changed. In patients with Moya-Moya-Syndrome, stenoses or obliterations of the inner carotid artery are found, shortly above the ophthalmic artery. This process causes the development of a subtle network of anastomoses that gives the impression of a "cloud of smoke" in the angiography (Scheid 1983). The pathomorphology of this disease corresponds to the signs of an impaired microcirculaton that can be derived from the distribution of cortical pO_2 values (Fig.1). From this single observation it can be tentatively assumed that Pentoxifylline had no vasomotoric effect within the tissue of disturbed microcirculation since vasomotoric changes would cause both an alteration of the position and of the shape of the histogram.

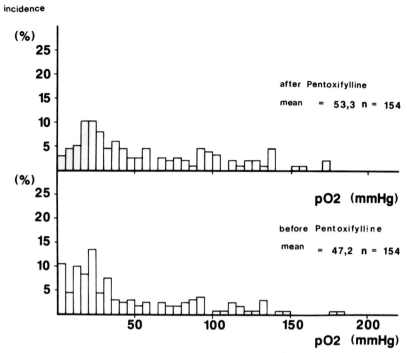

Fig. 1. Couple of pO₂ histograms from cortex of a patient with Moya-Moya-Syndrome, before and after intravenous injection of Pentoxifylline

In the 6 tumor patients, the effect of Pentoxiphylline injections on cortical pO₂ varied immensely (see Fig.2). The distinct rise of the cortical pO₂ after the injection of Pentoxifylline in patients with a marked brain edema (Pat.No. 2, 4, 6) was not observed in patients with little or missing edema (Pat.No. 1, 3, 5). The couple of histograms from patient No.5 even shows a slight drop of the mean pO₂ value in consequence of Pentoxifylline injection. However, this result does not imply an impairment of oxygen supply caused by the drug: the shape of the histogram as well as its position was not significantly changed. The results from tumor patients do not allow statistical evaluation, but they are compatible with the experiences of Hossmann et al. (1980). The authors examined the perifocal brain edema after xenotransplantation of suspensions of rat glioma cells into cats. They found that changes in blood flow of peritumoral tissue are correlated with the extent of brain edema in this region. They describe the peritumoral edema as vasogenous. A reason for the perifocal edema might be a disturbance of the blood-brain-barrier due to a structural and functional change in the endothelium cells of the tumor. Altogether the mechanism of the decrease in perfusion of edematous tissue is not clear. Miller et al. (1976) observed a drop of blood flow even in regions that were not directly impaired by brain edema. Grote and Schubert (1982) demonstrated a reduction of vascular autoregulation in brain edema. This first of

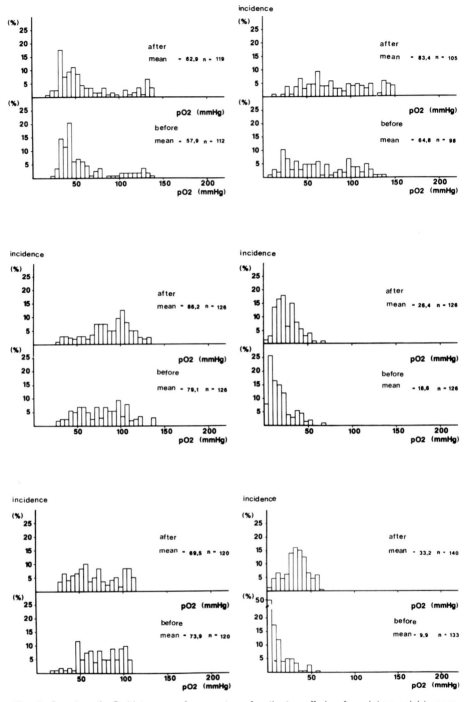

Fig. 2. Couples of pO₂ histograms from cortex of patients suffering from intracranial tumors, before and after intravenous injection of Pentoxifylline. The numbering of the coupled histograms corresponds to the patients' numbers in Tab. 1

all affects the pO$_2$-reactivity (Miller et al. 1975). The dependence of CBF on the extent of brain edema may explain the variability of the histograms that we observed. In patients with a marked brain edema, a decreased oxygen consumption in addition to the reduced blood supply is found (Gänshirt 1957). Hence, no direct conclusions can be drawn from cortical pO$_2$ distributions to the regional blood flow of the edematous cortical tissue. Assuming that an increase in tissue pO$_2$ after Pentoxifylline infusion is a sign of impaired microcirculation, in the cortex of patients with little edema the microcirculation was not impaired even despite the space occupying lesion.

Conclusions

Cortical oxygen pressure was increased by intravenous Pentoxifylline injections if the microcirculation of the cortex was impaired due to primary arterial vascular disease or due to severe brain edema in consequence of malignant growth.
In one patient suffering from Moya-Moya-Syndrome and in tumor patients with only little brain edema, cortical pO$_2$ distribution was not influenced by Pentoxifylline.

References

1. Assad F, Schultheiß R, Leniger-Follert E, Wüllenweber R (1984) Measurement of local oxygen partial pressure (pO$_2$) of the brain cortex in cases of brain tumors. In: Advances in Neurosurgery 12: 263-270
2. Gänshirt H (1957) Die Sauerstoffversorgung des Gehirns und ihre Störung bei der Liquordrucksteigerung und beim Hirnödem. Springer-Verlag Berlin, Göttingen, Heidelberg
3. Gänshirt H, Tönnis W (1956) Durchblutung und Sauerstoffverbrauch des Hirns bei intracraniellen Tumoren. Dtsch Z Nervenheilk 174: 305
4. Grote J, Schubert R (1982) Regulation of cerebral perfusion and pO$_2$ in normal and edematous brain tissue. In: Loeppky JA, Riedesel ML: Oxygen transport to human tissues. Elsevier Amsterdam, 169-178
5. Hossmann KA, Blöink M, Wilmes F, Wechsler W (1980) Experimental peritumoral edema of the cat brain. In: Cervòs-Navarro J, Ferszt R (eds) Advances in Neurology 28: Brain Edema. Raven Press, New York, 323-340
6. Kessler M, Lübbers DW (1966) Aufbau und Anwendungsmöglichkeiten verschiedener pO$_2$-Electroden. Pflügers Arch 291: 82
7. Leuwer R (1988) Die polarographische Messung von Veränderungen des pO$_2$ auf der Hirnoberfläche des Menschen unter dem Einfluß von Pentoxifylline. Med. Diss. Bonn
8. Miller JD, Garibi J, North JB, Teasdale GM (1975) Effects of increased arterial pressure on blood flow in the damaged brain. J Neurol Neurosurg Psychiatry 38: 657-665
9. Miller JD, Reilly RL, Farrar JK, Rowan JO (1976) Cerebrovascular reactivity related to focal edema in the primate. In: Pappius HM, Feindel W (eds) Dynamics of brain edema. Springer-Verlag, New York, 68-76
10. Reichardt M (1905) Zur Entstehung des Hirndrucks bei Hirngeschwülsten und anderen Hirnkrankheiten und über eine bei diesen beobachtete besondere Art der Hirnschwellung. Dtsch Z Nervenheilkunde 28: 306
11. Scheid W (1983) Lehrbuch der Neurologie. Thieme-Verlag, Stuttgart, 362-363

Influence of Intra-Arterial Prostaglandin E_1 Infusion on the Tissue pO_2 of the Tibialis Anterior Muscle in Patients with Diabetic Gangrene

H.-W. Krawzak, R. Heinrich, H. Strösche

Introduction

A humid gangrene of the foot is a common complication in patients suffering from diabetes for many years. It is a multicausal disease combining problems of neuropathy, macro- and especially micro-angiopathy. Surgical operations include vascular reconstruction, sympathectomy (with limited efficacy) and a whole range of local measures. But in spite of all therapeutic efforts, a major amputation is often unavoidable.

In patients for whom vascular reconstructive surgery is not indicated the aim of a conservative treatment is the reduction of local infection and above all the improvement of microcirculation. This can be achieved by hemodilution or application of vaso-active drugs.

Prostaglandin E_1 is a potent and short-lived vasodilative and antiaggregatory substance. It was first used by Carlson and Erikson in 1973 in the treatment of patients with severe arterial occlusive disease to make rest pain ease off and to produce a complete cure of the ulcers [2]. Because of the well-known deactivating effects of the lungs on this substance, intra-arterial infusion of PGE_1 is recommended as the most effective method of administration.

Investigations of muscle pO_2 using polarographic needle probes have so far only been reported for **intravenous** PGE_2 application [5, 7].

It was the aim of our preliminary study to verify the influence of intra-**arterial** PGE_1 on the tissue pO_2 of the tibialis anterior muscle in patients suffering from diabetic gangrene.

Patients and methods

We measured 9 patients with diabetic gangrene of the foot, 6 male and 3 female, between 63 and 84 years of age (mean: 71.3 yrs). All of them had been suffering from insulin-dependent diabetes for an average of about 19 years. In none of the cases was reconstructive vascular surgery indicated. 4 patients suffered from hypertonus. Furthermore we found 2 cases of myocardial insufficiency, 2 of renal failure and 1 of hepatic cir-

Clinical Oxygen Pressure Measurement II
A.M. Ehrly et al. (Eds.)
© Blackwell Ueberreuter Wissenschaft Berlin 1990

rhosis. All the patients were submitted to angiography. There were 3 cases with no vascular occlusion and 1 case with an obstruction of the superficial femoral arteria. 5 other angiograms showed occlusions of one or two of the lower leg arteries. The mean ankle/brachial pressure index was 0.87 (S.D. 0.32).

For the polarographic measurements of muscle pO_2 we used the "SIGMA-pO_2-Histograph/KIMOC" (Eppendorf Instruments, Hamburg, FRG) with a 300 µm needle probe according to the method developed by Flekkenstein et al. [6]. The probes were inserted through a short flexible vein catheter approximately 10 cm below the medial knee-joint cavity and about 3 cm to the side of the tibial margin. We measured in a cranial direction at an angle of about 30° to the longitudinal axis of the muscle fibers. The microprocessor-controlled probe advance was done according to the so-called "Pilgerschrittverfahren". Every pO_2 histogram was calculated out of 200 single values.

The examination of the patients took place shortly after their admission to hospital and before any specific conservative treatment had started. For the prostaglandin administration we used a totally implanted arterial access system (the so-called "port system") [8], the catheter having been operatively inserted into the superficial femoral arteria two days before.

After a rest period of 15 minutes blood gas analysis and basic hemodynamic parameters were recorded and the first pO_2 histogram was drawn up. After this the patients received Alprostadil (PGE₁-alpha-cyclodextrin) (Fa. Sanol Schwarz, Monheim, FRG) intra-arterially over a period of 45 minutes. The flow rate was 0.2 µg/min (corresponding to a dosage of approximately 3 ng/kg/min). The second pO_2 histogram was drawn up 30 minutes after the first one, and the final histogram was recorded 30 minutes after the end of the infusion (Fig. 1). For the purpose of statistical analysis we used the Wilcoxon test.

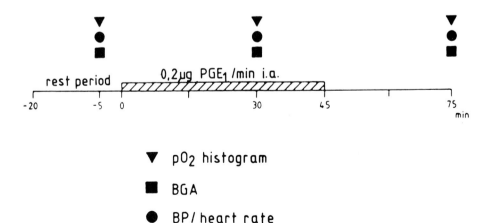

Fig. 1. Schematic presentation of the test procedure

Results

Regarding the individual courses, an increase of pO_2 during PGE_1 application could only be found in 3 out of the nine patients. In 6 cases tissue pO_2 of the tibialis anterior muscle actually decreased. The mean pO_2 figure for all patients went down from 20.3 to 18.2 mmHg.

30 minutes after the end of the infusion period tissue pO_2 again increased minimally to a mean value of 19.4 mmHg (Fig. 2, Table 1). None of these variations were significant below the 5 % level.

In order to demonstrate changes in the configuration of the histograms, single histograms were pooled.

Compared to a group of 15 healthy individuals (mean age 66 yrs) the cumulated results show a shift to the left of the histograms at the beginn-

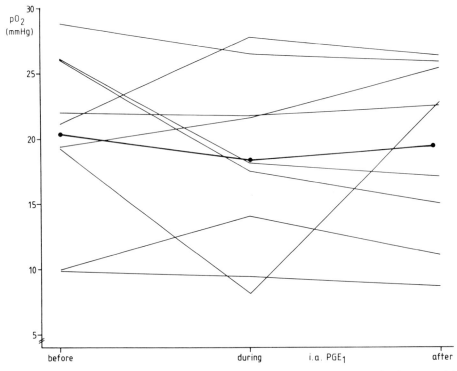

Fig. 2. Individual courses of tissue pO_2 of tibialis anterior muscle during and after intra-arterial PGE_1 (the line between the black points shows the mean pO_2 of all measurements)

Table. 1. Mean pO_2 of tibialis anterior muscle during the investigation

Tissue pO_2 (mmHg)	Before i.a.PGE_1	During i.a.PGE_1	After i.a.PGE_1
mean	20.3	18.2	19.4
S.D.	± 6.3	± 6.7	± 6.2

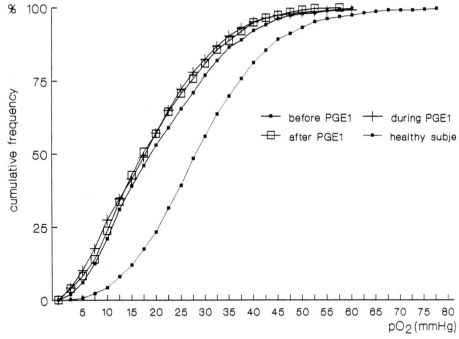

Fig. 3. Pooled histograms of tissue pO₂ of tibialis anterior muscle of healthy subjects and of diabetic patients before, during and after intra-arterial application of PGE₁

ing of the investigation. During and after PGE_1 infusion there is no change in the configuration of the histograms worth mentioning (Fig. 3).

Arterial blood gas analyses do not show any significant alteration during or after PGE_1 application. Blood pressure and heart rate too remain almost unaffected (Table 2).

During the infusion period 7 out of the 9 patients complained of strong tension and even pain in the treated leg. All of them showed a flush of the infused limb. Pain and flush disappeared shortly after the end of the infusion.

Table 2. Arterial blood gas analysis (BGA), blood pressure (BP) and heart rate (HR) before, during and after intra-arterial PGE₁ infusion

		Before i.a.PGE₁	During i.a.PGE₁	After i.a.PGE₁
BGA	pH	7.448	7.460	7.477
	pO₂ (mmHg)	69.8	66.7	71.5
	pCO₂ (mmHg)	37.5	37.2	36.0
	SBC (mmol/l)	25.2	25.7	25.9
BP	syst (mmHg)	138.3	137.2	136.6
	diast (mmHg)	70.0	68.3	70.5
HR	(min⁻¹)	81.3	82.2	80.8

Discussion

Our investigations show that there is, in comparison to healthy subjects, a decrease in the tissue pO_2 in the tibialis anterior muscle in patients suffering from a diabetic gangrene due to micro- and macroangiopathy. Several studies show an increase of transcutaneous pO_2 in normal subjects and in patients with POD stage II during intra-arterial PGE_1 administration [3, 4]. In our diabetics such positive effects could not be confirmed by means of muscular pO_2 measurements. Intra-arterial infusion of 0.2 µg prostaglandin E_1/min does not lead to any significant alteration of the muscle pO_2 of the lower leg.

As an augmentation of total blood flow to the limb is known to accompany intra-arterial infusion of PGE_1 [1, 9], the results may indicate a changed distribution of blood in favor of skin perfusion. A macroscopic manifestation of this might be the flush in the infused leg, which we observed during application.

Acknowledgements. We thank Ms G. Natterer for her skilful technical assistance.

References

1. Brecht Th, Ayaz M (1985) Circulation parameters during intravenous and intra-arterial administration of increasing doses of prostaglandin E_1 in healthy subjects. Klin Wochenschr 63:1201
2. Carlson LA, Eriksson I (1973) Femoral-artery infusion of prostaglandin E_1 in severe peripheral vascular disease. Lancet I:155
3. Creutzig A, Lux M, Alexander K (1984) Muscle tissue oxygen pressure fields and transcutaneous oxygen pressure in healthy men during intra-arterial prostaglandin E_1 infusion. Inter Angio (Suppl) 3:105
4. Creutzig A, Caspary L, Ranke C, Kiessling D, Wilkens J, Fröhlich J, Alexander K (1987) Transcutaner pO_2 und Laser Doppler Flux bei steigender Dosierung von intraarteriell und intravenös appliziertem Prostaglandin E_1. Vasa 16:114
5. Ehrly AM, Schenk J, Saeger-Lorenz K (1987) Einfluß einer intravenösen Gabe von Prostaglandin E_1 auf den Muskelgewebesauerstoffdruck, die transkutanen Gasdruckwerte und die Fließeigenschaften des Blutes von Patienten im Stadium III oder IV der chronischen arteriellen Verschlußkrankheit. Vasa Suppl 20:196
6. Fleckenstein W, Heinrich R, Kersting T, Schomerus H, Weiss C (1984) A new method for the bed-side recording of tissue pO_2 histograms. Verh Dtsch Ges Inn Med 90:439
7. Krawzak H-W, Strosche H, Heinrich R (1987) Zum Einfluß systemischer PGE_1-Infusion auf den Muskel-pO_2 bei Patienten mit arterieller Verschlußkrankheit. Klin Wochenschr 65:1004
8. Krawzak H-W, Strosche H (1988) Vollständig implantierbare Kathetersysteme zur arteriellen Extremitäteninfusion. Chirurg (in press)
9. Rexroth W, Amendt K, Römmele U, Stein U, Wagner E, Hild R (1985) Effekte von Prostaglandin E_1 auf Hämodynamik und Extremitätenstoffwechsel bei Gesunden und Patienten mit arterieller Verschlußkrankheit Stadium III-IV. VASA 14:220

Tissue pO_2 of Tibialis Anterior Muscle in Peripheral Occlusive Disease under Systemic PEG_1 Application in Relation to Fontaine's Stages

H.W. Krawzak, H. Strösche, R. Heinrich

Introduction

In 1973 Carlson and Erikson for the first time gave an account of the use of prostaglandin E_1 (PGE_1) in the treatment of severe circulatory disturbances [1]. In the beginning PGE_1 was applied only intraarterially in accordance to its specific pharmacokinetic properties. It has been the aim of this treatment – by means of improving microcirculation – to reduce rest pain and to induce a complete cure of the ulcers. To achieve this, various pharmacologically influencible factors are known, such as relaxation of arterioles and precapillary sphincters with consecutive reduction of peripheral resistance, inhibition of platelet activation, improvement of erythrocyte flexibility, inhibition of neutrocyte activation and increase of fibrinolytic activity. Moreover direct influence over cellular energetic metabolism is under discussion.

In 1976, it was again Carlson [2] who reported positive effects on the untreated side inspite of a 90% metabolism rate within the first lung passage. Thereupon PGE_1 was also applied intravenously. Up to now its efficacy and optimal dosage are points of controversy [6, 9].

The aim of the present study was to investigate the influence of intravenously applied PGE_1 on tissue-pO_2 of lower leg muscles in patients in different stages of chronic arterial occlusive disease.

Patients and Method

We measured 19 patients with chronic arterial occlusive disease, stages II-IV according to Fontaine. Their ages ranged from 33 up to 85 years. Most of them were male and smokers. 3 of them had been suffering from diabetes for many years. A further 3 patients suffered from hypertonus. Among the remaining ones there was one person with cardiac failure, one with silicosis, one with hyperuricemia and one with bronchial carcinoma. The 19 patients could be divided into two groups: 10 of them belonged to the compensated stage (stage II according to Fontaine) and 9 of them to the decompensated stage (Fontaine's stages III and IV). For the angio-

Clinical Oxygen Pressure Measurement II
A.M. Ehrly et al. (Eds.)
© Blackwell Ueberreuter Wissenschaft Berlin 1990

Table 1. Patients with chronic arterial occlusive disease in Fontaine's stages II-IV

	Total	State II	State III + IV
N	19	10	9
Age	63.3	63.4	63.1
Sex (male)	18	10	8
(female)	1	0	1
Smoker	11	5	6
Diabetic	3	1	2
Occlusion			
Pelvis	4	3	1
Thigh	7	2	5
Lower Leg	2	1	1
Combined	6	4	2
Doppler-Index	0.53	0.61	0.43*
	± 0.20	± 0.14	± 0.15

*$p < 0.05$

graphic type of vascular occlusion and the ankle/brachial pressure index (Doppler-Index) see Table 1.

To measure muscle pO_2 we used hypodermic needle probes and the "SIGMA-pO_2-Histograph KIMOC" (Eppendorf Instruments, Hamburg, FRG). The probes were inserted into the tibialis anterior muscle approximately 10 cm below the medial knee-joint cavity and about 3 cm to the side of the tibial margin. For description of technical details see [5].

The examination of the patients took place shortly after their admission to hospital, but before any surgical or conservative treatment had started. After a rest-period of 15 minutes blood gas analysis and basic hemodynamic parameters were recorded and the first pO_2-histogram was taken. Thereafter the patients received Alprostadil (PGE_1-alpha-Cyclodextrin) intravenously during a period of 45 minutes; delivering quantity 0.33 µg PGE_1/min. The second pO_2-histogram was taken 30 min after the first one. 30 minutes after the end of the infusion-period a final pO_2-histogram was recorded (Fig. 1). For the purpose of statistic analysis we used the Wilcoxon-test.

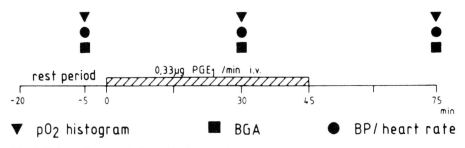

Fig. 1. Schematic presentation of test procedure

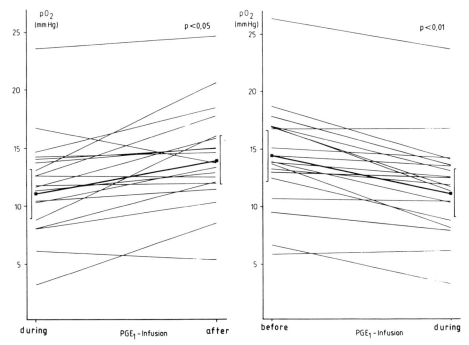

Fig. 2a, b. Individual course of tissue pO₂ of tibialis anterior muscle (**a**) during and (**b**) after infusion of PGE₁. The line between the rectangles shows the mean pO₂ of all measurements

Results

Examination of the individual courses yielded a decrease of the mean pO₂ under PGE₁ application in 17 out of 19 cases. In only 1 case did we record an increase of 0.5 mmHg. This is a significant difference (p<0.01). After the end of the infusion-period, pO₂ again rose in 16 cases, while only in 3 cases it further decreased. This change is also significant (p<0.05). The average muscular pO₂ calculated from all measurements, decreased from 14.4 mmHg to 11.9 mmHg under PGE₁, but the 14.2 mmHg at the end of the infusion period was up again and almost equivalent to the initial value (Fig. 2).

In order to estimate the levels of tissue pO₂ relative to the different stages the single histograms were pooled. Compared with a group of healthy individuals a shift of the histograms to the left is notable at the beginning of the examination. This effect is more marked in patients of stages III and IV than of stage II. Systemic application of PGE₁, as described before, causes a continuous shifting of the histograms to the left. Mean pO₂-figures decreased by about 2.4 mmHg (stage II) and by about 2.6 mmHg (stages III and IV). 30 min after the end of the infusion period the histograms looked more or less like they had done at the starting point (Fig. 3, Table 2).

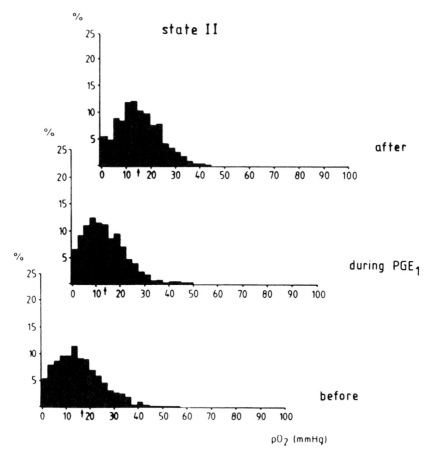

Fig. 3. Pooled histograms of tissue pO_2 of tibialis anterior muscle according to different Fontaine's stages before, during and after systemic application of PGE_1

Table 2. Mean pO_2 of tibialis anterior muscle

Tissue-pO_2 (mmHg)	Before	During PGE_1	After
State II–IV	14.4	11.9*	14.2**
II	16.3	13.9*	15.5**
III + IV	12.2	9.6*	12.9**

*p < 0.01
**p < 0.05

Arterial blood gas analysis didn't show any significant alteration due to PGE_1-application. Blood pressure and heart rate too remained almost unaffected (Table 3).

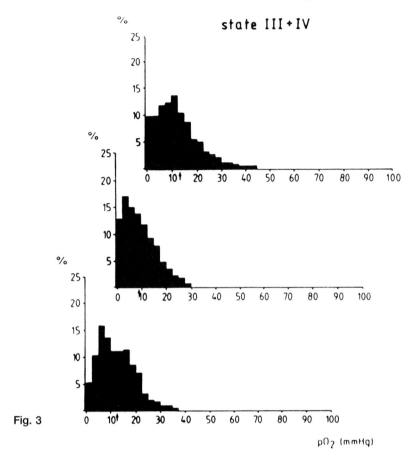

Fig. 3

Table 3. Arterial blood gas analysis (BGA), blood pressure (BP) and heart rate (HR) before, during and after intravenous PGE$_1$-infusion

	Before	During PGE$_1$	After
BGA			
pH	7.456	7.450*	7.450*
pO$_2$ (mmHg)	66.3	64.7*	68.2*
pCO$_2$ (mmHg)	36.7	36.6*	36.6*
SBC (mmol/l)	25.1	24.7*	24.9*
BP			
syst. (mmHg)	132.7	135.3*	136.7*
diast. (mmHg)	72.7	72.7*	73.3*
HR (min^{-1}	77.6	77.6*	75.2*

* no significant change

Discussion

As already mentioned at the beginning, PGE₁ has numerous pharmaco-logical influences, but their respective therapeutic importance is still largely unknown.

Fagrell and Heidrich reported a significant increase of transcutaneous pO_2 and a decrease of pathologic capillary conditions under intravenous PGE₁ application in patients with arterial occlusive disease [4, 7]. Such positive effects could not be substantiated by means of intramuscular pO_2 measurements [3, 8].

While measuring tissue pO_2 in the lower leg muscles with hypodermic needle probes, a low but constant decrease of tissue pO_2 became evident under systemic application of PGE₁. Consequently, no relationship be-tween muscular pO_2 and the stage of disease could be confirmed. We believe that the reason is a changed distribution of blood in favour of skin perfusion, especially when the results of transcutaneous pO_2-measure-ments are taken into account.

Longitudinal investigations would appear to be necessary to verify if long term intravenous PGE₁ therapy is capable of improving tissue pO_2 by acting on the different pharmacologically influencible factors.

References

1. Carlson LA, Eriksson I (1973) Femoral-artery infusion of prostaglandin E₁ in severe peripheral vascular disease. Lancet i:155
2. Carlson LA, Olsson A (1976) Intravenous prostaglandin E₁ in severe peripheral vascular disease. Lancet ii:810
3. Ehrly AM, Schenk J, Saeger-Lorenz K (1987) Einfluß einer intravenösen Gabe von Prostaglandin E₁ auf den Muskelgewebesauerstoffdruck, die transkutanen Gasdruck-werte und die Fließeigenschaften des Blutes von Patienten im Stadium III und IV der chronischen arteriellen Verschlußkrankheit. VASA Suppl. 20:196
4. Fagrell B, Lundberg G, Olsson A, Östergren J (1986) PGE₁ treatment of severe skin ischemia in patients with peripheral arterial insufficiency – The effect on skin micro-circulation. VASA 1:56
5. Fleckenstein W, Heinrich R, Kersting T, Schomerus H, Weiss Ch (1984) A new method for the bed-side recording of tissue pO_2-histograms. Verh Dtsch Ges Inn Med 90:439
6. Heidrich H, Dimroth H, Gutmann M, Helmis J, Peters A, Ranft J (1986) Long-term intravenous infusion of PGE₁ in peripheral arterial blood flow disorders. Results of an open screening study with patients in Fontaine's stages III and IV. In: Sinzinger H, Rogati W (eds) Prostaglandin E₁ in atherosclerosis. Springer, Berlin, p 92
7. Heidrich H, Lammersen T (1985) Vitalkapillarmikroskopische Untersuchungen und transkutane pO_2-Messungen bei intravenöser Prostaglandin E₁-Infusion. Dtsch med Wschr 34:1283
8. Krawzak H-W, Strosche H, Heinrich R (1987) Zum Einfluß systemischer PGE₁-Infusion auf den Muskel-pO_2 bei Patienten mit arterieller Verschlußkrankheit. Klin Wochenschr 65:1004
9. Schuler JJ, Flanigan DP, Holcroft JW, Ursprung JJ, Mohrland JS, Pyke J (1984) Efficacy of prostaglandin E₁ in treatment of lower extremity ischemic ulcers secondary to peri-pheral vascular occlusive disease. J Vasc Surg 1:161

Tissue pO$_2$ and Transcutaneous pO$_2$ in Patients with severe Renal Anemia before and During Erythropoietin-Treatment: Preliminary Results

H. Landgraf, Ch. Garcia-Bartels, P. Grützmacher, M. Bergmann, A.M. Ehrly, W. Schoeppe

One of the severe problems often associated with end stage renal disease is severe renal anemia. Until recently only symptomatic treatment, i.e. blood transfusion, was available. The development of recombinant human erythropoietin (rEpo), however, now provides the possibility to treat renal anemia effectively [2, 3, 7, 17].

With hematocrit levels corrected to about 30–35% most of the patients improved in their well-being and in their physical exercise tolerance [2]. On the other hand there were some adverse effects observed in the course of the treatment as for example the development of hypertension and thrombosis of arteriovenous fistulae [8, 13].

Hemodynamic investigations showed that the preexisting compensatory peripheral hyperperfusion was reduced when the anemia was at least partly corrected [10]. In contrast to this, an elevation of 2, 3 DPG levels, which can also be seen as a compensatory mechanism in anemia for sufficient oxygenation of tissue, did not return to normal after 10–12 weeks of treatment with rEpo; even an increase was observed. [2].

Transcutaneous oxygen pressure measurements in these patients revealed a marked increase after correction of anemia [10]. Measurements of tissue oxygenation during rEpo therapy, however, have not yet been reported.

For this reason we investigated the effect of rEpo treatment on muscle tissue oxygen pressure in patients with end stage renal disease and severe renal anemia.

The presented data are preliminary, they show the results of an investigation period of up to four weeks after onset of treatment.

Patients and Protocol

Nine patients (7 female, 2 male; average age 54 years, range 28 to 75 years) were investigated. They all suffered from end stage renal disease with severe renal anemia which required repeated blood transfusions (more than 6 transfusions/year). Additional diagnoses were coronary heart disease [3], arterial hypertension [2], history of cerebrovascular insult [1], diabetes mellitus [1].

Clinical Oxygen Pressure Measurement II
A.M. Ehrly et al. (Eds.)
© Blackwell Ueberreuter Wissenschaft Berlin 1990

Due to methodological reasons peripheral occlusive arterial disease of the lower extremities was considered an excluding factor.

rEpo was administered three times a week. During the correction phase the rEpo dosis (Boehringer Mannheim) was 80 or 100 IU/kg b.w. and during the maintenance phase 15–60 IU/kg b.w. Beside other measurements muscle tissue pO_2 and $tcpO_2$ values were determined about one week before, and then 4, 12, and 24 weeks after onset of treatment. Measurements were performed on the day after dialysis. In some cases blood transfusions interfered with the pO_2 measurements before treatment, so that the initial values may be slightly higher than they would normally have been.

Methods

Hematocrit values were determined with a micro hematocrit method in parallel to the tissue pO_2 measurements. For determination of muscle tissue pO_2 a polarographic method using micro Pt-needle-electrodes was performed in the anterior tibial muscle. This method is described in detail by Ehrly and Schroeder [5,14].

Transcutaneous pO_2 values were measured by means of a $tcpO_2$ measuring device by Radiometer, Copenhagen, Denmark. The core temperature of the electrode was 44°C, the electrodes were placed at the transition from the dorsum of the foot to the distal calf.

Tissue pO_2 values are given as medians as well as so called pooled histograms which include all the single histograms of each investigated patient. $TcpO_2$ values are given as mean values ± SD.

For statistical calculations the Wilcoxon test for paired values was applied [12].

Results

The mean hematocrit before treatment was 25.7 ± 2.9% and 30.6 ± 3.7% after four weeks of treatment.

$TcpO_2$ values were in the upper normal range before treatment and did not change: The mean value before therapy was 71.6 ± 6.5 mmHg and 71.0 ± 8.4 mmHg during medication (four weeks).

The median of the pooled tissue pO_2 histogram increased from 12.9 mmHg to 23.6 mmHg. The pooled histogram before treatment is shifted to the left and shows a high percentage of values in the hypoxic range from 0–4, and 5 to 9 mmHg.

Four weeks after onset of rEpo medication the pooled histogram is clearly shifted to the right and shows an almost normal configuration (see Table 1 and Fig. 1).

Table 1. Hematocrit, transcutaneous pO$_2$, and tissue pO$_2$ in 9 patients with severe renal anemia before and after 4 weeks of rEpo therapy. Tissue pO$_2$ values are given as medians of the pooled histograms, hematocrit and tcpO$_2$ values as mean values ± SD. Wilcoxon test for paired values (** = 2 α < 0.01, ns = not significant)

	Before therapy	After 4 week of therapy
Hematocrit (%)	25.7 ——— ** ——— 30.6	
SD	2.9	3.7
TcpO$_2$ (mmHg)	71.6 ——— ns ——— 71.0	
SD	6.5	8.4
Tissue pO$_2$ (mmHg) (medians)	12.9 ——— ** ——— 23.6	

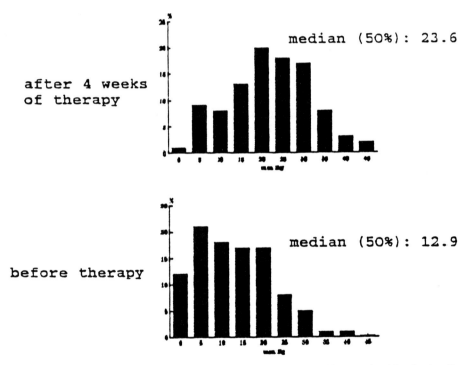

Fig. 1. Pooled histograms of tissue pO$_2$ values at rest in the anterior tibial muscle of 9 patients with severe renal anemia before (lower part) and four weeks after treatment (upper part) with recombinant human erythropoietin. Medians are given in mmHg. After four weeks of therapy a right shift of the histogram with a clear reduction of anoxic and hypoxic values can be found

None of the patients showed an increase in blood pressure during the first four weeks of medication and no other side effect or any complications were observed.

Discussion

The mean initial hematocrit value is relatively high for these patients but can be explained by the fact that three of the investigated patients had received transfusions shortly prior to the start of rEpo medication. Nevertheless there is a marked increase of hematocrit values after four weeks of treatment which is in good accordance to the results of other authors [2, 3, 7].

Muscle tissue pO_2 values before treatment are markedly reduced when compared to normals [4, 15]. This reduction and the marked left shift of the pooled histogram show that despite the compensatory mechanisms which can be found in severe renal anemia as e.g. peripheral hyperperfusion and elevated 2, 3 DPG levels [2, 10] tissue oxygen supply in these patients is impaired at rest. The degree of muscle tissue pO_2 reduction is close to that found in patients with peripheral occlusive arterial disease with severely impaired walking distances (according to stage IIb of Fontaine's classification) [5].

It must be underlined, however, that these low values are sufficient for tissue nutrition during resting conditions as these patients do not suffer from rest pain nor do they develop spontaneous necroses of the diseased limbs.

These results differ somewhat from the findings of Saborowski et al. [11] who describe normal tissue pO_2 histograms in 7 of 10 investigated patients with renal anemia and a left shift of the histogram only in 3 cases. These results, however, were obtained by means of multiwire surface electrodes and only 5 of the investigated patients had to undergo dialysis. It might be discussed therefore if these differences might be caused by methodological reasons or by different patients. The degree of anemia nevertheless was similar in both groups (the mean hct in our patients was $25.7 \pm 2.9\%$ vs 24.0 ± 4.7 in those investigated by Saborowski et al. [11].

After four weeks of rEpo treatment a marked increase of muscle tissue pO_2 values to almost normal pO_2 levels (despite the fact that hematocrit values of $30-35\%$ still have to be considered anemic) and a clear shift to the right of the histogram with an almost normal configuration can be found.

Even considering that these measurements were performed at rest and that pO_2 behaviour may be different during or after physical exercise [6] the improvement of muscle tissue oxygen supply is striking and has to be seen as an important factor in the improvement of physical exercise tolerance in these patients.

$TcpO_2$ measurements revealed different results: In contrast to the findings of Nonnast-Daniel et al. [10] our patients did not have reduced $tcpO_2$ values before rEpo medication and also did not show any significant changes during therapy.

The difference between pO_2 and muscle tissue pO_2 in these anemic patients at rest might be explained by a distribution phenomenon: In states of severe anemia muscle tissue perfusion at rest is reduced to the necessary minimum whereas skin perfusion is maintained for thermoregulation. This might be even more enhanced by the vasoparalysis and maximal vasodilation of the skin vessels caused by heating the tcpO$_2$ electrode to 44° C.

This explanation, however, does not apply to the findings of Nonnast-Daniel et al. [10]. These authors describe a marked reduction of tcpO$_2$ values (measured at electrode core temperatures of 37° and 44° C) in patients with renal anemia before rEpo therapy and a marked increase of both (37° and 44° C) values during medication.

Hematocrit values in these patients, however, were on average lower than in ours before therapy (20.7 ± 2.9 vs 25.7 ± 2.9 %) and higher after 10–12 weeks of treatment (33.1 ± 3.6 vs. 31.0 ± 3.7%). Furthermore these authors measured the tcpO$_2$ values on the forefeet of their patients which might be also a factor contributing to these differing results. Final statements concerning this point, however, can not be made at present.

Summary and Conclusions

Muscle tissue pO$_2$ values at rest were markedly reduced in patients with severe renal anemia when compared to normals. Even at rest compensatory mechanisms such as peripheral hyperperfusion and elevated 2, 3 DPG – levels were not sufficient to maintain normal muscle tissue pO$_2$ values.

After four weeks of rEpo treatment with an hematocrit increase from 25.7 to 31% a distinct improvement of tissue pO$_2$ values could be found.

This improvement of oxygen supply to the muscle tissue may be an important factor in the improvement of physical exercise tolerance in these patients.

TcpO$_2$ values were in the normal range already prior to treatment and did not show any significant changes during medication. This is in contrast to the results of other authors, the reasons for this difference, however, are still unclear.

References

1. Abendroth D, Sunder-Plassman L: Transkutante Sauerstoffdruckmessung bei arterieller Verschlußkrankheit. In: Ehrly AM, Hauss J, Huch R (eds.): Klinische Sauerstoffdruckmessung, Münchner Wissenschaftliche Publikationen, München 1985, p. 119
2. Böcker A, Reimers E, Nonnast-Daniel B et al.: Effect of erythropoietin treatment on O$_2$ affinity and performance in patients with renal anemia. In: Koch KM: Treatment of renal anemia with recombinant human erythropoietin. Contr. Nephrol. Karger, Basel 1988, vol. 66, pp. 165–175
3. Bommer J, Kugel M, Schoeppe W et al.: Dose-related effects of recombinant human erythropoietin on erythropoiesis. In: Koch KM: Treatment of renal anemia with recombinant human erythropoietin. Contr. Nephrol. Karger, Basel 1988, vol. 66, pp. 85.–93

4. Ehrly AM, Schroeder W: Kurzzeit- und Langzeitmessungen des mittleren Sauerstoffdruckes bei chronischen arteriellen Verschlußkrankheiten. In: Alexander K, Cachovan M (eds.): Diabetische Angiopathien. Witzstrock, Baden-Baden, Köln, New York 1977, p. 229

5. Ehrly AM, Köhler HJ, Schroeder W, Müller R: Sauerstoffdruckwerte im ischämischen Muskelgewebe von Patienten mit chronischen peripheren arteriellen Verschlußkrankheiten. Klin. Wschr. 53 (1975) p. 687

6. Ehrly AM, Dehn R, Saeger-Lorenz K: Verhalten des Muskelgewebesauerstoffdruckes (pO$_2$) bei Gesunden und Patienten mit Claudicatio intermittens nach definierter fußergometrischer Belastung. VASA Suppl. 14 (1986).

7. Eschbach JW, Egrie JC, Adamson JW: Correction of the anemia of end-stage renal disease with recombinant human erythropoietin. Results of a combined phase I and II clinical trial New Engl. J. Med. 316 (1987) pp. 73–78

8. Grützmacher P, Bergmann M, Weinreich T et al.: Beneficial and adverse effects of correction of anemia by recombinant human erythropoietin in patients on maintenance hemodialysis. In: Koch KM: Treatment of renal anemia with recombinant human erythropoietin Contr. Nephrol. Karger, Basel 1988, vol. 66, pp. 104–113

9. Lübbers DW: Die Beziehungen zwischen Gewebe-Sauerstoffdruck, Hautoberflächen-pO$_2$ und transkutanem pO$_2$. In: Ehrly AM, Hauss J, Huch R (eds.): Klinische Sauerstoffdruckmessung. Gewebesauerstoffdruck und transkutaner Sauerstoffdruck bei Erwachsenen. Münchner Wissenschaftliche Publikationen, München 1985, p. 3

10. Nonnast-Daniel B, Creutzig A, Kühn K et al.: Effect of treatment with recombinant human erythropoietin on peripheral hemodynamics and oxygenation. In: Koch KM: Treatment of renal anemia with recombinant human erythropoietin. Contr. Nephrol. Karger, Basel 1988, vol. 66, pp. 185–194

11. Saborowski F, Kessler M, Höper J, Greitschus F, Rath K, Dickmans HA, Thiele KG: Skeletal muscle oxygen pressure in patients with chronic renal insufficiency. In: Ehrly AM (ed.): Determination of tissue oxygen pressure in patients. Pergamon, Oxford 1983, p. 79

12. Sachs L: Angewandte Statistik, 6. Auflage. Springer, Berlin-Heidelberg-New York-Tokyo, 1984

13. Samtleben W, Baldamus CA, Bommer J et al.: Blood pressure changes during treatment with recombinant human erythropoietin. In: Koch KM: Treatment of renal anemia with recombinant human erythropoietin Contr. Nephrol. Karger, Basel 1988, vol. 66, pp.114–122

14. Schroeder W: Die Messung des Sauerstoffdrucks in der Skelettmuskulatur – eine quantitative Methode zur Kontrolle der Sauerstoffversorgung und der Funktion der terminalen Muskelstrombahn. Herz/Kreislauf 10 (1978) p. 146

15. Schroeder W, Treumann F, Ratschek W, Müller R: Muscle pO$_2$ in trained and untrained non anaesthetized guinea pigs and in men. Eur. J. Appl. Physiol. 35 (1976) p. 215

16. Steffen HM, Brunner R, Müller R et al.: Periphere Hämodynamik bei Hämodialysepatienten unter Therapie mit rekombinantem humanen Erythropoietin Nieren/Hochdruckkrh. 17 (1988) p. 374

17. Winearls CG, Pippard MJ, Downing MR et al.: Effect of human erythropoietin derived grom recombinant DNA on the anemia of patients maintained by chronic hemodialysis. Lancet ii (1986) pp. 1175–1177

Influence of Lumbar Sympathetic Nerve Blockade on Tissue pO_2 of the Anterior Tibial Muscle in Patients with Peripheral Arterial Occlusive Disease

G. Singbartl, R. Stögbauer, M. Gölzenleuchter, G. Metzger

Introduction

Patients with serious distal limb ischemia beyond the help of direct reconstructive vascular surgery are often considered for lumbar sympathectomy. Although this therapeutic measure has been practiced for more than 45 years, its efficacy in advanced atherosclerotic vascular disease remains controversial [1].

Some vascular surgeons advocate lumbar sympathectomy as a treatment for intermittent claudication [2] while others use it to supplement revascularisation procedures [3]. Others feel that it should be reserved for palliation of ischemic ulcers or rest pain when direct revascularisation is not feasible [4].

In the literature therapeutic results of lumbar sympathectomy vary greatly and the response to this treatment is different from patient to patient [5].

Many authors have attempted to predict the success of lumbar sympathectomy by using different variables, i.e. ankle pressure index, toe temperature, transcutaneous pO_2, etc.

Direct measurements of tissue pO_2 (tpO_2) in the anterior tibial muscle of patients with peripheral arterial occlusive disease (PAOD) under lumbar sympathectomy nerve blockade by continuous epidural anesthesia (EDA) is expected to yield useful information on tissue oxygen supply of the lower limb and help predict the clinical effects of operative lumbar sympathectomy.

Patients and Methods

This study was performed in 11 patients, all of them suffering from severe peripheral vascular disease stage III/IV according to Fontaine. Six patients had been suffering from diabetes for many years. In toto, measurements were done in 21 limbs, 13 of diabetic and 8 of non-diabetic patients. The patients' ages ranged from 56 to 81 years. Accompanying medication due to cardiovascular or pulmonary diseases was continued

Clinical Oxygen Pressure Measurement II
A.M. Ehrly et al. (Eds.)
© Blackwell Ueberreuter Wissenschaft Berlin 1990

during the study as well as the intake of substances with hemorheological activity.

The severity of vascular disease was demonstrated by an arteriographic study in every case. Patients were selected for lumbar sympathetic nerve blockade by the vascular surgeon. In no case was a suitable distal revascularisation possible.

The measurement of tpO_2 was obtained in the anterior tibial muscle by hypodermic needle probes based on the polarographic principle (SIGMA pO_2-Histograph KIMOC®, Fa. Eppendorf, Hamburg FRG) described by Fleckenstein et al. [6]. In every patient each measurement consisted of 200 single values which were cycled in form of a histogram and mean tpO_2 values by the integrated computer. The needle probe was inserted into the muscle tissue through a small catheter and moved forward automatically by means of a micromanipulator.

An epidural catheter was inserted at the third lumbar interspace, and after 30 minutes of rest the first measurement of tpO_2 in the anterior tibial muscle was performed, succeeded by a second tpO_2 measurement 30 minutes after the injection of 12 ml of bupivacain 0.25% through the EDA-catheter. Following this single shot dose bupivacain 0.25% was given continuously at a dosage of 4 ml/h for three days. During this time interval tpO_2 measurements were carried out every day at the same time in the afternoon. The presence of an effective lumbar sympathetic nerve blockade by EDA was inferred from the level of sensomotoric block and changes in foot skin's temperature.

Arterial blood gases, BP, HR were obtained as well.

Results

As no patient demonstrated significant changes in arterial blood gases, BP or HR during the investigation these data are not presented here.

In three patients the investigation was stopped after two days; one patient had a catheter complication, and in two patients a limb amputation had to be performed subsequently to local deterioration.

For the total of 21 limbs studied, we found only a slight rise in mean tpO_2 from 16.7 mmHg to 20.8 mmHg on the third day of continuous EDA (Fig. 1). The summarized histograms obtained from the 11 patients did not change in form either, in particular no left or right shifted histograms were obtained (Fig. 1).

In contrast to these findings and to the non-diabetic group (Fig. 2) the diabetic patients (Fig. 2b) demonstrated a marked rise in mean tpO_2 from 17.9 mmHg to 27.9 mmHg associated with a deformation (broadening) of the pO_2-histogram (Fig. 2b).

These changes in the diabetic group were mainly caused by the reaction of two patients with long term diabetes (Fig. 3). Compared to the overall group the five non-diabetic patients demonstrated no major changes either in mean tpO_2 values or in the summarized histograms (Fig. 2a).

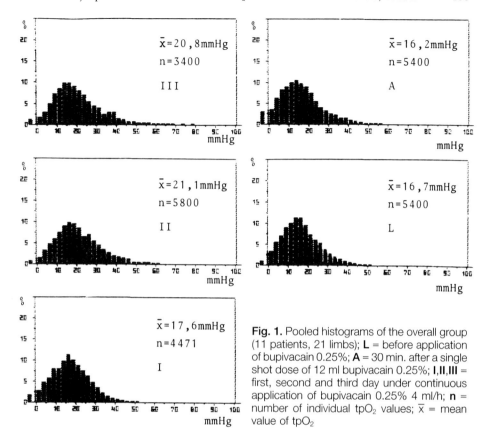

Fig. 1. Pooled histograms of the overall group (11 patients, 21 limbs); **L** = before application of bupivacain 0.25%; **A** = 30 min. after a single shot dose of 12 ml bupivacain 0.25%; **I,II,III** = first, second and third day under continuous application of bupivacain 0.25% 4 ml/h; **n** = number of individual tpO$_2$ values; $\bar{x}$ = mean value of tpO$_2$

Discussion

It is well established that lumbar sympathetic nerve blockade by EDA in patients with PAOD causes major changes in lower limb blood flow [7]. Blockade of sympathetic nerve fibres results in vasodilation especially in the skin with a concomitant increase in skin blood flow while muscle blood flow decreases [7].

The effects of lumbar sympathetic nerve blockade on collateral vessels and arterio-venous (av) shunts are unpredictable. Therefore, measuring pO$_2$ in the muscle tissue should yield reliable information on oxygen supply in the muscle tissue of patients with PAOD under EDA.

Our data show no major changes in muscle tpO$_2$ following lumbar sympathetic nerve blockade by EDA for the overall group. This supports the clinical experience that there is no benefit of lumbar sympathectomy to patients with intermittent claudication [8] and agrees with the findings of an unchanged or even decreased muscle blood flow following lumbar sympathetic nerve blockade [7, 9]. In contrast to our findings Sunder-Plassmann [10] demonstrated by means of the multiwire platinum surface electrode marked improved muscle pO$_2$ levels in patients with PAOD

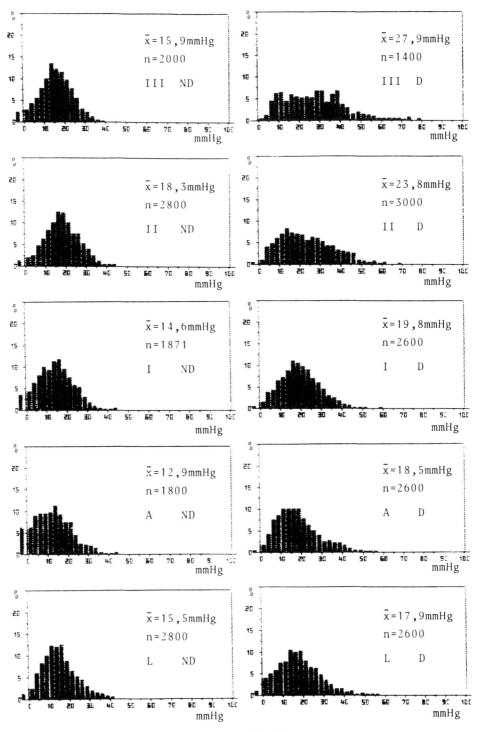

Fig. 2a   Fig. 2b

following lumbar sympathectomy. So far as known to us he is the only investigator who reports an increase in muscle blood flow of the lower limb following lumbar sympathectomy in animal studies using the microsphere technique.

Ebell et al. [11] demonstrated positive effects of EDA on transcutaneous pO$_2$ (tcpO$_2$) in patients with PAOD. In their study 49% of the patients selected for lumbar sympathectomy showed a statistically significant increase in tcpO$_2$ following lumbar EDA. As tcpO$_2$ reflects changes in blood flow of the underlying skin capillaries, rising tcpO$_2$ levels following lumbar sympathetic nerve blockade are caused by the increased blood flow. This might be helpful in patients suffering from gangrene or distal skin ulcers.

In our investigation diabetic patients showed a different reaction compared to the non-diabetic patients. They showed high tpO$_2$ levels which continuously increased following EDA and a deformation (broadening) of their histogram curves. The interpretation of the tpO$_2$ changes in the diabetic group becomes very difficult because the changes were mainly caused by the reaction of two patients only. Similar changes of muscle tpO$_2$ in long term diabetic patients could be demonstrated by Krönert et al. [12]. They found high tpO$_2$ values and right shifted histograms and discussed the influence of pre-existing neuropathic syndromes on the muscle tissue.

The presence of normal pO$_2$ levels in diabetic patients was also demonstrated with transcutaneous pO$_2$ measurings in patients with PAOD. In contrast to the non-diabetic patients the diabetic group showed no correlation between tcpO$_2$ levels and the clinical severity of the underlying vascular disease [13].

The high tissue pO$_2$ levels in diabetic patients may be due to a general vasodilation described in this group. It is still an open question whether there is an increase in nutritional blood flow or just an increase in av shunting (pre-capillary av shunt flow is a temperature control mechanism under sympathetic nerve control) without any nutritional benefit.

Considering the different responses of muscle tpO$_2$ under EDA in patients with peripheral atherosclerotic disease, the general application of this measure as a therapeutic tool has to be questioned.

Summary

The efficacy of lumbar sympathetic nerve blockade in the treatment of peripheral atherosclerotic vascular disease is highly controversial. We per-

---

Fig. 2a, b. a) Pooled histograms of the non-diabetic group (4 pat., 8 limbs) **ND** = non-diabetic group. **b)** Pooled histograms of the diabetic group (7 pat., 13 limbs); **D** = diabetic group; **L** = before application of bupivacain 0.25%; **A** = 30 min. after a single shot dose of 12 ml bupivacain 0.25%; **I, II, III** = first, second and third day under continuous application of bupivacain 0.25% 4 ml/h; **n** = number of individual tpO$_2$ values; $\overline{x}$ = mean value of tpO$_2$

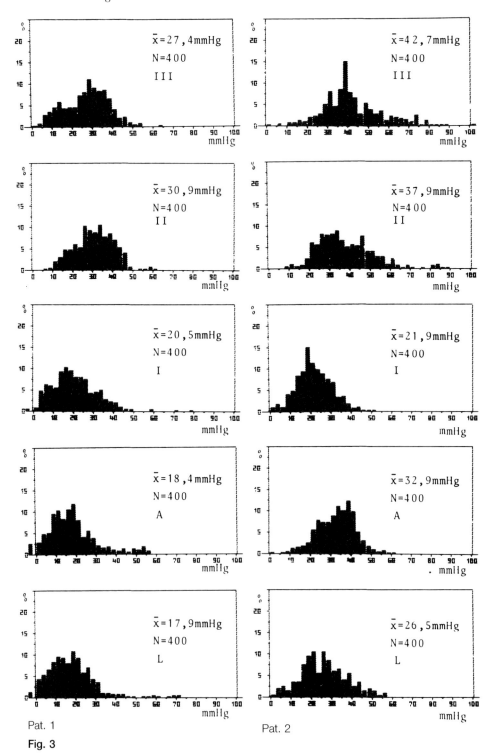

Pat. 1   Pat. 2

Fig. 3

formed lumbar sympathetic nerve blockade by EDA in 21 limbs of 11 patients with peripheral vascular occlusive disease and studied the changes of the tissue pO_2 in the anterior tibial muscle. We found no major changes in tpO_2 for the overall group studied. The diabetic patients showed an increase in mean tpO_2 under continuous EDA with a deformation of the pooled histograms. Our investigation reveals that major changes in muscle pO_2 due to EDA occur, if at all, only in diabetic patients with vascular occlusive disease. The general application of lumbar EDA in patients with PAOD is to be questioned.

References

1. Cotton LT, Cross FW (1985) Lumbar sympathectomy for arterial disease. Br J Surg 72:678
2. Taylor I (1973) Lumbar sympathectomy for intermittent claudication. Br J Clin Pract 27:39
3. Terry HJ, Allan JS, Taylor GW (1979) The effect of adding lumbar sympathectomy to reconstructive arterial surgery in the lower limb. Br J Surg 57:51
4. Smith RB, Dratz AF, Coberly JC, Perdue GD, Thoroughman JC (1971) Effect of lumbar sympathectomy on muscle blood flow in advanced occlusive vascular disease. Ann Surg 4:247
5. Walker PM, Johnston KW (1980) Predicting the success of a sympathectomy: A prospective study using discriminant function and multiple regression analysis. Surgery 87:216
6. Fleckenstein W, Heinrich R, Kersting Th, Schomerus H, Weiss Ch (1984) A new method for the bedside recording of tissue pO_2 histograms. Verh Dtsch Ges Inn Med 90:439
7. Cousins MJ, Wright CJ (1971) Graft, muscle, skin blood flow after epidural block in vascular surgical procedures. Surg Gynecol Obstet 7:59
8. Hirai M, Kawai S, Shionoya S (1975) Effect of lumbar sympathectomy on muscle circulation in dogs and patients. Nagoya J Med Sci 37:71
9. Fyfe T, Quin RO (1975) Phenol sympathectomy in the treatment of intermittent claudication: A controlled trial. Br J Surg 62:68
10. Sunder-Plassmann L (1984) Chirurgisch-therapeutisches Vorgehen bei Verschluß-krankheit der unteren Extremität. In: Arterielle Verschlußkrankheit und tiefe Bein-venenthrombose. Thieme, p 146
11. Ebell H, Abendroth D, Zehendner S, Sunder-Plassmann L, Noisser H (1987) Effekte der Sympathikusblockade durch Periduralanästhesie im forgeschrittenen Stadium der arteriellen Verschlußkrankheit. Anaesthesist 36 (Suppl) 400 (V 24.6)
12. Krönert K, Grauer W, Günderoth-Palmowski M, Schuler A, Heinrich R, Luft D, Egg-stein M (1988) Unterschiedliche Reagibilität von Muskelkapillaren insulinpflichtiger Diabetiker mit zunehmender Krankheitsdauer. "Theorie und Praxis der Gewebe pO_2 Messung" 11./12.03.88, Lübeck
13. Wyss CR, Robertson C, Love SJ, Harrington RM, Matsen FA (1987) Relationship between transcutaneous oxygen tension, ankle blood pressure, and clinical outcome of vascular surgery in diabetic and non diabetic patients. Surgery 101:56

Fig. 3. Pooled histograms of two patients with long term diabetes; **L** = before application of bupivacain 0.25%; **A** = 30 min. after a single shot dose of 12 ml bupivacain 0.25%; **I, II, III** = first, second and third day under continuous application of bupivacain 0.25% 4 ml/h; **n** = number of individual tpO_2 values; $\overline{x}$ = mean value of tpO_2

Drug Induced Variations of Muscle Tissue pO$_2$ after Pedalergometric Exercise in Claudicants

A. M. Ehrly, R. Dehn, K. Saeger-Lorenz

The quantification of therapeutic efficacy in patients with intermittent claudication is difficult, since pain-free walking distance is, in the final analysis, a subjective measure. Quantitative measurement of blood flow using, for instance, venous occlusion plethysmography, gives objective information on overall efficacy of treatment, but does not allow for differentiation between nutritive and non-nutritive capillary perfusion. Measurements of tissue oxygen pressure directly in the ischemic muscle tissue of patients with intermittent claudication make it possible to quantify the amount of oxygen actually supplied to the tissue, the aim and end of the long oxygen transport chain. Using this method, it is possible to judge if the capillary blood flow is mostly nutritive or non-nutritive [1].

In addition to the measurement of tissue oxygen tension (pO$_2$) under resting conditions, techniques have recently been developed that permit measurement of the pattern of tissue pO$_2$ in conjunction with muscular exercise. This technique of quantifying tissue oxygen supply appears especially important in the context of intermittent claudication because the cardinal clinical symptom (i.e., pain) occurs only on effort. Following earlier studies with nonstandardized exercise [2,3] tissue pO$_2$ can now be measured unter standardized exercise conditions with the aid of a pneumatic pedal ergometer with digital display of workload or work output [4].

On moderate exercise, patients with intermittent claudication display a far less pronounced and delayed increase in tissue pO$_2$ in the anterior tibial muscle (retarded reactive hyperoxia) than a group of age-matched subjects without vascular disease do. Thus, in addition to the level of the resting value, the kinetics of pO$_2$ after standardized pedal ergometer exercise are a measure of the dynamic changes in tissue oxygen supply during muscular effort [4].

Studies on the pattern of tissue pO$_2$ in patients with intermittent claudication have revealed marked differences in the behavior of this parameter before and after successful catheter dilation [4].

Former investigations have also shown that an intravenous application of the vasoactive drug pentoxifylline improves the muscle tissue pO$_2$ pattern after exercise [5,6].

Clinical Oxygen Pressure Measurement II
A.M. Ehrly et al. (Eds.)
© Blackwell Ueberreuter Wissenschaft Berlin 1990

The aim of the present two studies was to find out if 1. the intravenous application of the vasoactive drug buflomedil and 2. an oral administration of pentoxifylline can improve the excercise dependent pattern of muscle tissue oxygen pressure of patients with intermittent claudication.

Subjects and methods

Buflomedil versus placebo (i. v.)

The buflomedil investigations were performed in a placebo-controlled, simple-blind cross-over study including 13 patients with clinically and angiographically proven occlusions and stenoses in the femoral or pelvic arteries. The pain-free walking distance at the beginning of the study ranged between 50 and 200 m (as measured using a treadmill at a speed of 3.2 km/h and an inclination of 12.5 %). The known duration of the symptoms exceeded 1 year. The patients' age varied between 40 and 70 years. All patients were duly informed and gave their written consent.

Angina pectoris and/or myocardial insufficiency acute myocardial infarction, pregnancy, severe liver or kidney damage, diabetes mellitus, severe hyper- od hypotension were exclusion criteria. Washout period for vasoactive drugs was at least 2 weeks before onset of the study.

Muscle tissue pO$_2$ was measured in the tibial anterior muscle using microplatinum needle electrodes according to Ehrly and Schroeder [7,8]. The electrode with a tip diameter of about 1 to 3 µm was introduced into the muscle tissue to a depth of about 12 mm. During withdrawal of the electrode, oxygen tension was registered continuously.

After measuring the pO$_2$ values at rest, 400 mg buflomedil (Bufedil®, Abbott, Wiesbaden, FRG) dissolved in 50 ml or saline solution of 50 ml of pure saline solution as placebo were infused with a motor pump over a period of 10 min. The same procedure was repeated in every patient 2 or 3 days after the first examination, the infused liquid being switched from buflomedil to placebo or vice versa, as the case may be. What each infusion patient was given on the first day was determined randomly.

After the infusion, a 4-min standardized pedal ergometric exercise in the shape of a dorsal flexion of the foot 36 times per min was performed. The performance corresponded to 1.36 w/s, and the workload was 5.7 w [4]. Tissue pO$_2$ measurements were performed 3, 3 10, 20, 30, and 60 min after ending the 4-min exercise test. Details of the method have been described elsewhere [4]. In addition to tissue pO$_2$, the systemic blood pressure values according to Riva-Rocci as well as pulse frequency were registered. For statistical analysis, the Wilcoxon test was used.

Pentoxifylline versus placebo (orally)

This study was performed in an open randomized controlled prospective cross-over design including 17 patients with intermittent claudication stage IIb according to Fontaine. The selection of patients, the muscle tissue pO_2 measurement under exercise conditions and the other methods used were as described in study 1.

After measuring the pO_2 values at rest 1 tablet containing 600 mg pentoxifylline (Trental®, Albert Roussel-Pharma GmbH, Wiesbaden) or 1 tablet containing milk sugar (placebo) was administrered orally. According to the cross-over design of the investigation the test compound given first was assigned at random.

One hours after ingestion of placebo and/or verum a 4 min standardized pedal ergometric exercise in form of a dorsal flexion was performed. Tissue pO_2 readings were obtained 3, 10, 20, 30 and 60 min after ending the exercise test. The same procedure was repeated in every patient 2 or 3 days after the first examination in order to have a wash out phase in between the testings.

Results

Intravenous administration of buflomedil in claudicants

After a well-defined pedal ergometric exercise, patients with severe intermittent claudication stage IIb according to Fontaine, who had been infused with buflomedil, displayed an increase in tissue pO_2 values from an initial value of around 10 torr at rest to values around 15 torr. pO_2

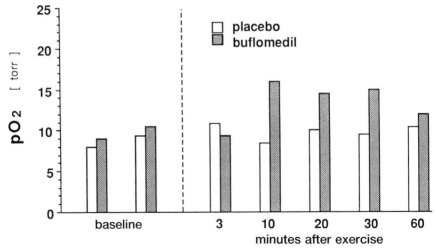

Fig 1. Behavior of exercise-induced muscle tissue pO_2 values (torr) after i. v. application of 400 mg buflomedil versus placebo in 13 claudicants (mean values) (modified from [9])

Table 1. Behavior of blood pressure, heart, rate, muscular tissue pO$_2$ after pedal ergometric exercise in patients with intermittent claudication (placebo) ($x \pm$ SD).

Parameter	values at rest		values after workload				
	RI	RII	3 min	10 min	20 min	30 min	60 min
Tissue pO$_2$ (torr) median	8.23	9.51	10.68	8.68	9.83	9.36	10.28
Heart rate (min)	65.5 ± 6.60	62.4 ± 5.49	71.1 ± 8.92	66.5 ± 6.57	63.4 ± 7.07	62.0 ± 5.44	62.1 ± 6.51
Blood pressure at the arm (mm Hg)							
systolic	132.4 ± 13.74	128.2 ± 13.11	144.8 ± 13.57	126.4 ± 12.59	129.2 ± 13.81	133.4 ± 13.47	136.8 ± 11.02
diastolic	78.3 ± 13.16	80.0 ± 12.31	85.9 ± 11.00	79.6 ± 13.17	81.9 ± 10.05	81.7 ± 9.73	82.9 ± 10.36

Table 2. Behavior of blood pressure, heart, rate, muscular tissue pO$_2$ after pedal ergometric exercise in patients with intermittent claudication (400 mg buflomedil i. v.) ($x \pm$ SD).

Parameter	values at rest		values after workload				
	RI	RII	3 min	10 min	20 min	30 min	60 min
Tissue pO$_2$ (torr) median	9.27	10.44	9.59	15.89	14.68	15.21	12.11
Heart rate (min)	65.3 ± 8.23	65.5 ± 9.26	75.1 ± 12.07	70.0 ± 9.43	67.2 ± 6.74	71.2 ± 7.95	71.2 ± 10.75
Blood pressure at the arm (mm Hg)							
systolic	134.2 ± 14.24	133.2 ± 17.12	153.8 ± 9.52	136.6 ± 17.56	136.4 ± 19.71	134.5 ± 18.90	137.5 ± 13.33
diastolic	77.44 ± 11.90	77.6 ± 10.88	91.3 ± 17.30	83.9 ± 11.46	86.7 ± 10.20	84.0 ± 12.19	87.6 ± 10.15

values were again close to starting point 1 h after the end of the exercise. In contrast, the placebo treated patients displayed no clear-cut changes in pO$_2$ median values. Comparison between the pO$_2$ medians of the buflomedil and the placebo groups yields a statistically significant difference versus placebo (2α<0.05) (Fig. 1) (modified from [9].

Tables 1 and 2 give data on the behavior of the systemic blood pressure as well as heart rate. Both in the placebo and the buflomedil group there is a limited increase in the systemic blood pressure and heart rate values, but the difference between the two groups is not statistically significant. These results have already published elsewhere (9).

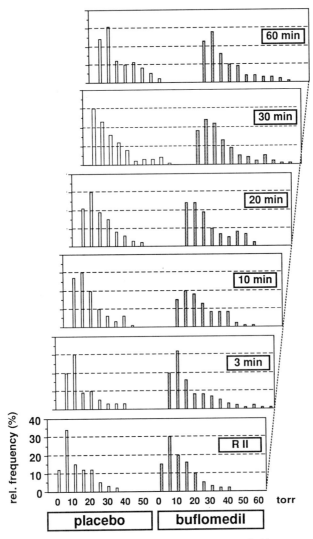

Fig. 2. Behavior of exercise-induced muscle tissue pO$_2$ histograms after i. v. application of 400 mg buflomedil versus placebo in 13 claudicants (modified from (9).

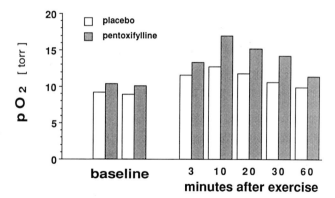

Fig. 3. Behavior of exercise-induced muscle tissue pO₂ values (torr) after oral application of 600 mg pentoxifylline versus placebo in 17 claudicants (medians)

Oral administration of pentoxifylline in claudicants

After a standardized pedal ergometric exercise, claudicants who had been treated with pentoxifylline displayed an increase in tissue pO₂ values from an initial value of around 10 torr at rest to values around 17 torr after exercise.

pO₂ values were again close to starting point 1 h after the end of the exercise. In contrast, the placebo 'group' displayed no clear-cut changes in pO₂ median values. Comparisons of the pO₂ medians of both treatment groups versus baseline revealed a statistically significant difference ($2\ \alpha < 0.05$) for the pentoxifylline group only (Fig. 3).

Comparison between the pooled histograms of the placebo and the pentoxifylline group taken at the various time intervals before and after the exercise yielded not significant differences between values at rest and pO₂ values 3 min after the end of the exercise. In contrast, between 10 and 30 min after the end of the exercise, the placebo group histogram displayed a shift to the left, whereas the pentoxifylline displayed a shift to the right with a tendency towards a more Gaussian distribution (see figure 4).

Tables 3 and 4 give data on the behavior of the systemic blood pressure as well as heart rate. Both in the placebo and the pentoxifylline group there is a limited increase in the systemic blood pressure and heart rate values, but the difference between the two groups is not statistically significant.

Discussion

Pedal ergometric exercise of the lower limb muscles in healthy subjects leads to a sudden increase in the flow rate as measured plethysmographically (reactive hyperemia) [10]. However, in patients with intermittent claudication and corresponding to the severity of their illness, reactive

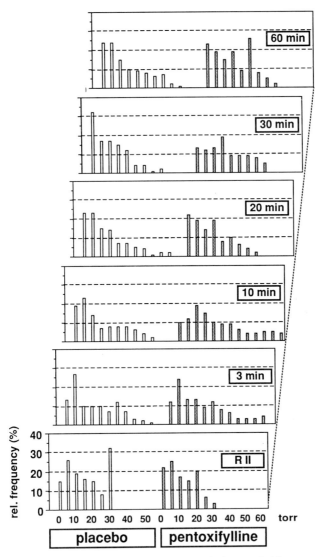

Fig. 4. Behavior of exercise-induced muscle tissue pO_2 histograms after oral application of 600 mg pentoxifylline versus placebo in 17 claudicants (medians)

hyperemia is increasingly delayed in time and less pronounced than in controls [2,4]. When measuring tissue supply instead of flow rate the results are similar.

Healthy volunteers display a sudden increase in pO_2 values followed by a sudden decrease in pO_2 values within less than quarter of an hour after the exercise (reactive hyperoxia) [4]. Patients with intermittent claudication, on the other hand, were not able to take such a high workload. We,

Table 3. Behavior of blood pressure, heart, rate, muscular tissue pO$_2$ after pedal ergometric exercise in patients with intermittent claudication (placebo) (x ± SD).

Parameter	values at rest		values after workload				
	RI	RII	3 min	10 min	20 min	30 min	60 min
Tissue pO$_2$ (torr) median	9.18	8.95	11.57	12.78	11.78	10.59	9.91
Heart rate (min)	71.1 ± 11.66	69.9 ± 10.45	76.4 ± 11.63	68.7 ± 7.94	67.9 ± 8.3	67.9 ± 8.15	68.0 ± 8.10
Blood pressure at the arm (mm Hg) systolic	137.1 ± 14.20	135.0 ± 14.16	151.0 ± 7.46	133.5 ± 17.59	138.1 ± 11.54	138.9 ± 9.04	140.4 ± 12.12
diastolic	84.6 ± 14.75	82.7 ± 12.80	86.0 ± 10.46	78.2 ± 11.99	82.2 ± 8.90	78.7 ± 7.58	78.0 ± 10.84

Table 4. Behavior of blood pressure, heart, rate, muscular tissue pO$_2$ after pedal ergometric exercise in patients with intermittent claudication (600 mg pentoxifyllin) (x ± SD).

Parameter	values at rest		values after workload				
	RI	RII	3 min	10 min	20 min	30 min	60 min
Tissue pO$_2$ (torr) median	10.48	10.10	13.32	16.98	15.19	14.23	11.34
Heart rate (min)	66.6 ± 5.88	65.1 ± 8.64	77.5 ± 9.54	68.1 ± 7.44	64.6 ± 6.63	66.4 ± 6.63	66.66 ± 8.32
Blood pressure at the arm (mm Hg) systolic	136.3 ± 21.93	132.2 ± 19.26	153.4 ± 14.96	133.7 ± 24.01	135.7 ± 20.56	136.7 ± 20.10	141.6 ± 17.27
diastolic	71.8 ± 8.52	72.2 ± 9.21	89.4 ± 14.88	77.1 ± 9.04	76.5 ± 9.39	76.1 ± 9.35	78.0 ± 8.01

therefore reduced their workload to a point where more than 90% of the patients in stage IIb were able to perform the exercise test [4]. The results show that the increase in tissue pO_2 was not only much less pronounced than in controls but its onset was also markedly delayed until the end of exercise (retarded reactive hyperoxia).

The optical display of the frequency distribution of the individual pO_2 measurements (between 0 and 5;5 and 10;10 and 15;15 and 20 torr, etc.) during continuous withdrawal of the electrode from the muscle tissue clearly indicates that there is a shift to the left in the direction of lowered pO_2 values immediately after the end of the exercise in patients with intermittent claudication (retarded reactive hyperoxia). Shifts to the left in pO_2 histograms are indicators of impaired tissue supply under exercise conditions. Therapeutic measures which influence these parameters in the direction of a shift to the right of the histogram and a more rapid and more pronounced reactive hyperoxia can be regarded as objective criteria for effective clinical improvement [4,5].

We decided on the cross-over design since former investigations have shown that the behavior of the muscle tissue oxygen pressure after standardized exercise can vary from patient to patient even within a very homogeneous group. The cross-over design even in a relatively small number of patients revealed that tissue oxygen pressure in the buflomedil group 20 min after the end of the exercise was statistically significantly higher than in patients treated with placebo.

When 600 mg pentoxifylline were given orally in claudicants there was a statistically significant increase in the muscle pO_2 values as compared to the initial values (at rest), whereas after placebo treatment these identical patients (cross-over design) revealed no statistically significant increase. There is a clear-cut shift to the right of the pO_2 histogram in the verum treated patients but no change or even a shift to the left in the placebo treated patients.

In spite of the fact that the tissue pO_2 measurement after exercise started immediately after the end of the 10 min infusion of buflomedil or 1 hour after the ingestion of pentoxifylline respectively the pO_2 response after exercise is comparable. This is true for the pO_2 medians (torr) as well as for the pattern of the pO_2 histograms.

The shift to the right of the pooled histograms in the verum treated patients as compared to the placebo treated patients 10, 20, and 30 min after the end of the exercise can be explained in terms of a more homogeneous nutritive capillary blood flow [11,12,13].

Tissue pO_2 results only give us information on the final results at the end of the oxygen transport chain. Therefore, from these results we cannot say anything about the mechanisms leading to an increase in tissue oxygen supply under exercise conditions. This could be vasomotion [14] in the case of buflomedil or hemorheologic improvement [15,16] in the case of pentoxifylline.

It should be mentioned that hemodilution is another therapeutic procedure to improve tissue supply in claudicants. These results are discussed in detail in the paper of Höffkes and co-workers in this book. Measurement of tissue oxygen pressure after exercise in patients with severe intermittent claudication seems to be a suitable method to quantify the effects of therapeutic measures on tissue oxygen supply.

Summary

Using micro-platinum needle electrodes, it is possible to measure tissue oxygen pressure directly in the ischemic muscle of the lower leg of patients with intermittent claudication under defined pedal ergometric exercise conditions. pO$_2$ values at rest as well as 3, 10, 20, 30, and 60 min after exercise were measured. In patients with intermittent claudication stage IIb according to Fontaine, not only reduced values at rest but also delayed recovery times after ending exercise (retarded reactive hyperoxia) were observed.

After performing catheter dilation, values at rest normalized, and rapid increase in oxygen pressure immediately upon terminating exercise with ensuing reduction towards initial value was observed.

An open study including 13 claudicants with ascertained occlusions or stenosis in the femoral artery or the pelvic region showed that the delayed increase in tissue pO$_2$ after exercise could be improved by i. v. infusion of 400 mg buflomedil. Comparison between the time-related pooled histograms confirmed improved oxygen supply under the influence of this drug.

In a second controlled, cross-over study in a comparable group of 17 patients the delayed increase in tissue pO$_2$ after exercise after placebo treatment could be improved by oral administration of 600 mg pentoxifylline. The pattern of mean pO$_2$ values after the end of exercise as well as the pO$_2$ histogram behaviour indicate an improved supply to the ischemic muscle tissue.

Refercences

1. Ehrly AM (1983): Verbesserung der nutritiven Durchblutung bei peripheren ischämischen Erkrankungen. Vasa 12 (suppl 11):2-21.
2. Ehrly AM, Landgraf H, Saeger-Lorenz K: Muskelgewebe pO$_2$ vor und nach fußergometrischer Belastung bei Patienten mit Claudicatio intermittens. In: Klinische Sauerstoffdruckmessung: Gewebesauerstoffdruck und transcutaner Sauerstoffdruck bei Erwachsenen, ed. by Ehrly AM, Hauss J, Huch R, Munich, MWP-Verlag, 1985, pp. 73-76.
3. Ehrly AM, Landgraf H, Saeger-Lorenz K: Muscle tissue pO$_2$ values in claudicants before and after pedalergometric exercise: Preliminary results. Int. Congr. Angiology Athens 1985 (abstract).
4. Ehrly AM, Dehn R: Verhalten des Gewebesauerstoffdrucks pO$_2$ bei Gesunden und Patienten mit Claudicatio intermittens nach definierter fußergometrischer Belastung. VASA, Suppl 14, pp. 1-48, 1986.

 5. Ehrly AM, Saeger-Lorenz K: Einfluß von Pentoxifyllin (Trental[R]) auf den Muskelge-
    webesauerstoffdruck von Patienten mit Claudicatio intermittens vor und nach fußer-
    gometrischer Belastung, Med. Welt 39, p 73, 1988.
 6. Ehrly AM, Saeger-Lorenz K: Influence of Pentoxifylline (Trental[R]) on the muscle tissue
    oxygen tension (pO$_2$) of patients with intermittent claudication before and after pedal-
    ergometer exercise. Angiology 38, pp. 93-100, 1987.
 7. Ehrly AM, Köhler H-J, Schroeder W, Müller R (1975): Sauerstoffdruckwerte im isch-
    ämischen Muskelgewebe von Patienten mit chronischen peripheren arteriellen Ver-
    schlußkrankheiten. Klin Wochenschr 53: p 687.
 8. Ehrly AM, Schroeder W: Oxygen pressure in ischemic muscle tissue of patients with
    chronic occlusive arterial diseases. Angilogy 28, p 101, 1977.
 9. Ehrly AM, Saeger-Lorenz K: Einfluß von Buflomedil i. v. auf den Belastungs-Sauer-
    stoffdruck im Muskelgewebe von Patienten mit Claudicatio intermittens. Med Welt 40,
    pp 912-915, 1989.
10. Shepherd JT (1950): The blood flow through the calf after exercise in subjects with
    arteriosclerosis and cludication. Clin Sci 9:49.
11. Kunze K (1969): Das Sauerstoffdruckfeld im normalen und pathologisch veränderten
    Muskel. Neurology Monograph Series, no 3. Springer, Berlin Heidelberg New
    York.
12. Ehrly AM, Schroeder W (1979): Zur Pathophysiologie der chronischen arteriellen Ver-
    schlußkrankheit. I., Mikrozirkulatorische Blutverteilungsstörungen in der Skelettmus-
    kulatur. Herz/Kreislauf 11: 275.
13. Ehrly AM (1980): New pathophysiological concept of ischemic disease: Microcircula-
    tory blood maldistribution (MBM). IN: Gaethgens P (ed) 11 th European Conference
    on Microcirculation, Garmisch-Partenkirchen. Bibliotheca Anatomica, vol 20. Karger,
    Basel, p 456.
14. Messmer K, Hammersen F (eds) (1983): Vasomotion und quantitative Kapillaroskopie.
    Karger, Basel.
15. Ehrly AM: Beeinflussung der Verformbarkeit der Erythrozyten durch Pentoxiphyllin.
    Med Welt 26 (N.F.) 2300, 1975.
16. Ehrly AM: The effect of pentoxifylline on the flow properties of human blood. Curr
    Med. Res Opin 5(8): 608, 1978.

Transcutaneous pO$_2$ versus Pulse Oximetry

R. Huch, F. Fallenstein, J. Bartnicki, A. Huch

A new method for the non-invasive monitoring of oxygenation has been in existence now for some years, and it seems appropriate to discuss the advantages and disadvantages of pulse oximetry in the light of the background knowledge we have about the possibilities and limitations of transcutaneous pO$_2$ (tcpO$_2$). Over the past five years, the use of pulse oximetry has spread widely. At first it was used mainly during anesthesia and in adults, but now it is available in most critical care units throughout the world. Pulse oximetry rapidly established itself in neonatal nurseries for monitoring the oxygenation of premature and term newborns, and it is especially in this area that it more or less competes with the only hereto available non-invasive method for continuous oxygen partial pressure measurements. It is known that the skin of the newborn is especially suitable for these measurements, since maximal perfusion, the result of stimulating the skin area under the tcpO$_2$ electrode through heating, seldom fails to take place [6].

In pulse oximetry, light absorption at two wavelengths when blood fills an arteriolar bed is compared to light absorption after that same blood has flowed out of the respective area. These data are then used to calculate the functional oxygen saturation of arterial hemoglobin, while the pulsatile characteristics of the signals allow the heart rate to be determined.

The idea of using pulsatile light variations to measure arterial oxygen saturation was first developed by the Japanese bioengineer T. Aoyagi [11]. His main thesis was that by restricting oneself only to the pulsatile changes in light transmission, one could register changes which were due exclusively to pulsatile alteration of the arterial blood volume flowing through the area measured. Thus, the absorption of light by different tissues, bones, skin, pigments etc. would be eliminated from the analysis, since it can be assumed to be constant in time. Thus it was possible to develop oximeters requiring no individual calibration, since all human blood is considered to display identical optical characteristics in the red and infra-red range used in oximetry.

However, direct application of the Lamdert Beer law for measuring transmitted light in a cuvette to the situation in body tissues soon revealed some of the pitfalls of the method. Body tissues lack the defined geometry of a

Clinical Oxygen Pressure Measurement II
A. M. Ehrly et al. (Eds.)
© Blackwell Ueberreuter Wissenschaft Berlin 1990

cuvette, blood is not a homogeneous solution, and the problem of light scattering is a substantial one [5]. Also, bodily movements decidedly make matters worse.

At the end of the 70s the first pulse oximeter manufactured by Minolta was tested by several groups [11]. Its extreme sensitivity to motion and the overestimation of saturation by 50 to 70 % of the actual value, due to scattering and the fact that theoretical equations did not apply to the reality of the situation, limited any rapid popularization of the technique. The breakthrough was achieved only after the technique had proved its usefulness in anesthesia with sedated or anesthetised patients, and after instruments with empirical algorithms to make the reported saturation fit a set of data had been developed [13]. Today, several firms manufacture oximeters, and the current models use tiny but powerful and highly efficient light-emitting diodes operating at wavelengths of 660 – 665 μm and 940 – 955 μm pulsed alternatingly at high frequency. The light intensity from both wavelengths is detected by a single photo-diode which generates signals proportional to the transmission.

Advantages

Clinical experience over the last 3-4 years seems to indicate that the advantages of this technique outweigh the disadvantages. Its rapid spread within such a short time seems to be proof of this. Compared to $tcpO_2$ measurements, pulse oximetry displays the following advantages, stemming from the sensor technique, the method of application and the underlying physiological basis of the method (see Table 1):

Table 1. Advantages of pulse oximetry compared with $tcpO_2$

- No sensor preparation (e.g. membrane)
- No drift
- No individual calibration necessary
- Inexpensive probes, allowing easy disposal
- No risk of burns
- No time needed for hyperemisation
  = rapid information about actual saturation
- Fast response time
- Reliability in a wide variety of clinical conditions in the motionless patient
- Relatively independent of changes in blood pressure and local blood flow
- Information about pulse rate

No sensor preparation/no drift

These first two aspects scarcely need comment; the advantages are self-evident.

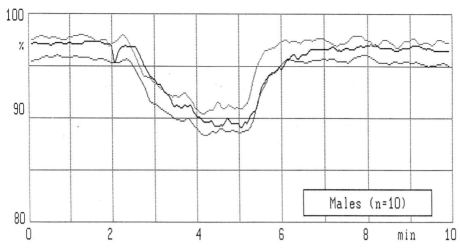

Fig. 1. Mean pulse oximetry saturation values during normoxemia and induced hypoxemia (3 mins 12 % O$_2$ in nitrogen) in 10 volunteers; measurements carried out simultaneously with three different oximetry machines

No individual calibration

None of the investigations on healthy probands with induced hypoxemia go far below 60 % arterial oxygen saturation [12]. Since, as we mentioned earlier, the built-in calibrations in the machines are empirically adjusted to the arterial saturation values measured, the statement "no individual calibration" applies to the range between 60 and 100 % saturation. In addition, if one uses machines of different manufacturers, as we did in fact do (Fig. 1), one can recognize both in the normoxemia and hypoxemia range systematic differences in the measured levels. However, it remains to be discussed whether the extent of these differences is of clinical relevance.

No heating

The fact that there is no need for carefully regulated and controlled heating of the sensor offers several advantages over the transcutaneous pO$_2$ technique. Manufacturing costs are substantially lower, there is less need for care and expertise in the use of the technique, and there is practically no risk at all of damage to the patient's skin. From the physiological point of view, a positive factor is that the 5-15 minutes which tcpO$_2$ usually requires for the arterialisation of the skin capillary area are done away with, and the time lapse from connection to the patient to obtaining a pulse oximeter reading amounts to only a few seconds.

Fast response time

Whether the possible faster response time is really an advantage for clinical management still needs to be discussed. In order to avoid false readings in either direction and to reduce the influence of motion, a certain amount of averaging out over several cardiac cycles might in fact be an advantage.

Reliability

The main advantage is the surprisingly good correlation between arterial and transcutaneous saturation values as long as the patient remains motionless, a situation which is found in sleep, during unconsciousness and during anesthesia. Numerous studies exist proving the high degree of reliability of pulse oximetry even in extreme clinical situations [1, 3, 4, 9, 10]. We too have noted similar positive results in such extreme situations [7]. In 12 children with a mean age of 2.5 years and in one adult, arterial-transcutaneous comparative measurements were taken before, during and after corrective surgery for cyanotic heart defects. Especially in the steady-state phases of the pulse oximetry registrations, the correlation is good down to the lowest arterial value of 48 % saturation, even though a certain tendency for the arterial value to be underestimated was observed. This good correlation, in line with observations by other investigators, could be seen in spite of varying blood pressure values in the phase when anesthesia was induced, as well as after the termination of the bypass phase. Thus, in contrast to the great sensitivity of the $tcpO_2$ technique in this respect, the relative independence of pulse oximetry from the circulatory situation, except during extreme shock, must be emphasized.

Heart rate

What could almost be termed a by-product of this method, which needs to detect every cardiac cycle in order to measure oxygen saturation, is the registration of the heart rate -though here too there are problems inherent in the measuring technique when averaging out is performed over several cardiac cycles in order to reduce the influence of motion artifacts and no separate analysis of the heart rate is done.

Disadvantages

Although the list of disadvantages (Table 2) is nearly as long as its counterpart, it does not carry as much weight when one considers that some of the current limitations can probably be eliminated through technical improvements.

Table 2. Disadvantages of pulse oximetry compared with tcpO$_2$

- Sensitive to movements
- Sensitive to ambient light
- Application limited to peripheral tissue because of light transmission
- Sensitive to skin pigmentation
- False saO$_2$ readings in the presence of dyshemoglobin
- Detection of hyperoxemia nearly impossible
- No local (skin) saturation measurements possible
- No dynamic changes due to cuff occlusion can be studied
- (Strong influence of peripheral vasoconstriction)

Motion artifacts

In contrast to tcpO$_2$, even the newest pulse oximeters are still highly sensitive to motion. The time-dependent component, which is crucial in pulse oximetry for the calculation of oxygen saturation, is comparatively small, representing only 1-5 % of the total signal [5]. Furthermore, the assumptions behind the calculations are that this pulsatile signal is due entirely to a new bolus of arterial blood introduced into the capillary circulation during systole, that the path lengths of the two wavelengths are identical and that both have the same wave shape. Motion on the part of the patient can cause the position of the sensor to shift, and not only changes in blood volume, but also other factors can cause variations in tissue volume. In each of these cases the optical density is altered and thus reliability of the saturation calculation is affected.

Different manufacturers use different signal processing techniques in an attempt to minimize the influence of motion. Our experience has shown these algorithms to vary greatly from model to model. When sensors from three different instruments were fixed to the fingers of one hand of a proband, clenching led to a constant decrease in saturation as recorded by Biox and to a one-time decrease as recorded by Nellcor, whereas sharp twisting motions resulted in a strong fall in saturation as recorded by Nellcor (Fig. 2). As can be seen, Novametrix shows a constant value over several minutes in the display, but in a monitoring situation this is scarcely a convincing solution.

The great sensitivity of pulse oximetry to motion has proved to be a crucial problem in both premature and term newborns. When the infants move, the saturation values fall, yet neither the speed of the saturation decrease nor the simultaneously displayed heart rate represent a criterium which allows the saturation values to be recognized as incorrect. The excerpt from a recording (Fig. 3) documents the apparent problem when a healthy baby, breathing spontaneously, moves frequently.

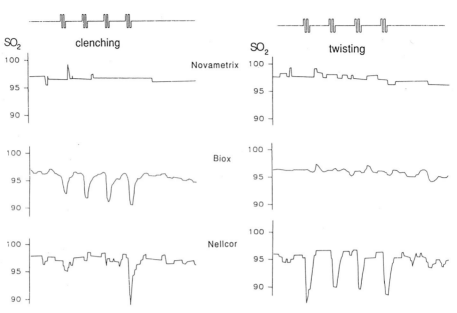

Fig. 2. Testing the sensitivity of three different pulse oximeters to motion by fixing each sensor to a different finger of the same hand

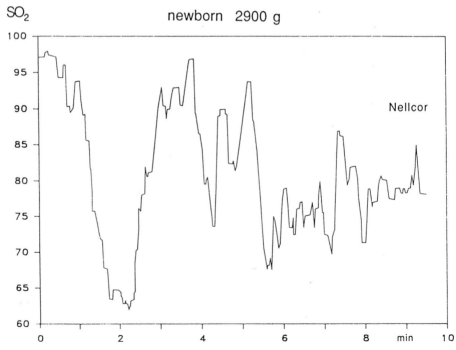

Fig. 3. Section of a 10-minute pulse oximetry saturation recording of a healthy newborn who was breathing spontaneously. Vigorous motions of the infant resulted in misleadingly low saturation value readings

Sensitivity to ambient light

Environmental factors can affect pulse oximeter functioning. Ambient light can mask the small changes in light transmission due to tissue volume variations and thus invalidate saturation calculations. Heat lamps have also been reported to interfere with pulse oximetry because of the high intensity infrared light they emit [2]. These problems can be avoided by shielding the photo diodes.

Site of application

All of the modern systems available commercially function in the light transmission mode, which means that fixation sites of the sensors are limited to peripheral areas of the body such as the ear, bridge of the nose, nasal septum, finger and, in infants, the palm of the hand or the foot. The main advantages of pulse oximetry in the reflection mode would be the possibility of central body fixation, which would probably result in fewer motion artifacts and more favorable conditions in shock and also allow application of the technique on the presenting part during labor. In addition it would permit combining pulse oximetry with other techniques, e.g. with transcutaneous pO$_2$.

Skin color

Skin pigmentation may have some effect on the functioning of the pulse oximeter, as it may be an additional factor affecting transmission of the red and infrared wavelengths differently [10].

Dyshemoglobins

The accuracy of the pulse oximetry technique is unavoidably diminished when Met-, CO-, or other pathological hemoglobins are present. Because the pulse oximeter uses only two wavelengths, the instrument interprets changes in absorption due to these hemoglobins either as reduced or increased oxygenated hemoglobin and calculates the saturation accordingly. Our calculations show that the presence of 10 % Methemoglobin can result in a pulse oximetry estimation of the arterial oxygen saturation 6 % below its true value.

Hyperoxemia

The very nature of the method and of the physiology precludes monitoring hyperoxemia with the desired degree of certainty. We tested the

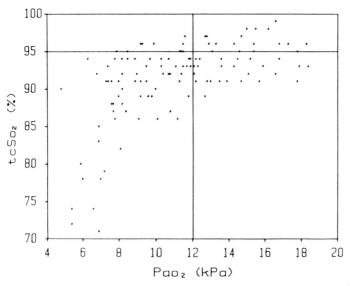

Fig. 4. Comparison between pulse oximetry (tcsO$_2$) and arterial oxygen tension (paO$_2$). Reproduced with permission from Baeckert et al, 1987

hypothesis that in neonates pulse oximetry, taking 95 % saturation as the upper limit, is reliable in detecting hyperoxemia, defined as arterial pO$_2$ above 12 kPa (90 mmHg) [1]. Fig. 4 shows the results. It illustrates the relationship between simultaneously measured pulse oximetry saturation and arterial pO$_2$. One line is drawn at a cut-off point for 95 % saturation and the other one for a paO$_2$ of 12 kPa. It can be seen that with pulse oximetry, only 14 out of a total of 46 hyperoxemic episodes were identified, which means that the sensitivity of pulse oximetry to detect hyperoxemia is 30 %. Normoxemia was correctly recognised in 68 out of 73 cases, that is, the specificity was 93 %. If the cut-off point is lowered, sensitivity could be increased at the expense of specificity, which of course would increase the false alarm rate. Our data indicate that pulse oximetry is not a reliable method for the detection of arterial hyperoxemia.

Local saturation

A further disadvantage of pulse oximetry is especially relevant for the study of microcirculation. The principle behind pulse oximetry is such that only arterial saturation can be measured, but never the local capillary condition, which is indeed possible with the tcpO$_2$ electrode at 37°C. The same limitation holds for the investigation of local vessel reactions or oxygen consumption during an arterial occlusion. Since the arterial occlusion also cuts off the pulsatile components, no measurement can take place.

Shock

The last point listed under the disadvantages, the strong influence of peripheral vasoconstriction, is set in brackets, since the question is open to discussion whether peripheral vasoconstriction affects tcpO$_2$ measurements to the same or even to a greater degree. The only difference is that the basic principle of pulse oximetry totally precludes the possibility of saturation measurements, while tcpO$_2$ at least permits an observation of the general pO$_2$ trend. Under severe shock with circulatory centralization, pulse oximetry must fail to function, in accordance with its underlying principle.

In our own investigations on infants immediately after delivery by Caesarean section, a similar limitation was observed, in addition to the difficulty of fixing the sensors in the first minute of life and the substantial motion artifacts immediately post partum [8]. When the probes were attached simultaneously both to the hand and to the foot of the newborn in the first minute of life, after three minutes there was still no signal detectable from the foot in 50 % of the newborns, and in the first 10 minutes of life in 10 % of the infants there was no measurement from the foot registered. Circulation in the extremities immediately post partum is not favorable for pulse oximetry. We also found that especially in the post partum situation, the reliability of heart rate measurements by pulse oximetry was quite low. The significant differences between the pulse oximetry and the actual heart rate as recorded by electrocardiography underlined the fact that the signal quality was too poor for correct processing.

In summary, pulse oximetry provides a new non-invasive method to reliably monitor arterial saturation, as long as clinicians are aware of its limitations and disadvantages and take these into consideration when using this technique and interpreting the results. Some of the disadvantages are of a technical nature, and improvements can certainly be expected in the future, e.g. by empirically improving the algorithms, by adding one or two additional wavelengths, or by improving the recognition of pulsatile components through external parameters such as electrocardiograms.

Some of the disadvantages simply cannot be eliminated, due to their very nature, as, for example, the impossibility of measuring local saturation or the difficulty in determining hyperoxemia with certainty. Especially in this last respect, the future will certainly not be concerned with the problem of pulse oximetry *versus* tcpO$_2$, but with the question of technical solutions allowing for improved monitoring by using both methods together.

References

1. Baeckert P, Bucher HU, Fallenstein F, Fanconi S, Huch R, Duc G (1987) Is pulse oximetry reliable in detecting hyperoxemia in the neonate? In: Huch A, Huch R, Rooth G (eds) Continuous transcutaneous monitoring. Plenum, New York, p 165
2. Brooks TD, Paulus DA, Winkle WE (1984) Infrared heat lamps interfere with pulse oximeters. Anesthesiology 61:630
3. Fanconi S (1987) Pulse oximetry and transcutaneous oxygen tension for detection of hypoxemia in critically ill infants and children. In: Huch A, Huch R, Rooth G (eds) Continuous transcutaneous monitoring. Plenum, New York, p 159
4. Fanconi S, Doherty P, Edmonds JF, Barker GA, Bohn DJ (1985) Pulse oximetry in pediatric intensive care: Comparison with measured saturations and transcutaneous oxygen tension. J Pediatr 107:362
5. Huch A, Huch R, Koenig V, Neumann MR, Parker D, Yount J, Luebbers DW (1988) Limitations of pulse oximetry. Lancet i:357
6. Huch R, Huch A, Luebbers DW (1981) Transcutaneous pO$_2$. Thieme, Stuttgart
7. Meier-Stauss P, Schmid ER, Weiss BM, Huch R (1989) Anwendbarkeit und Grenzen der Pulsoximetrie bei Korrektur zyanotischer Herzvitien. Der Anaesthesist (38, 302-308)
8. Meier-Stauss P, Bucher HU, Huerlimann R, Koenig V, Huch R. Critical dissection of pulse oximetry used for neonatal monitoring immediately after birth. Pediatrics (in print)
9. Mihm FG, Halperin BD (1983) Non-invasive monitoring of respiratory failure with pulse oximetry and capnography. Anesthesiology 59:3
10. Peabody JL, Jennis MS, Emery JR (1987) Pulse oximetry – an alternative to transcutaneous pO$_2$ in sick newborns. In: Huch A, Huch R, Rooth G (eds) Continuous transcutaneous monitoring. Plenum, New York, p 145
11. Severinghaus JW (1987) History, status and future of pulse oximetry. In: Huch A, Huch R, Rooth G (eds) Continuous transcutaneous monitoring. Plenum, New York, p 3
12. Severinghaus JW, Naifeh KH (1987) Accuracy of response of six pulse oximeters to profound hypoxia. Anesthesiology 67:551
13. Yelderman M, New W (1983) Evaluation of pulse oximetry. Anesthesiology 59:349

Transcutaneous versus Arterial pO_2 and pCO_2 During Exercise

H.-W. M. Breuer, H. Groeben, H. Worth

Introduction

Measurement of blood gas partial pressures is of importance for the analysis of pulmonary gas exchange during exercise. Usually arterial blood is sampled by multiple arterial or earlobe (capillary arterialized blood) punctures or an indwelling arterial cannula. Transcutaneous determination of blood gas partial pressures might make these procedures unnecessary, while at the same time ensuring uninterrupted pO_2 and pCO_2 monitoring during exercise. A number of studies [1 – 5] have demonstrated that transcutaneous oxygen monitoring under exercise conditions can be performed even in adults. However, the wide range of coefficients of correlation between pO_2 and $tcpO_2$ measurements obtained in these studies is striking (0.60 – 0.96). This variation is obviously related to the different test protocols and subjects under study as well as to the specific type of transcutaneous electrode used and to the site of electrode fixation on the skin. The purpose of the present study was to check reliability and practicability of transcutaneous blood gas measurements during exercise using an electrode allowing simultaneous pO_2 and pCO_2 measurements.

Subjects and methods

23 well trained, healthy, non-smoking male subjects were investigated. A bodyplethysmographic examination and determination of CO transfer factor was performed on all subjects prior to the test procedure (Table 1). The test consisted of a three minute pre-exercise resting phase, an incremental cycling test in the supine position and a post-exercise recovery phase of 9 minutes. The initial work load was between 60 and 90 Watts, which was then increased stepwise by 60 Watts every 6 mins until point of exhaustion was reached and exercise ended. Arterial blood gases from the hyperemized ear lobe were analyzed for blood gas determination in the 1st and 3rd minute of the pre-exercise resting phase, the 2nd and 5th minute of each added work load phase and the 3rd, 6th and 9th minute of the recovery phase using an ABL 300 (Radiometer, Copenhagen).

Clinical Oxygen Pressure Measurement II
A. M. Ehrly et al. (Eds.)
© Blackwell Ueberreuter Wissenschaft Berlin 1990

Table 1. Biometrical data, lung function indices and exercise characteristics of the 23 healthy subjects under study

Parameter	Mean values ± S.E.M.
Age (years)	21.7 ± 0.5
Broca index	93 ± 0.8
Max. heart rate (min^{-1})	181 ± 5.2
Achieved load (Watts)	267 ± 10
Max. lactate (mM/l)	14.4 ± 0.7
Achieved vO$_2$ (l/min)	3.42 ± 0.11
Vital capacity (l)	5.62 ± 0.1
(% predicted)	(106.5 ± 1.4)
Total lung capacity (l)	7.45 ± 0.12
(% predicted)	(100.8 ± 1.3)
Resistance (kPa*s*l^{-1})	0.22 ± 0.02
FEV$_1$ (l)	4.65 ± 0.07
(% predicted)	(113.9 ± 2)
FEV$_1$/VC (%)	83.6 ± 0.92
Transfer coefficient (mM*min^{-1}*mmHg^{-1}*l^{-1})	0.26 ± 0.00
(% predicted)	(88.3 ± 2.2)
Transfer factor (mM*min^{-1}*mmHg^{-1})	1.84 ± 0.03
(% predicted)	(107.6 ± 2.1)

Transcutaneous blood gas measurements were recorded continuously by means of the Radiometer combined tcpO$_2$ and tcpCO$_2$ electrode. The probe was fixed with self-adhesive rings to the right subclavian region, the skin beneath having been rinsed with ethanol and shaved when necessary. To achieve time constants as small as possible, the temperature of the probe was set to 45°C.

Results

162 parallel comparisons between transcutaneous values and pO$_2$ and pCO$_2$ were performed. On the average, pO$_2$ was underestimated by tcpO$_2$ (83 versus 93 mmHg), while pCO$_2$ was overestimated by tcpCO$_2$ (39 versus 36 mmHg). For the different phases of the exercise test see Table 2.

The overall correlation coefficient (r) between pO$_2$ and tcpO$_2$ was 0.55. The mean of the individual correlations was 0.66. The overall correlation between pCO$_2$ and tcpO$_2$ was 0.72, and the mean of the individual r was 0.80 (in all cases: $p < 0.001$). In addition separate analyses of linear regression were performed for the different phases of the exercise (see Table 2).

In order to check whether reliability of transcutaneous blood gas determination depends on individual factors, linear regression analysis was

Table 2. Transcutaneous blood gas values (tcpO$_2$, tcpCO$_2$ in mmHg) and the corresponding arterial blood gas values (pO$_2$, pCO$_2$ in mmHg) as well as the parameters of linear regression with respect to different phases of the exercise test (corr = coefficient of correlation; regr = coefficient of regression)

OXYGEN					
Rest		Cycling		Recovery	
pO$_2$	tcpO$_2$	pO$_2$	tcpO$_2$	pO$_2$	tcpCO$_2$
94.4	83.1	91.8	82.2	97.8	92.8
corr	regr	corr	regr	corr	regr
0.61	1.03	0.49	0.74	0.35	0.63
intercept		intercept		intercept	
− 13.9		14.7		31.2	

CARBON DIOXIDE					
Rest		Cycling		Recovery	
pCO$_2$	tcpCO$_2$	pCO$_2$	tcpCO$_2$	pCO$_2$	tcpO$_2$
38.7	40.6	37.2	40.6	32.1	35.2
corr	regr	corr	regr	corr	regr
0.33	0.28	0.65	0.59	0.58	0.77
intercept		intercept		intercept	
29.7		18.3		10.4	

performed between the individual r values of tcpO$_2$ measurements and the individual r values of tcpO$_2$ measurements. Both individual coefficients of correlation correlated significantly with each other (r=0.85, p<0.01).

Discussion

The well-established relationship between transcutaneous and arterial blood gas values, whereby tcpO$_2$ values are smaller than pO$_2$ values, and tcpCO$_2$ values higher than pCO$_2$ values [6 – 8] was confirmed by our study. However, it must be noted that in some instances during the recovery phase tcpO$_2$ values exceeded the corresponding pO$_2$ values. This phenomenon, which is also reported by Borgia and Horvath [9] and Kornum et al. [4], may be explained by post-exercise reduction in O$_2$ extraction by the cutaneous layers beneath the electrode. This is why the heat-induced increase in capillary pO$_2$, which is quite considerable (e.g. 100 to 130.8 mmHg in the presence of a skin surface temperature of 43°C [10]), may partly be registered by the transcutaneous probe, thus yielding higher tcpO$_2$ values than pO$_2$ values under these circumstances. In addition, the increase in body temperature during exercise may lead to an underestimation of arterial pO$_2$ values if no correcting factor is introduced (e.g. factor 1.05 for 38°C [11]). If a constant body temperature of

37°C is assumed, the pO_2 values measured towards the end of exercise may be systematically too low.

When performing linear regression analyses the $tcpO_2$ values exceeding pO_2 values were not taken into consideration, since these cases differed from the usual measuring situations. Nevertheless, the post-exercise r values were considerably lower than the r values measured during initial rest period and exercise (see Table 2). The assumption of reduced tissue consumption of O_2 is supported by the observation that during recovery phase the difference between pO_2 and $tcpO_2$ is smallest (5 mmHg). The overall coefficients of correlation were rather low, which may be explained by quite different individual coefficients of correlation. From former studies it is known that the divergence of $tcpO_2$ from pO_2 is constant at a specific site of the body and given that circulatory conditions are sufficient, but may vary between individuals [12, 13]. So it is necessary to look at the individual coefficients of correlation. As theoretically expected, these correlations were in the mean higher than the overall correlations (r=0.66, ranging from 0.46 to 0.84). Because of the insufficient number of samples taken during the different exercise phases (i.e. 2 values for each resting phase and 3 values for each recovery phase) the calculation of "individual" coefficients of correlation concerning those separate phases would be of doubtful validity.

The conformity between $tcpO_2$ and pCO_2 as well as the coefficients of correlation were higher than the corresponding values obtained for oxygen measurement. The overall correlation was 0.72. The best coefficient of correlation was found during the cycling phase (r=0.65), though the smallest mean difference between $tcpCO_2$ and pCO_2 was found in the resting phase before exercise (1.9 mmHg). From a statistical point of view it is not surprising therefore that the overall coefficient of correlation for this phase of the exercise was rather low (r= 0.33). The highest difference between $tcpCO_2$ and pCO_2 values (3.4 mmHg) was found in the cycling phase. This phenomenon is probably due to increased metabolism leading to increased CO_2 production in the layers beneath the probe. Again the mean individual coefficient of correlation for all values measured in one subject was superior to the overall correlation (r=0.80, ranging from 0.50 to 0.98).

Many individual factors affect $tcpO_2$ and $tcpCO_2$ measurements. Whether these factors influence both values in the same way or not could be answered by performing linear regression analysis between the different coefficients of correlation. The calculated coefficient of correlation was 0.85. Thus it may be concluded that the reliability of both $tcpO_2$ and $tcpCO_2$ measurements depends on similar factors. E.g. the two lowest coefficients of correlation, 0.17 and 0.10, were found in one and the same individual, and the two highest coefficients, 0.84 and 0.95, were found in another individual. Probably factors to do with the the electrode itself or to do with the patient's skin are responsible for these results. As the calibration procedures for the $tcpO_2$ and the $tcpCO_2$ measurements are independent of each other, the complex electrode/skin could explain the present results. Especially different time constants of the probe, depending also on individual skin factors such as the number of capillary loops or thickness of the layers beneath the probe, influence the measurement.

Reliability of transcutaneous blood gas determinations during exercise studies depends mainly on the optimal site of the sensor fixation on the body and optimal fixation. We often observed quite different values of the transcutaneous parameters when simply changing the site of the electrode. This is in accordance with former studies which stress the importance of the measuring site for performing such measurements [14]. Because the test subjects performed an exhaustion limited exercise, the extreme sweating caused problems in the fixation of the probe, which often lead to an abrupt increase in tcpO₂ values and a decrease in tcpCO₂ values due to contact with ambient air. As the loosening of the probe usually occurred during the period of maximum sweating, which was also the phase of maximal exercise, the course of the transcutaneous values in the post-exercise phase must be carefully interpreted so as to avoid wrong readings (measuring partial pressures of ambient air!).

In conclusion, transcutaneous measurements of blood gases during exhaustion limited exercise may be done with sufficient accuracy and reliability for monitoring blood gas course. Nevertheless, it must be stressed that it takes quite a lot of time to find the optimal site for fixation of the probe. Repeated comparisons of arterial blood gas values and transcutaneously achieved values are sometimes necessary before starting the test. Changing the fixation site always demands new heating of the probe, which again takes time. In addition, it is necessary to perform good fixation of the probe, usually with strips of adhesive tape over the electrode and the probe cable. All these preparatory steps will often take more than half an hour, which might prove too time-consuming for routine measurements. On the other hand, doing away with multiple arterial or ear lobe punctures or even an indwelling cannulla might, under special circumstances, e.g. monitoring blood gas course in children [15], be a sufficient justification for performing transcutaneous blood gas measurements during exercise.

References

1. Schonfeld T, Sargent CW, Bautista D, Walters MA, O'Neal MH, Platzker ACG, Keens TG (1980) Transcutaneous oxygen monitoring during exercise stress testing. Am Rev Respir Dis 121:457
2. McDowell JW, Thiede WH (1980) Usefulness of the transcutaneous pO₂ monitor during exercise testing in adults. Chest 78:853
3. Steinacker JM, Lohr P, Wodick RE (1982) Die transcutane Bestimmung des arteriellen pO₂ und ihre Einsatzmöglichkeiten bei der Spiroergometrie. Sport: Leistung und Gesundheit Kongressband Dtsch. Sportärztekongress, p 111
4. Kornum M, Oxhoj H, Nielsen G (1982) Transcutaneous versus arterial oxygen tension during exercise in chronic pulmonary disease. Clin Physiol 2:521

5. Kentala E, Repo UK (1984) Feasibility of cutaneous blood gas monitoring during exercise stress testing. Ann Clin Res 16:40
6. Lübbers DW (1979) Cutaneous and transcutaneous pO_2 and pCO_2 and their measuring conditions. Birth Defects 15:13
7. Eberhard P, Mindt W, Schäfer R (1981) Cutaneous blood gas monitoring in the adult. Crit Care Med 9:702
8. Wimberley PD, Pedersen KG, Thode J, Fogh-Andersen N, Moller Sorensen A, Siggaard-Andersen O (1983) Transcutaneous and capillary pCO_2 and pO_2 measurements in healthy adults. Clin Chem 29:1471
9. Borgia JF, Horvath SM (1978) Transcutaneous, noninvasive pO_2 monitoring in adults during exercise and hypoxemia. Pflügers Arch 377:143
10. Huch R, Huch A, Lübbers DW (1981) Transcutaneous pO_2. Thieme-Stratton Inc, New York
11. Löllgen H (1983) Kardiopulmonale Funktionsdiagnostik. Ciba-Geigy GmbH Wehr/Baden
12. Shoemaker WC (1981) Physiological and clinical significance of $ptcO_2$ and $ptcCO_2$ measurements. Crit Care Med 9:689
13. Tremper KK, Shoemaker WC (1981) Transcutaneous oxygen monitoring of critically ill adults, with and without low flow shock. Crit Care Med 9:706
14. Breuer H-WM, Niedtheidt E, Berger M, Breuer J, Loogen F (1985) Cutaneous oxygen supply in diabetics with known microangiopathy. Diabete Res Clin Pract, Suppl 1:177
15. Lindemann H, Bauer J (1984) Transkutane Bestimmung des Sauerstoffpartialdrucks unter standardisierter Belastung und Hyperoxie-Bedingungen bei Kindern. Prax Klin Pneumol 38:545

Biphasic Reactive Hyperemia Pattern Sensed by a Combined Laser Doppler and Transcutaneous Oxygen Device

U. K. Franzeck, B. Stengele, H. Tillmanns, W. Kübler

Introduction

The noninvasive evaluation of skin microcirculation has popularized itself since the introduction of transcutaneous oxygen tension (tcpO$_2$) measurements in the periphery [1, 2] and the development of Laser Doppler fluxmetry [3]. Whereas tcpO$_2$ depends on the amount of oxygen diffusing from the papillary capillaries to the skin surface, Laser Doppler fluxmetry measures perfusion of the nutritional and thermoregulatory microvasculature. The combination of both techniques into a single unit allows for simultaneous measurements under identical conditions and at one and the same location.

Subjects and method

Method

The recently designed combined Laser Doppler and tcpO$_2$ probe [4] is shown in Fig. 1. The Laser Doppler (LD) fiber optics are embedded in close proximity to the three platinum cathodes of the oxygen electrode.

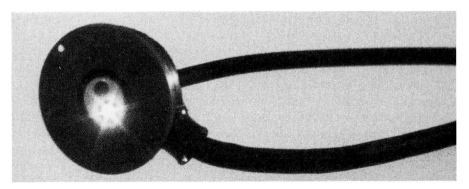

Fig. 1. Recently designed double probe with Laser Doppler fiber optics incorporated in a transcutaneous oxygen electrode (skin side)

Clinical Oxygen Pressure Measurement II
A. M. Ehrly et al. (Eds.)
© Blackwell Ueberreuter Wissenschaft Berlin 1990

The laser light (wavelength 632.8 nm) of a low-power (2.0 mW) helium-neon laser (Periflux PF2, Perimed, Stockholm) is scattered back from moving blood cells and is shifted in frequency (Doppler principle). The output of the LD-instrument is given in volts or perfusion units and reflects perfusion of the superficial skin layer. The sampling volume approximates a hemisphere with a radius of 1.0 mm. The oxygen electrode characteristics are the same as for conventional $tcpO_2$ sensors, and therefore an Oxymonitor SM 361 (Hellige GmbH, Freiburg, F.R.G.) can be used. An oxygen electrode core temperature of 37°C was used ($sspO_2$). Both recordings were registered on a two-channel stripchart recorder (Rikadenki, Hellige GmbH, Freiburg, F.R.G.).

The investigations were performed on subjects in the supine position. After attachment of a blood pressure cuff around the ankle the combined probe was fixed at the distal forefoot in the usual manner. After 10 minutes the initial recordings of $sspO_2$ and LD flux were made. Then a reactive hyperemia provocation test was performed. The suprasystolic occlusion lasted for 4 minutes.

Subjects

Ten healthy volunteers, 5 women and 5 men, were included in the study. The mean age was 25.1 ±1.9 years.

The ankle/arm pressure ratio was greater than 1.0. Six of the probands smoked regularly more than 15 cigarettes per day. All volunteers were normoglycemic.

Statistics

Statistical analyses were performed on a personal computer (Olivetti M28). From the statistical package of MS-DOS 2.11 (Microsoft Corporation) the Wilcoxon signed rank test was used. The data are expressed as means and one standard deviation.

Results

The results are listed in Table 1. The most interesting finding is the existence of a biphasic and a monophasic hyperemia response demonstrated by continuous Laser Doppler fluxmetry (Fig. 2). The biphasic hyperemia response of type A and B is present in 80 % of the probands, whereas the monophasic response of type C could be found in only 20 %.

The postocclusive reactive pO_2 response is delayed. However, the course of the postocclusion pO_2 reaction is always monophasic, reaching maximum $sspO_2$ when the LD flux hyperemia is already subsiding again.

Table 1. Laser Doppler (LD) flux and cutaneous pO_2 ($sspO_2$) values of healthy volunteers before and during postocclusive reactive hyperemia (PORH)

	initial			PORH	
	LD flux	$sspO_2$	LD flux	LD flux	$sspO_2$
			Max. 1	Max. 2	Max.
	[mV]	[mmHg]	[mV]	[mV]	[mV]
Controls	526.6	0.7	1129.9	1912.4	9.1
(n=10)	± 133.59	± 1.34	± 504.69	± 883.24	± 7.22

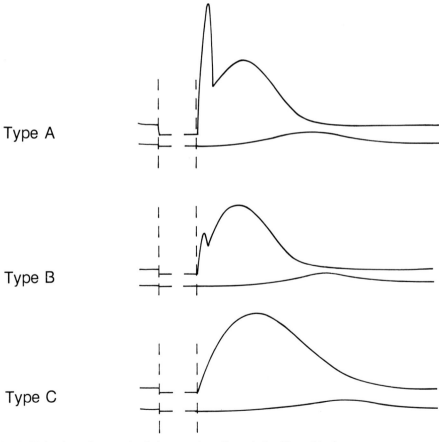

Type A

Type B

Type C

Fig. 2. Biphasic and monophasic hyperemia patterns in healthy subjects

Discussion

The combined Laser Doppler/tcpO$_2$ electrode [4] permits simultaneous recordings of superficial skin perfusion and tcpO$_2$. The most interesting finding of the study is the existence of a biphasic hyperemia pattern on the dorsum of the foot demonstrated by LD fluxmetry. A biphasic hyperemia has been found before on the forearm of healthy subjects [4] and on the big toe in patients with peripheral occlusive disease [5]. However, the sspO$_2$ response after 4 minutes arterial occlusion consistently displays a monophasic course. The longer oxygen diffusion times explain why pO$_2$ does not follow the biphasic course of the reactive hyperemia.

The biphasic hyperemia response results from an initial stretching of the myogenically active microvessels, mainly arterioles, which provokes a short vasoconstriction known as the Bayliss effect [6]. Thereafter, the pressure and tension on the vessel walls increases again, although to a lesser degree, which results in a second maximum. Superimposed on the mean LD flux are the oscillations resulting from arteriolar vasomotion [7]. The amplitude of these oscillations increases significantly during the hyperemia period ($p < 0.05$).

The hyperemic response pattern may depend mainly on the viscoelastic properties of the vessel wall [8].

Further investigations will possibly reveal any specific pattern in patients with diabetes mellitus or arterial hypertension.

References

1. Franzeck UK, Talke P, Bernstein EF, Golbranson FL, Fronek A (1982) Transcutaneous pO$_2$ measurements in health and peripheral arterial occlusive disease. Surgery 91:156
2. Franzeck UK, Bollinger A, Huch R, Huch A (1984) Transcutaneous oxygen tension and capillary morphologic characteristics and density in patients with chronic venous incompetence. Circulation 70:806
3. Tenland T (1982) On Laser Doppler flowmetry. Dissertation, Linköping University
4. Ewald U, Huch A, Huch R, Rooth G (1987) Skin reactive hyperemia recorded by a combined tcpO$_2$ and Laser Doppler sensor. Adv Exp Med Biol 220:231
5. Oestergren J, Schöps P, Fagrell B (1988) Evaluation of a Laser Doppler multiprobe for detecting skin microcirculatory disturbances in patients with obliteral arteriosclerosis. Int Angiol 7:37
6. Bayliss WM (1902) On the local reaction of arterial walls to changes in internal pressure. J Phys (Lond) 28:220
7. Funk W, Endrich B, Messmer K, Intaglietta M (1983) Spontaneous arteriolar vasomotion as a determinant of peripheral vascular resistance. Int J Microcirc Clin Exp 2:11
8. Wilkin JK (1987) Cutaneous reactive hyperemia: Viscoelasticity determines response. J Inv Derm 89:197

Transcutaneous Oximetry Monitoring During the Early Phase of Exercise Stress Test in Patients with Peripheral Artery Disease

P.A. Modesti, A. Taiti, T. Taddei, G.F. Gensini

Introduction

The functional evaluation of patients with peripheral arterial disease has its cornerstone in the assessment of the patients' capacity for walking before appearance of ischemic pain in the lower limbs. However, the quantitative assessment of intermittent claudication based on the evaluation of the walking distance is subjective and unreliable since tolerance to pain varies considerably depending on the personality. This method of measurement therefore yields a poor correlation between walking distance and hemodynamic changes [1, 2].

In recent years devices for measuring transcutaneous oxygen tension ($tcpO_2$) and transcutaneous carbon dioxide tension ($tcpCO_2$) have proved to be a useful tool for the evaluation of patients with peripheral artery disease [3, 4, 5]. This technique has made the continuous measurement of $tcpO_2$ during an exercise stress test possible [6], thus enabling an objective assessment of vascular perfusion under these conditions [7, 8]. However, early occurence of pain in the leg often meant that the test had to be interrupted, making an assessment of the vascular condition of the other leg unfeasible.

The purpose of the present study was to try to characterize the pauci-symptomatic arteriopathic patients on the basis of the early changes in transcutaneous oximetry pattern.

Patients and methods

Ten healthy subjects aged 46 ±5 years (31 to 51 yrs) displaying normal values under Doppler examination of the lower limbs and 18 non-diabetic patients aged 54 ±4 (46 to 62 yrs) suffering from atherosclerotic peripheral arterial disease were investigated. All patients were affected by intermittent claudication (stage II according to Fontaine), and their symptoms had been steady (walking distance within ±10 %) for at least 6 months. The patients were divided into 2 groups according to their walking capacity. The first group was composed of 10 patients with a walking

Clinical Oxygen Pressure Measurement II
A.M. Ehrly et al. (Eds.)
© Blackwell Ueberreuter Wissenschaft Berlin 1990

distance of over 1000 m (treadmill ergometer, 2.5 m.p.h., 10 % incline). Doppler examination for this group yielded a Winsor index (WI) of 81 ±14 % at tibialis posterior and 81 ± 17 % at dorsalis pedis. The second group was composed of 8 patients with a walking distance of 30 to 500 m; Doppler examination yielded a WI of 40 ±11 at tibialis posterior and 39 ±12 at dorsalis pedis.

None of the subjects had taken any drugs for at least 2 weeks or had smoked for at least 3 hours before the study. All the examinations were carried out in the morning in a quiet room at 20°C temperature.

The transcutaneous oxygen pressure ($tcpO_2$) values were monitored by a Clark-type electrode (Microgas 7640, Kontron) which was calibrated and applied to the skin according to the manufacturer's specifications.

The electrode was warmed to 44°C to produce maximal arterialization of the skin circulation. Recordings were made on the upper chest in the infraclaveolar area and in the pretibial region 5 cm above the malleolus lateralis of the lower extremity. The regional perfusion index (RPI) was calculated as the ratio between the value obtained at the foot and the value recorded at the upper chest.

Measurements were performed with subjects standing, all readings starting after the trace had stabilized for at least 10 mins. Subjects were then exercised on a treadmill at an incline of 10 % and at a speed of 2.5 mph.

Data were continuously recorded on graded paper both at rest and during exercise. The curves obtained were then compared by MANOVA test. The maximum percent increment of $tcpO_2$ and RPI at lower limbs after the start of exercise stress was calculated in control subjects and confidence limits of 95 % were defined. Specificity and accuracy of these limits in evaluating patients with initial peripheral arterial disease were assessed.

Data are given as mean ±SD, confidence limits at 95 % are reported in brackets.

Results

When subjects were standing, $tcpO_2$ did not discriminate between patients and controls, ie. there were no differences between the resting values of either group. In contrast, the difference in the percentage change in $tcpO_2$ under exercise conditions was highly significant and allowed for discrimination between the two groups (Fig. 1).

After starting the exercise test in the control subjects a brief $tcpO_2$ fall (-2 ±1 %) at the calf occurred within the first minute. However, this fall was shortlasting, and a rise of $tcpO_2$ above baseline values was soon observed reaching its maximum percentage increment (35 ±8 %, 19-50 %) after 7 ±2 (3-11) min, after which the values plateaued.

For values recorded at the chest, a time-dependent increase in $tcpO_2$ was also found. In fact, pulmonary ventilation increased, so that a 21 ±5.6 %

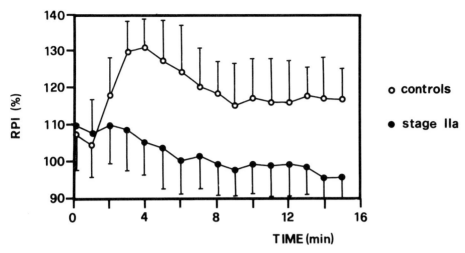

Fig 1. Regional perfusion index (RPI) at the lower limbs in controls and in arteriopatic patients in stage IIa during the early phase of an exercise stress test (treadmill ergometer, 2.5 mph, 10 % gradient) (p<0.001 for the whole curve)

(10-32) increase of tcpO$_2$ at chest was observed within 10 ±2 min (6-14). As a result, after an initial brief fall, RPI showed a steep percentage increment (22 ±5 %, 12-32) within 4 ±1 min (2-6), followed by a slow return to basal values (Fig. 1, 2).

In patients with initial stages of intermittent claudication a different pattern during the early phases of the exercise test was found. Although no actual fall in tcpO$_2$ at the lower limbs was observed in these patients, the increase in tcpO$_2$ after the first minute of the exercise test was significantly smaller than in the controls (8.7 ±5.4, -2/20, p<0.001), and the curve remained flat (p<0.001 vs. controls). The pattern of the curve recorded at chest was not different from that of the controls, so that the early increase in the RPI was lacking (1 ±4.8, -8/10, p<0.001). All the patients with stage IIa remained asymptomatic during the exercise test.

When the 95 % confidence limits of tcpO$_2$ in controls were used as normal limits, a sensitivity of 70 % and an accuracy of 85 % in discriminating paucisymptomatic patients with stage IIa peripheral arterial disease was obtained. The calculation of RPI improved both sensitivity and accuracy. In fact, RPI normal confidence limits allowed for a sensitivity of 90 % and an accuracy of 95 % (Fig. 2).

In patients with severe intermittent claudication a progressively deep fall in tcpO$_2$ was observed after the start of the exercise with a 50 % decrease in the RPI 5 ±1.5 min. The onset of pain occurred after 6 ±1.4 min. (4-10) (with an RPI decrement of -59 ±9 %). The maximum exercise load was reached after 8 ±2 min when RPI decreased by -80 ±8.6 %.

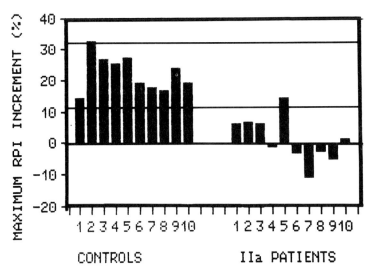

Fig. 2. RPI maximum percentage increase at lower limbs in controls and in stage IIa patients during the exercise stress test. Confidence limits at 95 % for control subjects are indicated.

Discussion

The earliest phases of exercise stress test are associated with a number of cardiac and peripheral vascular adjustments.

With the onset of exercise the resistance to blood flow through contracting muscles significantly decreases whereas other perfusion beds in non-working areas, mainly the splanchnic area, undergo significant vasoconstriction, thereby redirecting blood flow toward exercising muscles.

We observed an early transient decrease of $tcpO_2$ followed by a steady increase in $tcpO_2$. The behavior of the skin blood flow during an exercise test is quite peculiar. In fact, there is a minimal increase in total blood volume in the muscles during exercise, probably because the contracting muscles compress capacitance vessels and venoconstriction in this vascular bed is very active. In contrast, as a result of the relatively passive role played by the skin, an increase in skin blood flow at the lower limb during upright exercise occurs [9] since the compensatory mechanisms are overwhelmed by gravity [10].

Resting $tcpO_2$ values recorded at legs in patients were not different from control values. In contrast, during exercise the difference was highly significant and allowed for a much better discrimination between groups. Patients in stage IIb showed a rapid and progressive fall in $tcpO_2$ at legs under exercise conditions, the onset of pain occurring after about 6 min. and of intolerable pain after about 9 mins. In contrast, patients in stage IIa remained asymptomatic and $tcpO_2$ at the end of the test was only slightly reduced. However, on the basis of the $tcpO_2$ increment which follows the onset of exercise in controls, it was possible to discriminate with good accuracy and sensitivity between normal subjects and patients with initial peripheral arterial disease. Accuracy and sensitivity increased when RPI was also taken into consideration, because this made it possible to rule out the variability connected with breathing.

By carefully studying the first phase of an effort test in those patients with a short walking distance because of severe claudication in one leg, the condition of the other, apparently healthy lower limb can easily be assessed simultaneously.

In conclusion, the sensitivity of this technique makes it useful as a diagnostic tool not only in patients with severe intermittent claudication, but especially in patients who are still paucisymptomatic.

References

1. Lorentsen E (1973) Blood pressure and flow in calf in relation to claudication distance. Scand J Clin Lab Invest 31:141
2. Sasaki H et al. (1980) A planter ischemia test after walking as an index of walking exercise in the patients with buerger's disease. J Jap Coll Angiol 20:873
3. Hauser CJ, Shoemaker WC (1983) Use of transcutaneous pO$_2$ regional perfusion index to quantify tissue perfusion in peripheral vascular disease. Ann Surg 197:337
4. Smith DJ, Madison SA, Bendick PJ (1983) Transcutaneous pO$_2$ monitoring in the vascular laboratory. J Clin Engineering 8:141
5. Modesti PA, Boddi M, Poggesi L, Gensini GF, Neri Serneri GG (1987) Transcutaneous oximetry in evaluation of the initial peripheral artery disease in diabetics. Angiology 38:457
6. Ehrly AM, Dehn R (1986) Verhalten des Gewebesauerstoffdruckes pO$_2$ bei Gesunden und Patienten mit Claudicatio intermittens nach definierter fibergometrischer Belastung. VASA 14:1
7. Holdich TA, Reddy PJ, Walker RT, Dormandy JA (1986) Transcutaneous oxygan tension during exercise in patients with claudication. Br Med J 292:1625
8. Ohgi S, Ito K, Hara H, Mori T (1986) Continuous measurement of transcutaneous oxygen tension in stress test in claudicants and normals. Angiology 37:27
9. Roberts MF, Wenger CB (1979) Control of skin blood flow during exercise: Thermal and non-thermal factors. J Appl Physiol 46:780
10. Bjurstedt H et al (1983) Orthostatic reactions during recovery from exhaustive exercise of short duration. Acta Physiol Scand 119:25

Transcutaneous Oxygen Tension During Treadmill Exercise in Patients with Mild Arterial Occlusive Disease

J. A. Schmidt, C. Bracht, A. Leyhe, P. von Wichert

Summary

We examined transcutaneous oxygen tension ($tcpO_2$) on the foot during treadmill exercise in 27 patients with arterial occlusive disease (AOD) stages I and IIa.
$tcpO_2$ indices differentiated these patients easily from normal controls, since their mean $tcpO_2$ foot index was 34 compared to 94 for the controls. The parameters were stable on repeated measurements. Sensitivity and specificity were 100 % and 88 % respectively.
Unlike Doppler indices, $tcpO_2$ foot indices correlate well with pain-free walking distance (R $= +0,73$; $p<0,001$).

Introduction

In the mild stages of arterial occlusive disease (AOD) too there is the need for objective quantification in order to describe the natural history of the disease and to monitor noninvasive therapeutical measures.
Oscillography is only semiquantitative, and Doppler analysis is very often not sensitive enough in stages I and IIa, at least not for monitoring conservative therapeutical measures.
Pain as the primary leading symptom in AOD is the result of a biochemical cascade beginning with tissue hypoxia. Since reduction in transcutaneous oxygen tension ($tcpO_2$) has so far only been described for the higher stages according to Fontaine but not for the very mild stages, we aimed at measuring this parameter during treadmill exercise. This was done in order to be able to differentiate between normal and impaired states of circulation and to find a parameter correlating with the sensation of pain which might allow one to follow the course of AOD more objectively.

Patients and methods

27 patients were compared with 24 normal controls. In line with the epidemiology of the disease the majority were male, 21 and 20 persons in

Clinical Oxygen Pressure Measurement II
A. M. Ehrly et al. (Eds.)
© Blackwell Ueberreuter Wissenschaft Berlin 1990

the two groups respectively. The median age of the patient group was 56 years, ranging from 39 to 74; the corresponding figures for the control group were 35 years ranging from 22 to 58.

Referal of the subjects to the patients' group was done according to the following criteria for AOD: 1. typical history of claudication with a lower limit of pain-free walking distance of 200 m on even ground; 2. clinical examination yielding reduced pulse on palpitation and typical arterial bruits; 3. Doppler analysis at arm and ankle before and 1 to 5 mins after treadmill exercise; 4. oscillography at rest and after exercise; 5. angiography (in 2 patients). Normal controls had to be negative on all these counts. Subjects with a major orthopaedic or neurologic disease of the lower limbs or severe cardiac or pulmonary insufficiency were excluded from the study.

All the subjects carried out the treadmill exercise at 5 km/h and at an inclination of 10 % for up to 750 m or until they became symptomatic. $tcpO_2$ was measured using an Oxymonitor and a Transoxode (Hellige, Freiburg, FRG) at 44°C. Equilibration before measurment was allowed for 20 mins. Measuring sites were the dorsum of the foot of the more severely symptomatic leg and the frontal thorax. Measurement was repeated at an interval of 2 to 8 days.

Apart from standard conventional data, the following parameters were measured and calculated:

1. $tcpO_2$ value on the foot at rest in mmHg
2. $tcpO_2$ value on the thorax at rest in mmHg
3. minimal $tcpO_2$ value on the foot during or after exercise in mmHg
4. minimal $tcpO_2$ value on the thorax during or after exercise in mmHg
5. $tcpO_2$ foot index (= 3/1 x 100) in %
6. $tcpO_2$ thorax index (= 4/2 x 100) in %
7. $tcpO_2$ foot/thorax index (5/6 x 100) in %.

Additionally, coefficients of correlation were calculated:

1. between $tcpO_2$ foot/thorax index and Doppler index during exercise
2. between Doppler index during exercise and pain-free walking distance
3. between $tcpO_2$ foot index and pain-free walking distance
4. for repeated measurements of $tcpO_2$ foot index and of $tcpO_2$ foot/thorax index.

Statistical calculations were carried out using the Mann-Whitney-U-Test and the Spearman-Rank-Correlation-Test, with a significance at $p < 0.05$.

Results

All the controls could walk 750 m without experiencing any pain or discomfort. As to the patients, their average pain-free walking distance was 376 m, ranging from 116 to 750 m; 11 of them experienced no claudication and were therefore classified as Fontaine stage I.

Comparative data for Doppler and $tcpO_2$ values are given in Table 1. The lack of correlation between $tcpO_2$ indices and age had already been shown in former studies [4, 5].

Comparison between $tcpO_2$ foot/thorax index and Doppler index during exercise shows a coefficient of correlation of $R = +0.6164$ ($p<0.001$). Comparison between a) Doppler index during exercise and b) $tcpO_2$ foot index on the one hand and pain-free walking distance on the other yields coefficients of correlation of $R = +0.3727$ (p:n.s.) for a) and $R = +0.7315$ ($p<0.001$) for b).

Table 1

	controls	patients
Doppler value on the foot at res in mmHg	x̄ 138	112
	R 110–176	70–162
	p=0.0003	
Doppler index at rest in %	x̄ 110	72
	R 99–118	52–102
	p<0.0001	
Doppler index during exercise in %	x̄ 86	48
	R 58–110	22– 79
	p=0.0003	
$tcpO_2$ value on the foot at rest in mmHg (1)	x̄ 66	66
	R 50– 80	41– 80
	p=0.5693	
$tcpO_2$ value on the thorax at rest in mmHg (2)	x̄ 59	54
	R 44– 84	42– 68
	p=0.1844	
minimal $tcpO_2$ value on the foot during or after exercise in mmHg (3)	x̄ 52	11
	R 39– 69	0– 32
	p<0.0001	
minimal $tcpO_2$ value on the thorax during or after exercise in mmHg (4)	x̄ 52	52
	R 33– 76	40– 67
	p=0.7716	
$tcpO_2$ foot index (= 3/1 × 100) in % (5)	x̄ 94	34
	R 73–114	0– 79
	p<0.0001	
$tcpO_2$ thorax index (= 4/2 × 100) in % (6)	x̄ 90	96
	R 75–100	85–100
	p=0.0136	
$tcpO_2$ foot/thorax index (= 5/6 × 100) in % (7)	x̄ 92	18
	R 66–116	0– 53
	p<0.0001	

Correlation between two measurements at different times yields almost identical R values for tcpO$_2$ foot index with R = 0.9270 (p<0.0001) and for tcpO$_2$ foot/thorax index with % = 0.9193 (p<0.0001).
Sensitivity and specificity were calculated for the tcpO$_2$ foot index with values of 100 % and 88 % respectively.

Discussion

The present study confirms that tcpO$_2$ measured at the foot at rest does not distinguish patients with AOD from normal controls.
However, when this diagnostic device is used before, during and after treadmill exercise, patients with AOD stages I and IIa were easily distinguishable from normal controls (see Table 1). Ohgi et al. were not able to achieve this with their foot-stamping exercise test [3], whereas Hauser et al. and Holdich et al. included stage IIb in there studies [1, 2].
For diagnosing mild AOD stages in our study, tcpO$_2$ stress test performed slightly better than conventional Doppler analysis, besides having the advantage of giving information during and directly after exercise.
Sensitivity and specificity of the tcpO$_2$ foot index of 100 % and 88 % respectively make the test clinically useful.
Repeated measurements within a few days' interval disclosed a very high stability of the tcpO$_2$ indices calculated.
Simultaneous measurement on the frontal thorax as a reference site was done to exclude tcpO$_2$ changes due to systemic alterations in oxygen pressure, e.g. in cardiac or pulmonary diseases. In our study, where any such disease at an advanced stage was excluded on clinical grounds, systemic pO$_2$ changes under exercise were not great enough to make the tcpO$_2$ indices with thoracic reference values look any different from those without.
The most promising result of this study, however, was the high correlation between tcpO$_2$ foot index and pain-free walking distance with a significant coefficient of correlation of R = +0.73, whereas there was no significant correlation between conventional Doppler index and pain-free walking distance.
This means that a valid parameter has been found for objective quanitification of the functional severity of AOD. It should be of particular interest in pharmacological studies by doing away with sole reliance on pain-free walking distance as the only available parameter. However, its value remains to be established in further studies.

References

1. Hauser CJ, Shoemaker WC (1982) Use of a transcutaneous pO$_2$ perfusion index to quantify tissue perfusion in peripheral vascular disease. Ann Surg 197:337
2. Holdich TAH et al (1986) Transcutaneous oxygen tension during exercise in patients with claudication. Brit Med J 292:1625

3. Ohgi S et al (1986) Continuous measurement of transcutaneous oxygen tension in stress test in claudicants and normals. Angiology 37:27
4. Schmidt JA, Leyhe A, Wichert P von (1987) Transcutaner Sauerstoffdruck unter Belastung bei Patienten mit arterieller Verschlußkrankheit der Beine im Stadium I und IIa nach Fontaine. Vasa 16, suppl 20:306
5. Schmidt JA, Leyhe A, Wichert P von (in press) Transcutaner Sauerstoffdruck unter Laufbandbelastung bei Patienten mit milder arterieller Verschlußkrankheit der Beine. Innere Medizin

Transcutaneous Oxygen Pressure Measurements in Type I Diabetic Patients

H.-W. M. Breuer, B. E. Strauer, M. Berger

Introduction

As a consequence of vascular changes oxygen supply to peripheral tissues may be impaired in patients with diabetes mellitus. Using transcutaneous oxygen tension measurements as a means to determine oxygen flux through the skin [1], an attempt was made to study cutaneous oxygen supply and from this draw possible conclusions about microcirculation in different regions of the body in a cross-sectional analysis of Type I (insulin dependent) diabetic patients free of large vessel disease.

Subjects and methods

76 Type I diabetic patients were studied. Their diabetes duration ranged from some weeks to 30 years (median 6.0 yrs). Their mean HbA_{1c} was 8.9 % Hb, and their mean daily insulin dosage 47 U. Patients with abnormalities on a 6-lead ECG, with any clinical evidence of macroangiopathy, venous diseases, edema or skin ulcers were excluded from the study. For comparison, 82 age-matched healthy volunteers were studied.

Clinical data of the subjects investigated are presented in Table 1. As an index of sensoric neuropathy, the vibration sense at the right ankle was measured using a vibration fork and an 8-point sensitivity scale – values below 0.75 were considered as pathological (n=3). The investigation of autonomic neuropathy was done by assessment of beat-to-beat variation and by measuring heart response to standing [2] (n=13).

Retinopathy was diagnosed on fundoscopic examination through dilated pupils (n=13). Diabetic nephropathy was diagnosed when at least two of the following four symptoms were present: elevated levels of serum creatinine, decreased creatinine clearance, clinically manifest proteinuria (i.e. 400 mg/d), arterial hypertension (n=7).

Study design

Investigations were performed with the test subjects lying in a supine position. The transcutaneous oxygen measurements were done by the

Clinical Oxygen Pressure Measurement II
A. M. Ehrly et al. (Eds.)
© Blackwell Ueberreuter Wissenschaft Berlin 1990

Table 1. Clinical data of the test persons studied; mean values ±S.D. are given, except when otherwise indicated; + = not measured

	Controls	Diabetics	p-value
Males	44	38	
Females	38	38	
Age (years)	23 ±4	24 ±8	0.184
Body-mass-index (kg/m²)	21.4 ±2.7	22.0 ±2.5	0.106
Smoking habits (packyears, median)	1.5	3.2	
Heart rate (min⁻¹)	75 ±10	78 ±11	0.079
Syst. blood pressure (mmHg)	124 ±12	126 ±15	0.324
Diast. blood pressure (mmHg)	81 ±8	83 ±11	0.166
Blood glucose (mmol/l)	4.75 ±0.07	9.55 ±0.40	0.001
Cholesterol (mmol/l)	4.9 ±1.0	5.2 ±1.5	0.209
HDL-cholesterol (mmol/l)	1.3 ±0.3	1.3 ±0.4	0.595
Triglycerides (mmol/l)	1.2 ±0.5	1.6 ±1.4	0.021
Uric acid (μmol/l)	280 ±65	239 ±62	0.001
Creatinine (μmol/l)	93 ±15	96 ±24	0.380
Creatinine clearance (ml/min, median)	+	93.0	
Proteinuria (g/die, median)	+	0.065	
pO₂ (mmHg, finger tip)	77.5 ±8.4	77.7 ±10.3	0.937

TCM unit of Radiometer (Copenhagen, Denmark) equipped with two TCM2 oxygen monitors and a TCM200 chart recorder. The skin beneath the electrode membrane was heated by the sensor thermistor set at 44°C. One sensor was attached just below the midpoint of the right clavicula (c), and the other just above the right inner malleolus (m).

Basal values of transcutaneous oxygen pressure ($tcpO_2$) were evaluated after establishing steady state conditions. Then the subjects were asked to breathe 5 l O_2/min ($tcpO_25$) and 10 l O_2/min ($tcpO_210$) by means of a facial mask until reaching a stable maximum. The sequence of breathing 5 and 10 l O_2 was randomized.

Besides the maximum transcutaneous oxygen pressure values, the following parameters were obtained graphically from the recordings during inhalation of oxygen: i) rate of rise of transcutaneous oxygen pressure at 50 % amplitude of maximal transcutaneous oxygen pressure achieved ($dp_{50}/dt5$ and $dp_{50}/dt10$); ii) half-time elapsed between the beginning of the increase in oxygen pressure and achievement of its maximum ($T_{50}5$ and $T_{50}10$). Furthermore, the ratio of limb-to-trunk tcp values, i.e. the regional perfusion index (RPI), was calculated [3].

Finally, occlusion of the proximal calf by means of a 12 cm sphygmomanometer cuff was carried out. The cuff pressure used was about 250 mmHg. When $tcpO_2m$ had declined to 5 mmHg, the compression was released, and the half-time up to full tcpO$_2$ amplitude was recorded (T$_{50}$OCCL); dp$_{50}$/dt value after cuff occlusion was also measured (dp$_{50}$/dtOCCL).

Statistics

When data were normally distributed, results are expressed as means ±S.E.M. or ±S.D., respectively, otherwise the median value is given. Where a normal distribution was present, two-sided Student's t-tests were applied. A p-value below 0.05 was considered statistically significant.
The next step included a reduction of the transcutaneous parameters to the main factors by factor analysis [4]. The required condition was that all the factors should account for at least 90 % of data space, and that each factor taken seperately should be mainly represented by a single variable. The extracted variables were used for analysis of variance [5], regression analysis [4] and discriminant analysis [6]. Finally, discriminant analysis was performed to find out whether it was possible to identify a discriminant function for correct classification of patients and controls based upon the transcutaneous parameters. The discriminant function stemmed from a random sample of 80 % of the patients and was verified with the remaining 20 %.

Results

Except for the RPI, T$_{50}$ values and dp$_{50}$/dtOCCL, all the variables obtained by transcutaneous oxygen measurements display significant differences between diabetic and control subjects (Table 2). The transcutaneous oxygen pressure readings were significantly diminished in the diabetic patients. On discriminant analysis, we found that pressure readings which were obtained during oxygen inhalation and which may be regarded as "dynamic parameters", were able to discriminate more reliably between diabetic and control subjects than the baseline values (Fig. 1).
The discriminatory power of the transcutaneous oxygen pressure parameters is characterized by the following function constructed by discriminant analysis:

$$y = 4.8797 - 0.03482 \cdot tcpO_2m - 0.01005 \cdot tcpO_2c10 - 0.74866 \cdot dp_{50}/dtm10$$

where y-values above zero are indicative of diabetic patients and below zero of non-diabetic subjects. This equation allowed to perform the correct classification into diabetic and control subjects in 75 % of cases. The specificity and sensitivity for the classification according to this formula were likewise 75 %.
By factor analysis, the following parameters accounting for approximately 94 % of data space were extracted: tcpO$_2$c, tcpO$_2$m, tcpO$_2$c10,

Table 2. Measured transcutaneous values of the test persons studied; mean values ±S.E.M. are given; p-value = statistical difference of the measured parameter between both groups.
c: subclavian region; *m*: supramolleolar region; *tcpO₂ (mmHg)*: transcutaneous oxygen pressure; *5*: breathing 5 l O₂/Min through facial mask; *10*: 10 l of the same; *dp₅₀/dt (mmHg)*: rate of rise in tcpO₂ at 50 % of the amplitude achieved when breathing 5 resp. 10 l O₂/min through facial mask; *T₅₀ (s)*: half-time between beginning of increase of tcpO₂ and achievement of its maximum; *OCCL*: cuff occlusion of the calf; *bOCCL*: before occlusion; *aOCCL*: after occlusion; *T₅₀OCCL (S)*: half-time up to maximal amplitude after ending of occlusion; *dp₅₀/dtOCCL (mmHg/s)*: rate of rise in tcpO₂ at 50 % of the amplitude achieved after cuff occlusion of the calf; *RPI*: regional perfusion index = limb-to-trunk ratio of tcpO₂ values

	Controls	Diabetics	p-value
$tcpO_2c$	66.3 ±1.8	59.8 ±1.6	0.010
$tcpO_2m$	66.6 ±1.2	55.8 ±1.6	0.001
$tcpO_2c5$	166.8 ±4.8	125.1 ±4.4	0.001
$tcpO_2m5$	142.0 ±4.3	98.0 ±3.1	0.001
$tcpO_2c10$	249.9 ±6.4	186.8 ±7.1	0.001
$tcpO_2m10$	204.5 ±6.8	135.5 ±6.1	0.001
$dp_{50}/dtc5$	0.81 ±0.04	0.58 ±0.04	0.001
$dp_{50}/dtm5$	0.56 ±0.04	0.36 ±0.02	0.001
$dp_{50}/dtc10$	1.35 ±0.07	0.95 ±0.07	0.001
$dp_{50}/dtm10$	0.90 ±0.07	0.52 ±0.04	0.001
$T_{50}c5$	75.3 ±3.0	75.6 ±4.3	0.950
$T_{50}m5$	106.9 ±3.6	96.7 ±3.7	0.053
$T_{50}c10$	83.9 ±3.1	83.8 ±4.0	0.700
$T_{50}m10$	122.5 ±4.2	111.3 ±4.4	0.067
TcbOCCL	70.4 ±1.2	58.5 ±1.5	0.001
TcaOCCL	70.1 ±1.3	58.1 ±1.4	0.001
$T_{50}OCCL$	41.4 ±3.8	40.9 ±2.3	0.904
$dp_{50}/dtOCCL$	1.29 ±0.08	1.11 ±0.07	0.072
RPI	1.09 ±0.04	1.00 ±0.04	0.143
RPI5	0.88 ±0.034	0.84 ±0.03	0.255
RPI10	0.83 ±0.02	0.76 ±0.03	0.069

$dp_{50}/dtm5$, $dp_{50}/dtc10$, $T_{50}c5$, $T_{50}m10$, $dp_{50}/dtOCCL$, RPI5. These factors were used for analysis of different subgroups of diabetic patients defined by metabolic and clinical characteristics. The transcutaneous oxygen pressure readings $tcpO_2c$, $tcpO_2c10$ and $dp_{50}/dtm5$ are significantly associated with sex, as almost invariably higher values were recorded in female subjects. Overall, there were no significant differences between subgroups of patients defined according to their body mass index, blood pressure, smoking habits, actual glycemia, glycosylated hemoglobin, total serum cholesterol, and triglyderide levels when evaluated by analyses of variance. Even patients with diabetes a duration of less than one year and free of any detectable microangiopathic complication did not differ significantly from those patients suffering from diabetes for many years.

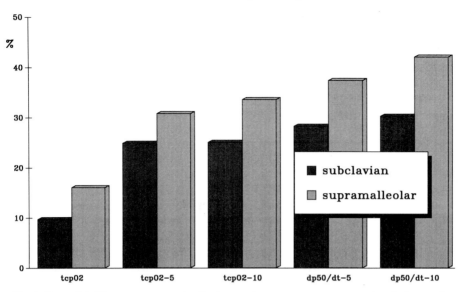

Fig. 1. Percental differences concerning the transcutaneous pressure parameters between diabetic patients and control subjects (for abbreviations, see Table 2)

However, on performing stepwise discriminant analysis to estimate Mahalanobis distances, significant differences could be demonstrated between patients with and without diabetic complications.

Discussion

This study demonstrates diminished transcutaneous oxygen pressures associated with Type 1 diabetes mellitus. It is noteworthy that diminished transcutaneous oxygen pressure readings were observed even in those patients who were free of any signs of microvascular, macrovascular or neurological complications at the time of examination, and further that no independent relationship between this phenomenon and the duration of the patient's diabetes became apparent. In addition to the transcutaneous oxygen pressures at baseline conditions ("static parameters"), we have developed and standardized dynamic parameters of transcutaneous oxygen pressure changes following oxygen breathing and during the recovery from peripheral arterial occlusion ("functional parameters") [7]. In general, these functional parameters appeared to be more sensitive in discriminating between diabetic and non-diabetic individuals (Fig. 1).

Despite the substantial diminution in maximal transcutaneous oxygen pressure values during inhalation of oxygen, the time required for the transcutaneous pressure to reach half of its maximum value (T_{50} values) did not differ between diabetic patients and controls. This indicates a faster delivery of oxygen in controls compared to the diabetic patients. Transcutaneous oxygen pressure readings vary depending on the site of the body where the measurement is taken. This phenomenon is compatible with the observations of differences in capillary diameters in diabetic patients by Karlander et al. [8], who described heterogeneous capillary patterns at different toes even of the same foot. Nearly all of the transcutaneous oxygen pressure parameters obtained in this study were smaller when recorded in the malleolar region than in the subclavian region, resulting in a limb-to-trunk ratio (RPI-values) of less than 1 in most instances (Table 2). Although the absolute values of transcutaneous oxygen pressure at any time of the measurement phase were lower in the diabetic patients, the comparable RPI-values exclude any particular deterioration of oxygen delivery in the limb of diabetic patients.

All the measurements were carried out at an electrode temperature of 44°C. At this ambient temperature, periodic microcirculatory changes are suppressed due to maximal hyperemia [9, 10, 11], as confirmed by the lack of any reactive shoot-over hyperemia following the cuff occlusion of the distal calf. Thus, due to this particular detail of the experimental protocol, neurocirculatory phenomena affecting the periodic changes of peripheral blood flow [10] or significant arteriovenous shunts accounting for increased blood flow in patients with diabetic neuropathy at lower ambient temperatures [12] can be widely excluded as causative factors for the observed differences.

The results may indicate the occurrence of an early functional abnormality in peripheral oxygen delivery due to microcirculatory disturbances. Functional parameters of microcirculation, such as maximum cutaneous blood flow [13] or transcutaneous oxygen pressure changes during oxygen inhalation (Table 2) are superior for discovering early disturbances in the regulation of cutaneous circulation in diabetic patients. LoGerfo and Coffman [14] have pointed out that there is no evidence of an occlusive microvascular disease in diabetic patients, but that there may be functional abnormalities at the level of the capillaries. It may be that such abnormalities in oxygen diffusion at the level of the capillaries are responsible for the alterations of transcutaneous oxygen delivery observed in the diabetic patients of this study.

Although there was no strong correlation between transcutaneous oxygen delivery and acute or chronic degree of disfunction in glycemic control and although there was no independent correspondence with duration of diabetes, an influence of metabolic control and thus the reversibility of the observed changes cannot be excluded. In fact, the subgroup of 13 patients with a diabetes duration of less than one year and already displaying – on the whole – characteristic disturbances in transcutaneous oxygen delivery were, at the time of the investigation, in particularly bad metabolic control (HbA$_{1c}$ 9.42 ±0.85 %, glycemia 8.97 ±1.23 mmol/l).

Although clearly reduced, transcutaneous oxygen delivery in the diabetic patients was still sufficient for appropriate oxygenation of cutaneous layers so as not to lead to manifest skin diseases. Whether a further deterioration of oxygen delivery might, at least in part, become responsible for the induction of skin lesions or for impaired wound healing remains to be determined [12]. Likewise, it is not known whether determination of transcutaneous oxygen pressure will prove helpful in the early detection of patients prone to develop microangiopathy, i.e. whether the changes observed in this study might signify early functional abnormalities, or whether the reduction in transcutaneous oxygen pressures are merely due to microcirculatory alterations precipitated by metabolic alterations. At present, the findings only demonstrate a deterioration of oxygen supply to the skin during heat induced hyperemia in Type 1 diabetes mellitus independent of manifest diabetic vascular complications.

Acknowledgement. We are indebted to M. Daniel and U. Schlaghecken for their technical assistance.

References

1. Huch A, Huch R (1979) The development of the transcutaneous pO$_2$ technique into a clinical tool. Birth Defects 15:5
2. Ewing DJ, Clarke BF (1982) Diagnosis and management of diabetic autonomic neuropathy. Br Med J 285:916
3. Hauser CJ, Shoemaker WC (1983) Use of a transcutaneous pO$_2$ regional perfusion index to quantify tissue perfusion in peripheral vascular disease. Ann Surg 197:337
4. Berenson ML, Levine D, Goldstein M (1983) Intermediate statistical methods and applications – a computer package approach. Prentice-Hall, Englewood Cliffs
5. Iversen GR, Norpoth H (1976) Analysis of variance. Sage Publications, Beverly Hills
6. Deichsel G, Trampisch HJ (1985) Clusteranalyse und Diskriminanzanalyse. Fischer, Stuttgart
7. Breuer H-WM, Breuer J, Berger M (1988) Transcutaneous oxygen pressure measurements in type I diabetic patients for early detection of functional diabetic microangiopathy. Europ J Clin Invest 18:454
8. Karlander SG, Hermansson IL, Hellström K (1985) Nutritive toe skin capillaries in middle-aged patients with diabetes mellitus. Diabete Metab 2:165
9. Huch R, Huch A, Lübbers DW (1981) Transcutaneous pO$_2$. Thieme-Stratton Inc, New York
10. Gaylarde PM, Sarkany I (1985) Periodic skin blood flow. N Eng J Med 312:1194
11. Ewald U, Tuvemo T, Rooth G (1981) Early reduction of vascular reactivity in diabetic children detected by transcutaneous electrode. Lancet i:1287
12. Gaylarde PM, Fonseca VA, Llewellyn G, Sarkany I, Thomas PK, Dandona P (1988) Transcutaneous oxygen tension in legs and feet of diabetic patients. Diabetes 37:714
13. Fagrell B, Östergren I (1985) Clinical use of capillary flow velocity measurements. Microcirculation, a new dimension in clinical angiology. Int Congress of Angiology, Athens, p 23
14. LoGerfo FW, Coffman JD (1984) Vascular and microvascular disease of the foot in diabetes. N Eng J Med 311:1615

Significance of Transcutaneous Oxygen Pressure in Diabetic Microangiopathy

T. Maeda, J. Ogawa, K. Kuchiba, M. Akiyama, S. Ikemoto, T. Yokose, Y. Isogai

Introduction

Diabetic microangiopathy is a vascular disease characteristic of diabetes mellitus. Due to the substantial decline in mortality from diabetic coma, complications connected with microangiopathy are now the major problem in diabetes therapy.

Despite the various approaches available to describe the etiology and mechanism of the progression, much still remains unknown. However, metabolic disorders due to lack of insulin, particularly in persistent hyperglycemia, are considered to be a major cause. Here symptoms include thickening of the basal membrane of capillaries, proliferation of mesangial and endotherial cells and degeneration of pericytes. Extensive morphological and biochemical research has been done to discover the source of these lesions. Attracting much attention as the primary location of these symptoms in diabetics is the microcirculatory area. Special importance has been attached to hemorrheological parameters and circulatory disorders investigated in connection with impaired oxygen supply to the affected area [1].

In the present study, oxygen pressure of the skin surface was measured without heating the skin, i.e. at $37°C$, by polarography. It was assumed that the oxygen pressure of the skin surface could be taken to equal oxygen pressure in the tissues (tissue pO_2) [2]. The effects of HbA_1 and 2,3-DPG on oxyhemoglobin dissociation, red cell filterability and whole blood viscosity – responsible for microcirculatory disturbances in diabetics – were studied.

Subjects and methods

31 diabetics, 19 male and 12 female of average age 43.4 ±9.1 years, were studied. 15 had no retinopathy, 11 had nonproliferative retinopathy and 2 had proliferative retinopathy. All the subjects were NIDDM and had relatively stable control over blood glucose. The control group consisted of 7 subjects, 5 male and 2 female of average age 39.5 ±6.2 years. Transcutaneous oxygen pressure at $43.5°C$ and $37°C$ as well as local perfusion were measured using an adapted PO-200 transcutaneous pO_2

Clinical Oxygen Pressure Measurement II
A.M. Ehrly et al. (Eds.)
© Blackwell Ueberreuter Wissenschaft Berlin 1990

sensor (Sumitomo Electric Industries Co). This apparatus utilized an oxygen sensor of 16 mm in diameter, 8 mm thickness and weighing less than 10 g. The oxygen sensor, consisting of a heater, a thermister for temperature control and an electrode, detected oxygen pressure using the polarographic principle.

In order to assess arterial oxygen pressure, the skin was heated by the electrode to 43.5°C so as to dilate the capillaries, thus causing arterial blood to flow into them and to diffuse from there to the surface of the skin. The resultant transcutaneous oxygen pressure (tcpO₂) was measured. Then the sensor was reset to 37°C so as to measure tcpO₂ at normal skin temperature.

Using the sensor we were also able to measure local blood perfusion, which was indicated by the consumption of electric power needed by the sensor in order to maintain the skin at a temperature of 43.5°C: where power consumption is lower, local perfusion is greater. Measurements were taken in the right subclavicular region of the anterior wall of the chest.

Whole blood viscosity was measured at 37°C, at 115 sec^{-1}, using a Wells-Brookfield cone plate viscometer. Whole blood viscosity index was obtained by dividing the subject's whole blood viscosity value by the whole blood viscosity value of a normal subject displaying the same hematocrit value. Plasma viscosity was measured at 37°C using a capillary viscometer.

Red cell filterability was measured using a negative pressure filtration system, consisting of a Nuclepore membrane of 5 μm diameter [3]. Using 10 cm H_2O of negative pressure, red cells were suspended in phosphate buffered saline (PBS) of pH 7.4 and 295 mOsm so as to obtain a red cell concentration of 9000 RBC/mm³. The number of red cells passing through the membrane in one second determined the red cell filterability (RCF). HPLC was used to measure HbA_1, and a Boerhinger-Yamanouchi kit was used to measure 2,3-DPG.

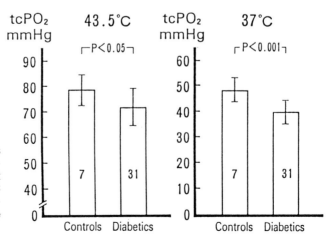

Fig. 1. Transcutaneous pO₂ in controls and diabetics. Both the tcpO₂ at 43.5°C and tcpO₂ at 37°C on the skin surface of diabetics were found to be reduced

Results

1. Both tcpO₂ at 43.5°C and tcpO₂ at 37°C on the skin surface of diabetics were found to be reduced (Fig. 1).
2. There was significant positive correlation between tcpO₂ at 43.5°C and tcpO₂ at 37°C (r=0.603) (Fig. 2).
3. There was significant negative correlation between tcpO₂ at 43.5°C and whole blood viscosity. There was a tendency towards negative correlation between tcpO₂ at 37°C and whole blood viscosity (Fig. 3).

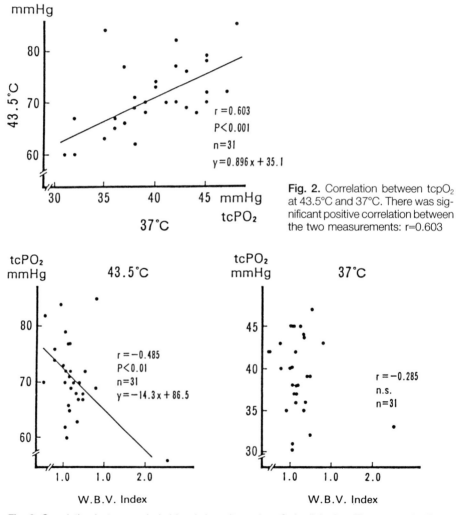

Fig. 2. Correlation between tcpO₂ at 43.5°C and 37°C. There was significant positive correlation between the two measurements: r=0.603

Fig. 3. Correlation between whole blood viscosity and tcpO₂ in diabetics. There was significant negative correlation between tcpO₂ at 43.5°C and whole blood viscosity. There was a tendency towards negative correlation between tcpO₂ at 37°C and whole blood viscosity

4. There was a significant negative correlation between HbA_1 and $tcpO_2$ at 37°C.
5. $tcpO_2$ at 43.5°C and $tcpO_2$ at 37°C of the diabetic subjects showed a reduction already at a stage where no retinopathy was present. Especially $tcpO_2$ at 37°C of the proliferative retinopathy group tended to be lowest.
6. Local perfusion in diabetics tended to increase, particularly in the proliferative retinopathy group. Reduction of $tcpO_2$ at 37°C was in apparent contradiction to the observed increase in local perfusion.
7. There was no uniform correlation between red cell filterability, whole blood viscosity or 2,3-DPG on the one hand and $tcpO_2$ at 43.5°C or $tcpO_2$ at 37°C on the other.

Conclusions and discussion

As retinopathy progresses, the number of shunts increases, thereby increasing circulation, but decreasing $tcpO_2$ at 37°C. It is believed that microcirculation in diabetic retinopathy groups is actually more active than in normal subjects. This is due to the fact that diabetic neuropathy, in conjunction with microangiopathy, causes many shunts to be formed, thus connecting arterioles to venules. As retinopathy progresses, the increase in the number of shunts leads to increase in circulation on the one hand but a decrease in tissue pO_2 on the other [4]. This study shows that, using the methods described above, $tcpO_2$ at 37°C gives an indication of tissue pO_2.

References

1. Isogai Y, Iida A, Mochizuki K, Abe M (1974) Hemorrheological studies on the pathogenesis of diabetic microangiopathy. Thromb Res (Suppl) 8:17
2. Ewald U, Rooth G, Tuvemo T (1987) Transcutaneous pO_2 measurement at 37°C in children with diabetes. In: Ehrly AM (ed) Clinical oxygen pressure measurement. Springer, p 184
3. Kikuchi Y, Arai T, Koyama T (1983) Improved filtration method for red cell deformability measurement. Med & Biol Eng & Comput 21:270
4. Maeda T, Kuchiba K, Akiyama M, Ikemoto S, Yokose T, Isogai Y (1988) Transcutaneous oxygen tension and tissue oxygen tension in diabetic microangiopathy. In: Tsuchiya M (ed) Microcirculation an update. Proceedings of Fourth World Congress for Microcirculation. Tokyo, Japan 1978. Elsevier Science, vol 2, p 607

Evaluation of Skin Microcirculation Reactivity in Pregnancy by cpO_2, $tcpO_2$ and Laser-Doppler Flux (LDF)

E. Beinder, A. Bollinger, R. Huch, A. Huch

Introduction

The measurement of cutaneous oxygen pressure at 37°C, of Laser-Doppler Flux and of thermoclearance based on the relative heating power of a $tcpO_2$ probe at 45°C are all methods for evaluating changes in skin microcirculation. However, absolute blood flow values cannot be measured, as is possible with venous occlusion plethysmography. The advantages of the above-mentioned methods lie in their ability to detect changes in blood flow using provocative procedures and in their non-invasiveness, thus permitting their unproblematic use during human pregnancy.
It was the aim of our study to examine functional changes in the microcirculation of the maternal skin in humans during pregnancy.

Patients

There were 3 groups of patients:
- Group I: 12 pregnant women (gestational age 15-17 weeks)
- Group II: 12 pregnant women (gestational age over 32 weeks)
- Control Group (CG) of 12 non-pregnant women.

The age distribution in all 3 groups was quite similar: Group I: 28.3 (22-35), Group II: 30.1 (24-37), Control Group: 27.7 (20-41) years. All patients were non-smokers with no indications of hematologic or vascular disorders or diabetes. The pregnancies were free of complications.

Methods

The following measuring principles were used:
- cutaneous pO_2 with an electrode temperature of 37°C: cpO_2
- transcutaneous pO_2 with an electrode temperature of 45°C: $tcpO_2$
- relative heating power of the $tcpO_2$ probe: RHP
- Laser-Doppler flux: LDF

Clinical Oxygen Pressure Measurement II
A.M. Ehrly et al. (Eds.)
© Blackwell Ueberreuter Wissenschaft Berlin 1990

The probes were attached on the volar distal forearm. After a constant signal was received, venous occlusion was induced using a blood pressure cuff on the upper arm of 50 mmHg for 2 mins. After pressure release and receipt of a constant signal, an arterial occlusion was brought about using a cuff pressure of 250 mmHg for 3 mins. The measurements were registered simultaneously on a multichannel recorder.

The following parameters were measured:

– Δ RHP: Decrease of blood flow during venous occlusion compared to the decrease during arterial occlusion as measured by RHP
– $tcpO_2$ 45°C (mmHg)
– $t\frac{1}{2}\,tcpO_2$ (sec): Time necessary to reach half the original level of $tcpO_2$ after release of the arterial occlusion
– t RH (sec): Time to peak flux after release of arterial occlusion as measured by LDF
– RH cpO_2 (mmHg): Maximal cutaneous pO_2 during reactive hyperemia
– RH LDF (AU): Peak flux during reactive hyperemia measured by LDF

For statistical analysis we used the Whitney-Mann U Test. The results are documented with box plots (median, 10th, 25th, 75th and 90th percentile) [1].

Results

1. Δ RHP: The decrease of blood flow during venous occlusion compared with the decrease during arterial occlusion is in both groups of

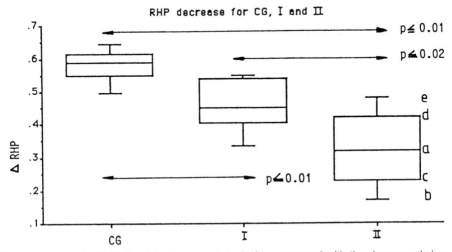

Fig. 1. Decrease in RHP signal during venous occlusion compared with the decrease during arterial occlusion (Δ RHP) in the control group (CG) and the two patient groups (I, II); the box plots show the median (a), the 10th (b), 25th (c), 75th (d) and 90th (e) percentile

pregnant women significantly lower than in the Control Group (p≤0.01) (Fig. 1).

2. tcpO$_2$ 45°C and t$\frac{1}{2}$ tcpO$_2$: No significant difference in tcpO$_2$ among all three groups was found (Fig. 2a).
t$\frac{1}{2}$ tcpO$_2$ is significantly shorter in Group II compared with Group I and the Control Group (p≤0.02) (Fig. 2b).

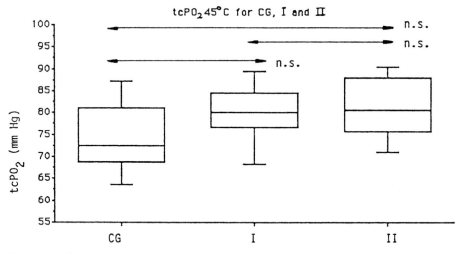

Fig. 2a. tcpO$_2$ in all three groups (7.5 mmHg = 1 kPa)

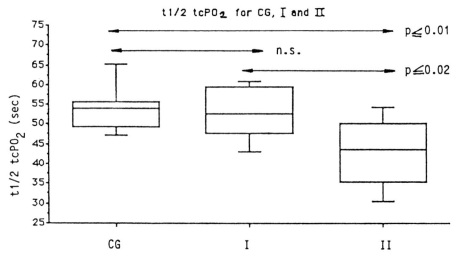

Fig. 2b. Time to reach half of the original level of tcpO$_2$ signal after release of the arterial occlusion (t1/2 tcpO$_2$)

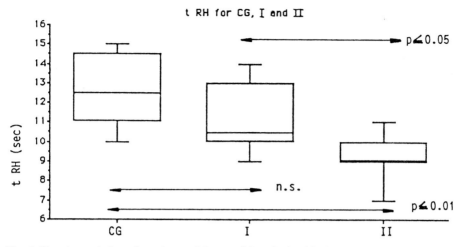

Fig. 3. Time to peak flux after release of the arterial occlusion (tRH); measurement with LDF

3. Time to peak flux (t RH) after release of the arterial occlusion measured by LDF is significantly shorter in Group II than in the other two groups ($p \leq 0.05$) (Fig. 3).
4. RH LDF and RH cpO_2: The peak flux value in late pregnancy (Group II) is significantly higher than in the non-pregnant state ($p \leq 0.01$) (Fig. 4a).

    cpO_2 during reactive hyperemia shows a different pattern: The values in late pregnancy are significantly lower than in the Control Group ($p \leq 0.01$) (Fig. 4b).

Discussion

Investigations have shown that the techniques under discussion measure skin blood flow over areas of various extent and at different depths of the dermis [2, 3]. The measurement of cutaneous pO_2 primarily detects the microcirculation in the subepidermal papillary capillaries, whose main task is the nutrition of the upper dermis and the epidermis [4].
Laser-Doppler Flux can detect blood flow changes in an area of ca. 1.5 mm² and up to a depth of 0.6 mm [5]. Other authors are of the opinion, however, that measurement signals can be obtained up to a depth of 1.2 or even 3 mm [6]. This would mean that LDF measures not only the nutritive capillary bed but also the plexus shunt blood flow as well as the arterio-venous shunt blood flow [3].
The fact that LDF and cutaneous pO_2 measurements are done at different depths of the skin may explain the different findings obtained by the two

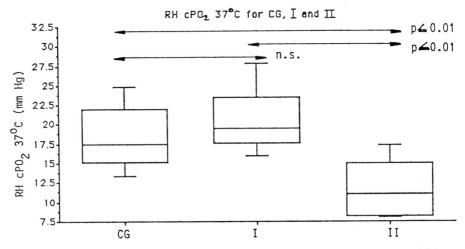

Fig. 4a. Maximal reactive hyperemia, measured by cPO$_2$ (RH cPO$_2$) (7.5 mmHg = 1 kPa)

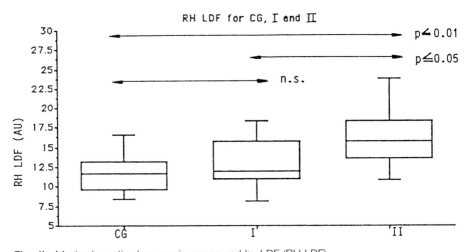

Fig. 4b. Maximal reactive hyperemia, measured by LDF (RH LDF)

methods. In pregnancy, peak flux during reactive hyperemia as measured by LDF increases, whereas maximal cutaneous pO$_2$ decreases. The cause of this could be the dilation of arteriolar resistance vessels and arteriovenous anastomoses, resulting in a shift of the skin blood flow from the nutritive-capillary level to the plexus and arteriovenous shunt blood flow level. From a physiological point of view this redistribution makes sense since the primary purpose of arteriovenous shunt flow is thermoregulation and elimination of the increased heat production during pregnancy.

In Group II, that is women in late pregnancy, a statistically significant shorter time span from occlusion release to maximal reactive hyperemia (t RH) compared to the Control Group of non-pregnant women was observed. Other authors, using video capillary microscopy instead of LDF, have shown that the time to peak flow velocity was longer in patients with increased blood viscosity due to polycythemia or sickle-cell disease and also in patients with diabetes and proximal arterial stenosis [7, 8, 9].

Not only blood viscosity may influence t RH, but also the myogenic reaction of the vessels to the sudden increase of the intraluminal pressure after release of the arterial occlusion. During pregnancy the viscosity of the maternal blood is diminished, since the relative increase in blood plasma volume is greater than that of the blood cell volume [10].

These rheologic changes as well as the diminished myogenic contractility and increased elasticity of smaller arterioles proved in animal experiments [11] may be the explanation for the reduction in time peak flow in pregnancy.

A diminished contractility of arteriolar resistance vessels is also indicated by the less pronounced decrease in perfusion during venous occlusion. The diminished blood flow during venous blockage is probably caused by a local arteriolar mechanism which prevents an increase in pressure and thus hyperfiltration in the capillary area [12].

Yet clinical experience indicates that precisely during pregnancy the skin is especially prone to edema, and the capillary filtration rate is increased [13]. Direct measurements of pressure have shown an elevated intracapillary pressure in late pregnancy [14].

Although the $tcpO_2$ values did not vary significantly among the three groups, the reincrease rate of $tcpO_2$ after release of the arterial occlusion is higher in Group II, that is in late pregnancy, than in the non-pregnant state. This higher reincrease rate could be due to the elevated skin blood flow in pregnancy.

Our results seem to indicate that in pregnancy a redistribution of skin blood flow occurs, from the superficial capillary bed to the plexus and arteriovenous shunt blood flow deeper within the dermis. The cause might be a decrease in myogenic contractility or an increase in elasticity of the arteriolar resistance vessels. Certain clinical findings, such as a disposition to skin edema or a decrease in the frequency of functional vasospastic syndromes in pregnancy might thus be explained.

References

1. McGill R, Tukey JW, Larsen WA (1978) Variations of blox plots. American Statistician 32:12
2. Saumet JL, Dittmar A, Leftheriotis G (1986) Non-invasive measurements of skin blood flow: Comparison between plethysmography, Laser-Doppler flowmeter and heat thermal clearance method. Int J Microcirc Clin Exp 5:73

3. Tooke JE, Ostergren J, Fagrell B (1983) Synchronous assessment of human skin microcirculation by Laser Doppler flowmetry and dynamic capillaroscopy. Int J Microcirc Clin Exp 2:277

4. Rooth G, Ewald U, Caligara F (1987) Transcutaneous pO_2 and pCO_2 monitoring at 37°C. Cutaneous pO_2 and pCO_2. In: Huch R, Huch A, Rooth G (eds) Continuous transcutaneous monitoring. Plenum, New York, p 23

5. Nilsson GE, Tenland T, Öberg PA (1980) Evaluation of a Laser Doppler flowmeter for measurement of time blood flow. IEEE Trans Biomed Eng 27:597

6. Kvietys PR, Shepherd AP, Granger DN (1985) Laser Doppler, H_2 clearance and microsphere estimates of mucosal blood flow. Am J Physiol 249:221

7. Tooke JE, Lins PE, Ostergren J, Fagrell B (1985) Skin microvascular autoregulatory response in Type I diabetes: The influence of duration and control. Int J Microcirc Clin Exp 4:249

8. Fagrell B, Ostergren J (1981) Influence of isovolaemic hemodilution on skin microcirculation in patients with polycythemia. 2nd Eur Conf Clin Haemorh, Abstract 156, London

9. Lipowsky HH, Firrell JC, Usami S, Chien S (1957) Intravital microscopy of human nailfold capillaries in sickle cell disease. Microvasc Res 25:245

10. Heilmann L (1986) Die Veränderungen der Fließeigenschaften des Blutes während der Schwangerschaft. Zentralbl Gynakol 108:393

11. McLaughlin MK, Keve TM (1986) Pregnancy-induced changes in resistance blood vessels. Am J Obstet Gynecol 12:1296

12. Levick JR, Michel CC (1978) The effects of position and skin temperature on the capillary pressure in the fingers and toes. J Physiol (Lond) 274:97

13. Goodlin RC (1986) Venous reactivity and pregnancy abnormalities. Acta Obstet Gynecol Scand 65:345

14. Tooke JE, Williams SA (1987) Capillary blood pressure. In: Huch R, Huch A, Rooth G (eds) Continuous transcutaneous monitoring. Plenum, New York, p 209

The Contribution of Inflammation to Hyperemia, Hypoxia and Hypercapnia in Human Skin

F. M. T. Carnochan, N. C. Abbot, J. Swanson Beck, V. A. Spence, W. F. Walker

Abstract

This study examined the sequence of changes in transcutaneously measured respiratory gases (O_2 and CO_2) that result from the experimental introduction of inflammation to a normal skin site. The inflammation was induced by a tuberculin skin test, which has proved to be a useful model for investigating the metabolic consequences of chronic inflammation. Hyperemia was quantified daily, for 4 days, by Laser Doppler flowmetry, and the effects of hyperoxia and inflammatory hypercapnia were investigated using a combined transcutaneous pO_2/pCO_2 electrode.

Hyperemia was present over all skin test sites, being most significant in the stronger reactions, but there was a paradoxical 'central relative slowing' (CRS) of blood flow velocity over the centre of the most intense reactions with respect to flow at their periphery. Over the centre of the reaction, $tcpO_2$ fell progressively; the extent of hypoxia was inversely related to the degree of hyperemia, with the lowest oxygen levels being observed in those reactions exhibiting CRS. $tcpO_2$ was raised only in those reactions with CRS.

These results highlight the metabolic impact of the migration of inflammatory cells into skin with a normal arterial oxygen supply, and they provide a qualitative index of the severity of the respiratory debt which might result from the infection of an ischemic limb.

Introduction

Oxygen is an essential ingredient in the healing process [1, 2, 3]. The healing capacity of an ischemic ulcer will therefore be compromised by a regional perfusion deficiency. Edema will further impair normal aerobic respiration by increasing gas diffusion distances, but the greatest effect on respiratory imbalance may result from infection.

Infiltrating inflammatory cells have a high demand for oxygen, and the objective here was to determine the extent of local hypoxia and hypercapnia in the developing delayed-hypersensitivity reaction (DHS).

Clinical Oxygen Pressure Measurement II
A. M. Ehrly et al. (Eds.)
© Blackwell Ueberreuter Wissenschaft Berlin 1990

The tuberculin skin test is a widely used model of this type of reaction which can be evoked without too much inconvenience in human volunteers [4]. There have been quantitative histological studies describing the time course of cellular immigration into the various sub-compartments of the dermis during the course of the reaction [5]. Also, the pattern of change in dermal blood flow is well documented [6]. The pH in the dermis falls during the development of the reaction in healthy subjects, and concurrently transcutaneous measurements of pO_2 and pCO_2 have shown local hypoxia and hypercapnia [7, 8]. With this background information we have studied the relation between the changes in blood flow velocity and those in local dermal repiratory gas tensions.

Subjects and methods

20 subjects (9 males, 11 females) aged between 22 and 27 years gave their informed consent to the test procedure, which was approved by the local ethical committee. All subjects were healthy, normotensive and free from medication. Subjects were seated comfortably in an ambient temp. of 22 $\pm 1°C$, with the left arm resting at heart level.

Measurements on undisturbed skin

Control measurements were initially performed on undisturbed skin from the mid-volar forearm on 3 seperate occasions after calibration of the sensor at 44°C. The transcutaneous sensor was applied to the skin and left in place for 25 mins to obtain stable $tcpO_2/pCO_2$ values. Following stabilization, subjects were given 100 % O_2 to breathe via a mouthpiece (nose-clipped) until a $tcpO_2$ level of 200 mmHg was reached. Forearm blood flow was then arrested for 4 minutes by applying an upper arm cuff, and the subsequent changes in respiratory gases were recorded.
The following parameters were obtained:
$tcpO_2$ (ss) – the steady-state $tcpO_2$ measurement
$tcpCO_2$ (ss) – the steady-state $tcpCO_2$ measurement
$d/dt\ pO_2$ – the rate of fall of $tcpO_2$ on cuff occlusion

The mean and SD of 3 replicate values obtained on the undisturbed skin of each subject was used as a control ('pre'-values for the subsequent experiments). $tcpO_2$ (ss) measurements were temperature-corrected to 37°C using the Siggaard-Andersen formula.

Measurements on inflammatory reactions

10 IU of tuberculin (PPD, Evans Medical) was injected intradermally into the left volar forearm of each of the subjects, the bolus of fluid being

deposited approx. 1 cm from the site of needle entry, and respiratory gas measurements repeated over the centre of the reaction at 24, 28, 72 and 96 hours following injection.

On each day prior to transcutaneous measurements, erythema and induration were measured along the long axis of the forearm. The longitudinal skin blood flow profile of the reaction was also obtained with a Laser Doppler (PF2b, Perimed, Sweden) using a specially designed probe holder consisting of 12 probe orifices each 1 cm apart [6].

Results

Blood flow measurements

In most subjects, the Laser Doppler signal was maximal over the site of deposition of the tuberculin bolus i.e. at the centre of the reaction (Fig. 1a). However, in the clinically very strong reactions, the laser flux was maximal at the periphery, and there was central relative slowing (CRS) (Fig. 1b). The 20 subjects were divided into 3 groups depending on the severity of the reaction as determined by the Laser Doppler flux and the degree of saturation:

"negative" reaction (4 subjects) – induration < 5 mm
strong reaction (12 subjects) – induration > 5 mm
strong reaction with CRS (4 subjects) – induration > 5 mm

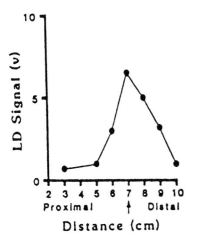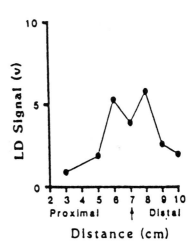

Fig. 1. Laser-Doppler measurement of blood flow velocity at 1 cm intervals along the long axis of the forearm. The holder has been positioned so that orifice 7 overlies the antigen injection site. **a)** Usual pattern in strong tuberculin response with velocity maximal at the center of the reaction. **b)** Reaction where blood flow velocity is greatest at the periphery and submaximal at the center – this response is seen in the most intense reactions and is named "central relative slowing" (CRS)

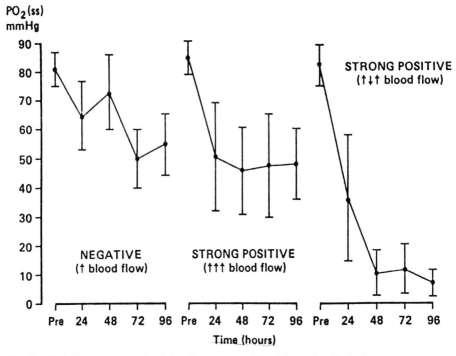

Fig. 2. pO₂ (ss) measurements during the course of the tuberculin skin test response

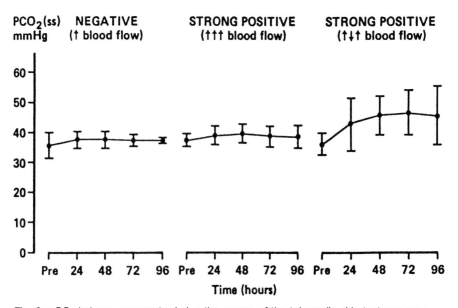

Fig. 3. pCO₂ (ss) measurements during the course of the tuberculin skin test response

Respiratory gas measurements

In most subjects, stable pO_2 (ss) values were obtained after 20-25 mins, and after breathing 100 % O_2 a $tcpO_2$ level of 200 mmHg was reached in 2-3 mins. On occlusion, the O_2 level fell to 7-8 mmHg within the first 2 or 3 mins.

Fig. 2 and Fig. 3 summarize the mean $tcpO_2$ and $tcpCO_2$ steady-state measurements for each of the 3 groups during the course of the reaction.

In the subjects with "negative" reactions, the pO_2 (ss) fell progressively over the first 3 days to about 2/3 of the resting level; in those with strong reactions, where blood flow was maximal at the centre, a similar pattern was seen, but there was an earlier fall prominent by 24 hours; subjects with a strong reaction and CRS had a much greater fall in $tcpO_2$ (ss) to about 10 % of the pre-skin testing values.

The tissue metabolism was estimated by $d/dt\ pO_2$. There was a small but statistically significant increase in O_2 consumption in the "negative" reactions over the period of the study; in the strong reactions, O_2 consumption was much greater and continued to rise up to 96 hours; in the subjects with CRS, $d/dt\ pO_2$ could not be measured at 48 and 72 hours because $tcpO_2$ (ss) could not be increased despite breathing 100 % O_2.

pCO_2 (ss) values did not differ significantly from the control values in the "negative" subjects over the 96 hour period. In both the strong positives and the strong positives with CRS, there was a small but significant rise in $tcpO_2$ at 24 hours, which continued up to the 72 or 96 hour point.

Discussion

This study has reemphasized that severe hypoxia and hypercapnia can arise in normally perfused tissue when it is the site of an intense inflammatory reaction provoked experimentally by an immunologically delayed hypersensitivity reaction. There is no reason to suspect that other types of inflammation give rise to any different response. The respiratory changes were most marked in those subjects showing CRS, a vascular response which appears to be an indication of incipient gangrene [Beck and Kardjito, unpublished observations]. The present study confirms that the main factor causing the respiratory imbalance has been the large scale migration of inflammatory cells. The diffusion barrier created by the inflammatory edema plays a relatively minor role [Abbot, unpublished data]. In the most severe reactions with CRS there are other factors. As well as an increased metabolic load, the flow at the center of the reaction is decreased, and this may affect the supply of nutrients. In severe inflammation, there is marked edema, perivascular infiltrates of inflammatory cells and associated pavementing of the endothelium by lymphocytes, so that flow is reduced.

The respiratory debt seen in the uninfected skin of limbs affected by PVD shows a similar respiratory imbalance which makes the assessment of the ischemic limb difficult [9, 10], and the situation becomes exaggerated by the onset of low-grade infection. The failure of ulcers to heal in PVD and the devolopment of gangrene may occur due to this respiratory imbalance, since under conditions of very low tissue oxygen tensions wound healing cannot occur as there is an impairment of fibroblast division, collagen synthesis and protein synthesis.

Oxygen is essential to healing, and the formation tissue consumes oxygen. In the presence of low oxygen tensions, limited anaerobic metabolism can occur with an accumulation of lactid acid. Molecular oxygen is also needed for the hydroxylation of proline and lysine during collagen synthesis, and collagen cannot be released from fibroblasts unless this important step has taken place. In the healing wound the development of a collagen/fibroblast scaffold is essential for capillary budding so that revascularization of the area can occur.

In these experiments we have shown that in cases of severe inflammation there is a gross imbalance between oxygen supply and demand which cannot be redressed by breathing 100 % oxygen. If this metabolic oxygen debt could be corrected, the critically ischemic limb might be returned to a stable state and the limb salvaged. Preliminary experimental work in this laboratory suggests that hyperbaric therapy may be helpful in achieving this.

Acknowledgement. The authors are grateful for the invaluable assistance given by Mr. Faisel Khan in the preparation of all manuscripts.

References

1. Hunt TK, Zederfeldt BH, Goldstick TK (1969) Oxygen & Healing. Am J Surg 118:521
2. Hunt TK, Pai MP (1972) The effect of varying ambient oxygen tension on normal metabolism and collagen synthesis. Surg Gynecol Obstet 135:561
3. Silver IA (1969) The measurement of oxygen tension in healing tissue. In: Herzoy H (ed) Progress in respiration research. Karger, Basel 3:124
4. Beck JS (1988) Editorial: The tuberculin skin test. J Pathol 155:1
5. Gibbs JH, Ferguson J, Brown RA, Kericer KJA, Potts RC, Coghill G, Beck JS (1984) Histomatic study of the localisation of lymphocyte subjects and accessory cells in human Mantoux reactions. J Clin Path 37:1227
6. Beck JS, Spence VA (1986) Patterns of blood flow in the microcirculation of the skin during the course of the tuberculin reaction in normal human subjects. Immunology 58:209
7. Harrison DK, Spence VA, Beck JS, Lowe JG (1986) pH changes in the dermis during the course of the tuberculin skin test. Immunology 59:497
8. Spence VA, Beck JS (1988) Transcutaneous measurement of pO_2 and pCO_2 in the dermis at the site of the tuberculin reaction in healthy human subjects. J Pathol (in press)
9. Franzeck UK, Talke P, Golbranson (1983) Transcutaneous oxygen tension of the lower extremity as a guide to amputation level. In: Huch R, Huch A (eds) Continuous transcutaneous blood gas monitoring. Marcel Dekker Inc, New York, p 709
10. Spence VA, McCollum PT (1985) Evaluation of the ischaemic limb by transcutaneous oximetry. Diagnostic techniques and assessment procedures in vascular surgery. Graine & Stratton ISBN 0-8089-1721-8

Relevance of tcpO$_2$ Measurements for Amputation Level of the Ischemic Leg

K. Ktenidis, Ph. de Vleeschauwer, H. Nigbur, U. Requa, R. Rausch, S. Horsch

Abstract

In 54 patients with peripheral occlusive arterial disease of the lower limb, transcutaneous pO$_2$ for determination of the optimal level of amputation was measured. We wanted to define the optimal borderline-isobar as a patient-specific function of tcpO$_2$ measured at the limb over the individual's reference value measured at the anterior axillary line in the 5th or 6th intercostal space.
In line with the published literature we found tcpO$_2$ measurement to be a useful diagnostic technique for the determination of the amputation level of the ischemic limb.
So far, comparison between the so-called "standard-borderline-isobar" and an individually calculated tcpO$_2$ index has not proven to be of statistical significance.

Introduction

Thanks to continuous progress in vascular surgery and conservative therapy of occlusive arterial disease, the rate of major limb amputations has been reduced by 50 % over the last years.
In order to attain optimal postoperative function of limb in combination with the prescribed prosthesis, it is necessary to strive for an amputation at the lowest level possible still ensuring primary healing.
According to Burgess [1], perfusion of the skin is the most important factor for the determination of the amputation site. Apart from the familiar criteria of clinical findings, angiography and Doppler ultrasound we now have an additional device at our disposal, namely transcutaneous pO$_2$ measurement, which permits indirect evaluation of local skin perfusion, is objective and reproduceable, and can be performed at any location on the limb.
In the literature we consulted we found no "standardized-borderline-isobar" which ought to be exceeded in order to guarantee primary healing. Studies in Japan recommended a value between 30 and 35 mmHg [7],

Clinical Oxygen Pressure Measurement II
A. M. Ehrly et al. (Eds.)
© Blackwell Ueberreuter Wissenschaft Berlin 1990

while a German group around Vollmar required at least 45 mmHg [4]. Nor did we find any standard values for "borderline-isobar" in the American literature [5, 6].

The aim of our study was to give transcutaneous oxygen pressure the task of determining the amputation level more exactly than has been possible up to now.

Taking into account that there are patients with cool, pale skin displaying "pathological" tcpO$_2$ values but who at the same time have no rest pain, we wanted to find out whether the borderline-isobar hadn't better be individually determined instead of using fixed standards.

Materials and methods

Between May 1986 and April 1988 we examined 54 patients (35 male and 19 female) of mean age 71 years.

The necessary amputation level was determined with the patients in a lying position. Fig. 1 shows the points of tcpO$_2$ measurement and the standard amputation sites. Beginning at the patella we moved the probe up- and downwards in steps of 5 cm at the front and back of the extremity. In this way we determined the standard-borderline-isobar for group B of our patients, which, according to the consulted publications, should reach at least 45 mmHg below and 35 mmHg above knee. In the 19 cases of group A we determined the amputation level using an individual index obtained by correlating the transcutaneous oxygen pressure at the extremity with a reference value measured on the chest, at the front axillary line

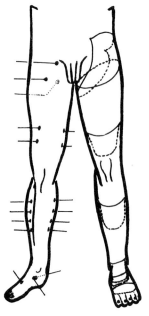

Fig. 1. Sites of tcpO$_2$ measurements and standard amputation

in the fifth or sixth intercostal space. The $tcpO_2$ index was to be calculated in the following way: the sum of the transcutaneous oxygen pressures at the front and the back of the chosen level divided by two and then related to the above-mentioned reference-value. The index ought not to be smaller than 0.66 for below-knee and 0.33 for above-knee amputation. The reliability of this index was judged by comparision with the intraoperative findings such as muscle perfusion and contraction, and the postoperative course (stump healing, re-amputaion, lethality).

$tcpO_2$ measurements were performed using an Oxykapnomonitor SMK 363 from Hellige Company, which consists of a pO_2 measuring module, a registering module, a receiver for the $tcpO_2$ value and a transoxode. It performs continuous registration of $tcpO_2$ as a function of pO_2 in blood. The temperature of the electrode was 45°C.

Results

In 21 cases (39 %) out of the 54 patients, we had to perform above-knee amputations. 26 patients (48 %) were amputated below the knee. In the remaining cases we could restrict ourselves to forefoot or even borderline amputation (Table 1).

Table 1. Comparison between "standard borderline isobar" and $tcpO_2$ index

Amputation Level		
above knee	13	8
below knee	18	8
forefoot	3	–
borderline	1	3
	35	19

In 13 of the above-knee amputations we found primary stump healing, in 3 cases secondary healing and in 1 case re-amputation was necessary. The below-knee amputation group showed primary healing in 18 cases, secondary healing in 3 cases, and no healing at all requiring re-amputation in a further 3 cases (Table 2).

Table 2. Stump healing after amputation

Stump Healing	primary	secondary	no*
above knee	13	3	1
below knee	18	3	3
forefoot	—	3	–
borderline	1	3	–

* second amputation

In the "tcpO$_2$-index" group (n=19) the 8 above-knee amputations performed led to 4 cases of primary stump healing and 1 case of secondary stump healing.No re-amputations were performed. The 8 below-knee amputations led to 5 cases of primary healing, 1 case of secondary healing and 1 case of no stump healing. 3 patients were amputated at borderline of necrosis. 3 patients with above-knee and 1 patient with below-knee amputation died.

In the "standard-isobar" group of 35 patients we performed above-knee amputation in 13 and below-knee amputation in 18 cases. 4 operations could be confined to forefoot or borderline amputation. We achieved primary healing of the above-knee stump in all but 2 cases. 1 patient had to undergo re-amputation. Here, 2 patients died.

The correspondence of tcpO$_2$ values with the intraoperative findings was as follows: In 2 cases we found intraoperatively a distinct reduction in muscle tissue perfusion. Histopathological findings yielded advanced inflammatory alteration of the muscle combined even with necrosis. Stump healing in both these cases was secondary. 1 case showed advanced necrosis of muscle during operation, though the transcutaneous pO$_2$ measurement seemed to allow below-knee amputation.

Lethality during the first two operative weeks was 11.1 % (6 patients).

The rate of re-amputation for the tcpO$_2$ index group was 5.3 % (1/19) and for the standard-isobar group 8.6 % (3/35).

Discussion

Transcutaneous pO$_2$ measurement is now established as a standard procedure in numerous branches of medicine (neonatology, intensive care medicine, angiology, etc). Without doubt, tcpO$_2$ is of some help in amputation surgery too. Being objective and reproduceable it might in one or the other case encourage the surgeon to opt for a lower level of amputation than clinical findings would otherwise suggest.

In our view, the distinguishing feature of the tcpO$_2$ method is its non-invasivity, which is especially important for patients in Fontaine's stages III and IV. In combination with the familiar parameters of local perfusion,it can contribute to a more accurate determination of amputation level. However, the subject of "borderline-isobar" needs to be discussed further.

Some years ago a German group around Vollmar [4] published convincing results with an augmented value of 45 mmHg for below-knee amputation. Nevertheless, we think it is of some use to determine the individual index in the way described above [5, 6].

As in the literature quoted, we too found that it is possible to transfer the amputation site of a severely ischemic limb to a lower level by using transcutaneous pO$_2$ measurement, without having to cope with a higher rate of re-amputation. Nor did numbers of disturbed stump healing or lethal outcome increase.

Comparing the so-called "standard-isobar" with an individually calculated index we have so far found no statistically significant differences regarding intraoperative findings, stump healing, rate of re-amputation and lethality. At present we are continuing our study.

References

1. Burgess EM (1974) Major lower extremity amputation following arterial reconstruction. Arch Surg 108:655
2. Burgess EM et al (1982) Segmental transcutaneous measurements of pO$_2$ in patients requiring below-the-knee amputation for peripheral vascular insufficiency. J Bone Joint Surg 64A:378
3. Byrne P et al (1983) Transcutaneous oxygen tension measurement as a predicative parameter for successful primary healing in above- and below-knee amputations. J Cardiovasc Surg 24:366
4. Cyba-Altunbay S et al (1986) Transkutane Sauerstoffpartialdruckmessung zur prä-operativen Bestimmung der optimalen Amputationshöhe im Endstadium der arteriellen Verschlußkrankheit. Chir Praxis 36:667
5. Katsamouris A et al (1984) Transcutaneous oxygen tension in selection of amputation level. Am J Surg 147:510
6. Malone JM et al (1987) Prospective comparison of non-invasive techniques for amputation level selection. Am J Surg 154:179
7. Oghi S et al (1981) Quantitative evaluation of skin circulation in ischaemic legs by transcutaneous measurement of oxygen tension. Angiology 32:833

Measurements of Transcutaneous Oxygen Tension for Selection of Amputation Level in Patients with Atherosclerotic Leg Ischemia

S. Zapalski, G. Oszkinis, T. Lyczkowski

Introduction

Proper evaluation of tissue blood flow for selection of amputation level in patients with peripheral vascular disease constitutes an important problem the surgeon has to deal with in his daily routine.

It seems particularly difficult to qualify patients for so-called peripheral amputations, i.e. of one or more toes or metatarsus, which don't require use of a prosthesis after rehabilitation. This advantage has to be weighed up against the risk of an amputation performed within an area of inappropriate blood flow, which may expose the patient to unnecessary pain, prolong hospitalization and rehabilitation and even lead to death.

There are many methods for measuring tissue blood flow at the site of amputation. Commonly used techniques combine clinical and peri-operative evaluations based on extent of necrosis, symptoms of infection, presence or absence of pulse, skin temperature, vasa reflects and location of dolorigenic zone, besides which much attention during actual surgery is paid to the quantity of tissue bleeding.

However, the assessment of post-amputational healing prospects based on these clinical and peri-operative evaluations seems rather inadequate. More objective diagnostic tools facilitating decision making as to level of amputation include: Xe-133 clearance, thermometry, plethysmographic and ultrasound examination and measurement of tissue pH. In recent years, a non-invasive method for measurement of percutaneous oxygen tension ($tcpO_2$) using a Clark's polarographic electrode has been added to the diagnostic methods available. This method is based on two commonly known physiological phenomena:

1. Local heating of skin leads to so-called blood arterialization of the surface network of capillary skin vessels located in the area immediately under the epidermis. Oxygen tension in the blood of these vessels approximates oxygen tension in the arterial blood.
2. Oxygen molecules may diffuse freely through the epidermis, whereby degree of perfusion depends above all upon the molecule pressure gradient.

Clinical Oxygen Pressure Measurement II
A.M. Ehrly et al. (Eds.)
© Blackwell Ueberreuter Wissenschaft Berlin 1990

Prolonged ischemia is always accompanied by skin capillary blood flow disorders leading to a decrease in oxygen partial pressure, which in turn reflects degree of tissue ischemia.

The main objective of the present study was to evaluate the usefulness of percutaneous measurements of oxygen tension at the amputation site and to estimate the critical values of $tcpO_2$ and foot-to-chest transcutaneous oxygen ratio values which might warrant good healing prospects. This method was then compared to the commonly used evaluation of tissue blood flow based on ultrasound examinations.

Patients and methods

From January to December 1987 peripheral and below-knee amputations were performed on 148 patients at the Clinic of General and Vascular Surgery in Poznań. These included 63 amputations of one or more toes, 19 amputations of metatarsus and 66 below-knee amputations.

The indications qualifying for amputation were necrosis of toe or toes or of metatarsus, or ulceration resulting from atherosclerosis, which occurred despite earlier attempts to improve blood flow. The ages of the patients ranged from 35 to 70 years (average age: 57).

Blood flow at ankle level was measured in all patients using an ultrasound flow meter, and the ankle-brachial index was calculated. At the same time, $txpO_2$ measurements were taken using a Hellige SM 361 Oxymonitor, and the foot-to-chest ratio was calculated. The measurements of $tcpO_2$ were taken along the line of amputation.

Results

The data obtained indicated significant differences in the healing of post-amputational wounds depending on $tcpO_2$ values and foot-to-chest transcutaneous oxygen ratio. In 119 patients (80.4 %) amputation was successful. The highest proportion of patients with poorly healed stumps was observed when $tcpO_2$ values exceeded 45 mmHg (94.0 % of the patients; mean value 50.4 mmHg) and foot-to-chest ratio was above 0.50 with a mean value of 0.82 (in 96.6 % of patients; see Table 1). The lowest proportion of patients with poorly healed stumps (15.0 %) was observed when $tcpO_2$ values were lower than 40 mmHg (mean value 31.7 mmHg) and foot-to-chest transcutaneous oxygen ratio lower than 0.45 (in 21.1 % of patients).

In 72 patients (48.6 %) peripheral vascular disease was accompanied by diabetes mellitus. Only 40 patients (27 %) indicated proper healing of wounds. The mean value of $tcpO_2$ in patients with properly healed stumps was 51.2 mmHg and foot-to-chest transcutaneous oxygen ratio was 0.79 (Table 2).

Table 1. Effect of some parameters on stump healing. $tcpO_2$ = transcutaneous oxygen pressure; PTP = absolute posterior artery doppler systolic pressure; ABI = ankle-brachial index; SD = standard deviation

	HEALED Mean ± SD	n	FAILED Mean ± SD	n
$tcpO_2$ (mmHg)	50.4 ± 9.1	119	31.7 ± 6.2	29
foot-to-chest $tcpO_2$	0.82 ± 0.68	119	0.31 ± 0.17	29
PTP (mmHg)	52 ± 9	99	43 ± 5	39
ABI	0.78 ± 0.68	96	0.64 ± 0.2	42

Table 2. Effect of parameters on stump healing in patients with diabetes mellitus; $tcpO_2$ = transcutaneous oxygen pressure; PTP = absolute posterior tibial artery doppler systolic pressure; ABI = ankle-brachial index

	HEALED Mean ± SD	FAILED Mean ± SD
$tcpO_2$ (mmHg)	51.2 ± 8.7	47.3 ± 7.2
foot-to-chest $tcpO_2$	0.79 ± 0.43	0.73 ± 0.38
PTP (mmHg)	53.0 ± 8.0	48.0 ± 5.0
ABI	0.82 ± 0.36	0.81 ± 0.42

Discussion

Ultrasound examinations yielded no statistically reliable correlation between blood pressure value at the ankle level or ankle-brachial index and healing of stump. Values for patients with healed stumps were 52 mmHg and 0.78, and for patients with unhealed stumps 43 mmHg and 0.64. Inaccuracies in blood pressure measurements resulted either from medial calcification of peripheral vessels causing artificially increased systolic pressures, particularly in patients with associated diabetes, or from measurement difficulties in older patients or patients with distal small vessel disease, e.g. Berguer's disease.

Out of the 148 patients examined, 12 (8,1 %) died, including two with a healed and ten with an unhealed stump. The main causes of death were pulmonary embolism, myocardial infarction and infection.

A particularly important problem was qualification for amputation in the case of patients with associated diabetes. Our experience indicates that the data based on ultrasound and tcpO$_2$ measurements have no bearing on amputation results. Even ,high values of the above parameters did not always lead to stump healing.

The lack of correlation regarding the ultrasound examinations can be explained, as already mentioned, in terms of an increase in systolic pressure. However, the lack of correlation regarding tcpO$_2$ measurements is difficult to explain and requires further research.

Finally, it must be noted that despite certain limitations the method of transcutaneous oxygen measurements in patients with peripheral vascular disease facilitates appropriate decision making as to amputation of extremities.

References

1. Dowd GSE, Linge K, Bentley G (1983) Measurement of transcutaneous oxygen pressure in normal and ischemic skin. J Bone Joint Surg 65B:79
2. Hauser CJ, Shoemaker WC (1983) Use of transcutaneous pO$_2$ regional perfusion index to quantify tissue perfusion in peripheral vascular disease. Ann Surg 197:337
3. Mustapha NM, Redhead RG, Jain SK, Wielegórski JWJ (1983) Transcutaneous partial oxygen pressure assessment of the ischemic lower limb. (1983) Surg Gynecol Obstet 156:582
4. Rabkin JM, Hunt TK (1987) Local heat increases blood flow and oxygen tension in wounds. Arch Surg 122:221
5. White RA (1982) Noninvasive evaluation of peripheral vascular disease using transcutaneous oxygen tension. Am J Surg 144:68
6. Wyss CR, Robertson C, Love SJ, Harrington RM, Matsen III FA (1987) Relationship between transcutaneous oxygen tension, ankle blood pressure, and clinical outcome of vascular surgery in diabetic and nondiabetic patients. Surgery 101:56

Transcutaneous Oxygen Pressure in Chronic Venous Incompetence: Behavior Pattern and Potential Uses

E. Mannarino, G. Maragoni, L. Pasqualini, S. Tucci

Summary

Transcutaneous oxygen pressure (tcpO$_2$) was measured in patients suffering from chronic venous incompetence (CVI) of the lower limbs to see if trophic lesions are associated with a reduced local oxygen delivery.
The tcpO$_2$ behavior pattern was charted in 60 limbs affected by CVI (20 stage I, 20 stage II and 20 stage III) and then compared to the pattern observed in the 20 limbs of 10 healthy controls.
Local oxygen delivery on the dorsum of the foot, and even more so in the internal ankle region, was significantly reduced in limbs affected by CVI. This was the case not only in the presence of ulcers and/or cutaneous atrophy (stages II and III CVI) but also in the early stages of CVI when only dilated subdermal venules are present.
The determination of tcpO$_2$ can therefore be considered a valid tool in the staging of CVI.

Introduction

The large number of different factors believed to be involved in the clinical manifestation of chronic vein incompetence (CVI) of the lower limbs has meant that studies on and treatment of this disease have not been systematic. Few controlled studies have indeed been carried out because of the difficulty in establishing standard instrumental parameters to evaluate both quantitatively and qualitatively the efficacy of any given therapy.
Over the last twenty years the development of Doppler velocimetry as well as improvements in and standardization of plethysmographic techniques have led to important advances in the field of non-invasive diagnosis of CVI in the lower limbs. Today the measurement of transcutaneous oxygen pressure (tcpO$_2$) can be added to these techniques.
This latter technique was originally developed to monitor oxygen pressure in the newborn [Eberhardt et al., 1976] but is currently employed in the study of peripheral vascular disease (PVD) [Tönneson et al., 1978] and is a useful tool in the evaluation of the ischemic damage caused by PVD

Clinical Oxygen Pressure Measurement II
A. M. Ehrly et al. (Eds.)
© Blackwell Ueberreuter Wissenschaft Berlin 1990

[Borzykowski et al., 1981; Byrne et al, 1984; Kram et al., 1985; Holdich et al., 1986; Mannarino et al., 1987].

It is well known, however, that PVD is not the only factor responsible for tissue hypoxia. Cutaneous lesions such as trophic skin changes and ulcers frequently observed in patients suffering from CVI are often the cause of local hypoxia.

This explains the observation made by Piulacks et al. (1953) that venous blood reflowing from a limb affected by varicose veins or a post-phlebitis syndrome, whether varicose ulcers are present or not, has a higher oxygen saturation than venous blood reflowing from a healthy limb. Venous hypertension in both the profound and superficial vessels appears to be the cause of this local hypoxia.

Furthermore, according to recent reports this hypertension enhances leucocyte plugging of the capillary loops and leads to the release of proteolytic enzymes and oxygen-free radicals which can, in turn, stretch the endothelial pores. The resulting increase in permeability permits the passage of larger molecules such as fibrinogen which, when polymerized, determine the formation of pericapillary cuffs of fibrin [Thomas et al., 1988] thus constituting an obstacle to the delivery of oxygen and nutrients to the epidermic cells [Browse et al., 1982].

Biopsies on skin from areas affected by chronic vein stasis indeed reveal pericapillary deposits of fibrin [Bournand et al., 1982].

Hypertension, moreover, also appears to modify the mechanism of hemostatic regulation by the endothelial cells, as can be seen from a reduced profibrinolysis [Hach et al., 1985], increased platelet adhesiveness [Hoak I.C. 1979], and disturbances in prostacyclin synthesis (PGI_2) [Moncada et al., 1977; Serneri et al., 1980]. The latter disturbance is also responsible for microthrombosis – a frequent occurrence – which conditions oxygen delivery to the tissues.

Since hypoxia is therefore the expression of ischemic damage induced by CVI which is easiest to evaluate and quantify we decided to monitor its behavior at different stages of the disease in a group of CVI patients and to evaluate the usefulness of $tcpO_2$ in determining the stages of this disease and for better follow-ups.

Materials and method

39 CVI patients (30 females and 9 males of average age 61.63 ±8.34) were recruited to the study and 60 limbs tested. 11 CVI cases were caused by primary varicose veins with incompetent perforating veins, and 28 by deep venous thrombosis.

Dilated subdermal venules were present in the medial ankle region in 20 limbs (Stage I CVI), pigmentation and white atrophy in another 20 (stage II CVI), while the remaining 20 had open or healed ulcers (stage III CVI). CVI was diagnosed on the basis of the case history, clinical findings and the results of Doppler ultrasound examination. None of the patients admitted to the study presented any evidence of peripheral arterial occlusive disease.

A control group of 10 healthy subjects (8 females and 2 males of average age 59.42 ±9.62, ie. 20 lower limbs) was also recruited.

The clinical examination and the Doppler velocimetry revealed no evidence of venous or arterial disease in the lower limbs of any of these controls.

TcpO$_2$ was determined using a polarographic method (Kontron Cutaneous pO$_2$ Monitor Module 632) after the electrode had been heated to a temperature of 44°C in a controlled environment (25°C, 40-60 % humidity).

The sites selected to determine the tcpO$_2$ values in each patient were the sub-clavical chest area (to exclude hypoxia resulting from any heart, lung or hematologic pathologies), the ankle area (2 cms. above the upper level of malleolus) and the dorsum of the foot (at the first intermetatarsal space). Where ulcers were present the electrode was placed on non-ulcerated skin at the edge of the lesion.

After the three selected measuring sites had been shaved and cleaned with alcohol tabs and the patients had rested for 40 mins. in the supine position, the electrode was applied. The reading taken 20 mins. after electrode application was considered valid.

Student's "t" test for unpaired data was used for the statistical analysis.

Results

The results of our study showed that the average tcpO$_2$ values registered in the medial ankle region were significantly lower in CVI patients at each stage of the disease and correlated clearly with the stage of venous incompetence. The mean tcpO$_2$ values were: 51.60 ±5.48 mHg in stage I CVI (p<0.01), 34.80 ±17.40 mmHg in stage II CVI (p<0.001), 26.60 ±17.00 mmHg in stage III CVI (p<0.001), and 58.93 ±7.45 mmHg in the controls (Table 1).

The average tcpO$_2$ values measured on the dorsum of the foot were also significantly lower in CVI patients compared to the control group

Table 1. Average basal tcpO$_2$ values in mmHg measured in the chest area, on the dorsum of the foot and in the internal ankle region in Stages I, II, and III CVI patients and healthy subjects

	Controls	CVI Stage I	CVI Stage II	CVI Stage III
tcpO$_2$ chest	60.07 ± 9.30	56.03 ± 6.03 NS	59.21 ± 5.88 NS	59.10 ± 4.30 NS
tcpO$_2$ dorsum of the foot	59.81 ± 9.30	52.98 ± 4.05 p<0.05	52.12 ± 3.35 p<0.05	52.83 ± 3.60 p<0.05
tcpO$_2$ internal ankle region	58.93 ± 7.45	51.60 ± 5.48 p<0.01	34.80 ± 17.40 p<0.001	26.60 ± 17.00 p<0.001

(p<0.05): 52.98 ±4.05 mmHg in stage I CVI, 52.12 ±3.35 mmHg in stage II CVI, 52.83 ±3.60 mmHg in stage III CVI, and 59.81 ±9.30 mmHg in the controls (Table I).
On the other hand, no significant difference was observed in the average tcpO$_2$ chest values in the patients affected by any of the three CVI stages compared to the normal subjects (Table 1).

Conclusions

In CVI patients tcpO$_2$ is significantly reduced in the internal ankle region (Fig. 2) (where trophic lesions most frequently occur), and to a lesser extent on the dorsum of the foot (Fig. 1). These results confirm that the origin of hypoxia lies in trophic lesions caused by CVI.
The registration of low tcpO$_2$ values even in stage I CVI patients where only dilated subdermal venules are present confirms the presence of tis-

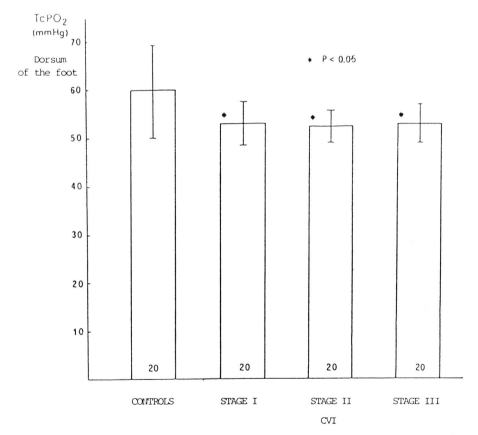

Fig. 1. Average basal tcpO$_2$ values measured on the dorsum of the foot in Stage I, II, and III CVI patients and healthy controls

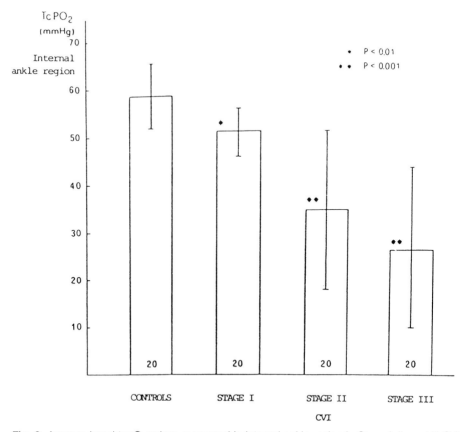

Fig. 2. Average basal tcpO$_2$ values measured in internal ankle region in Stage I, II, and III CVI patients and healthy controls

sue hypoxia even in the earliest stages of this disease. This may be due to the formation of fibrin loops on the pericapillary loops [Thomas P.R.S. et al., 1988] and concurs with the most recent theories on the genesis of venous trophic lesions.

Our study shows furthermore a correlation between the stages of the disease and the values of tcpO$_2$ taken in the inner ankle region. This suggests that the determination of tcpO$_2$ might be usefully employed in the staging of CVI and in the early identification of subjects at risk of ulceration.

Since tcpO$_2$ determination is non-invasive and reliable, it should also be considered a valid method for the monitoring of changes resulting from therapy aimed at improving the condition of CVI patients.

Acknowledgements. The authors would like to thank Ms. G.A. Boyd B.A. (Hons) for her translation of this paper.

References

1. Eberhard P, Mindt W, Jann F (1976) Continuous pO_2 monitoring in the neonate by skin electrodes. Med Biol Eng 13:436
2. Tönnesen KH (1987) Transcutaneous oxygen tension in imminent foot gangrene. Acta Anaesthesiol Scand, Suppl. 68:107
3. Borzykowski M, Krahenbul B (1981) Mesure non invasive de l'oxygénation cutanée en cas d'ulcères chroniques des membres inférieurs. Schweiz Med Wochenschr III 50:1972
4. Byrne P, Proven GL, Ameli FM, Jones DP (1984) The use of transcutaneous oxygen tension measurement in the diagnosis of peripheral vascular insufficiency. Ann Surg 200:159
5. Kram HB, White RA, Tabriski J, Appel PL, Fleming AW, Shoemaker WC (1985) Transcutaneous oxygen recovery and toe pulse reappearance time in the assessment of peripheral vascular disease. Circulation 72: 1022
6. Holdich TA, Reddy PJ, Walker RT, Dormandy JA (1986) Transcutaneous oxygen tension during exercise in patients with claudication. Br Med J 292:1625
7. Mannarino E, Maragoni G, Pasqualini L, Sanchini R, Rossi P, Orlandi U (1987) Transcutaneous oxygen tension behavior in the different stages of peripheral vascular disease and its correlation with ankle/arm pressure ratio and calf blood flow. Angiology 38:463
8. Burgess EM, Matsen FA, Wyss CR, Simmons CW (1987) Segmental transcutaneous measurements of pO_2 in patients requiring below-the-knee amputation for peripheral vascular insufficiency. J Bone Joint Surg 64:377
9. Piulacks P, Vidal Barraquer F (1953) Pathogenic study of varicose veins. Angiology 4:59
10. Warren R, White EA, Belcher CB (1949) Venous pressure in the saphenous system in normal, varicose and post-phebitic extremities. Surgery 26:435
11. Hach V (1985) Fibrinolytic activity in tissue of different varicose veins in comparison to normal vein tissue. I U.K. Meeting, London 16-20 September 1985
12. Hoak IC, Smith GB, Fry GL, Czervionke RL, Hycraft DL (1979) Prostacyclin and platelet adherence to vascular cells. Thromb Haemost 42:173
13. Moncada S, Higgs EA, Vanne JR (1977) Human arterial and venous tissues generate prostacyclin, a potent inhibitor of platelet aggregation. Lancet i:18
14. Neri Serneri GG, Masotti G, Poggesi L, Galanti G (1980) Release of prostacyclin into the bloodstream and its exhaustion in humans after local blood flow changes (ischaemia and venous stasis). Thromb Res 17:197
15. Browse NL, Burnand KG (1982) The cause of venous ulceration. Lancet ii:243
16. Thomas PRS, Nash GB, Dormandy JA (1988) White cell accumulation in dependent legs of patients with venous hypertension: A possible mechanism for trophic changes in the skin. Br Med J 196:1693
17. Burnand KG, Whimster I, Naidoo A, Browse NL (1982) Pericapillary fibrin in the ulcer bearing skin of the leg: The cause of lipodermatosclerosis and venous ulceration. Br Med J 285:1071
18. Franzeck UK, Bollinger A, Huch R, Huch A (1984) Transcutaneous oxygen tension and capillary morphologic characteristics and density in patients with chronic venous incompetence. Circulation 70:806
19. Bollinger A, Speiser D, Haselbach P, Jager K: Microangiopathy of mild and severe chronic venous incompetence (CVI) studied by fluorescence videomicroscopy. Schweiz Med Wochenschr, in press

Transcutaneous and Venous Oxygen Measurements during Provoked Venous Stasis in the Forearm of Normal Subjects

S. Forconi, M. Guerrini, R. Cappelli, P. Sani, L. Domini

Introduction

In some previous experiments we observed that changes in microcirculation, due to variations in arterial blood pressure and velocity, were responsible for rheological impairment [1]. In order to determine whether changes on the venous side might possibly have similar effects on microvessels, we prepared an experimental model of venous stasis in man. We did this with a view to studying also blood gas equilibrium.

Subjects and method

Venous stasis was obtained in volunteers using a pneumatic cuff inflated around one arm to a pressure of just 10 mmHg less than diastolic pressure for a period of 10 min. This model was conceived with the purpose of stopping the venous blood flow only for a limited amount of time since we observed that under these experimental conditions pressure in the veins reaches levels 5-10 mmHg above those of the cuff after no more than 30 seconds. After this first reaction blood continues to flow in the venous bed under stasis, even though at a higher pressure (and possibly at a lower velocity), and the venous blood we collected distally at the cuff stemmed directly from the microcirculatory bed.

This experimental model showed [2, 3] that important changes occur in the venous blood flowing from the area under stasis and that they are characterized by an important decrease in blood fluidity, which in our opinion is due to a complex interplay of factors released by the blood cells and the endothelium under conditions of ipoxic acidosis. The behavior of the blood gas is characterized by a reduction of venous pH and pO_2 and a slight increase in pCO_2.

We also performed transcutaneous measurements. Variations in $tcpO_2$ and in $tcpCO_2$ were parallel to those observed in the veins, even though the levels were different, although it must be pointed out, $tcpO_2$ values were higher – though of course lower than in the arteries.

Aiming at controlling this aspect of oxygen transfer we prolonged the stasis up to the 30th min in a group of 10 volunteers, collecting venous

Clinical Oxygen Pressure Measurement II
A.M. Ehrly et al. (Eds.)
© Blackwell Ueberreuter Wissenschaft Berlin 1990

blood before and at the end of the stasis. pO_2, pCO_2 and pH in the venous samples were measured by means of an I.L. 1302 Gas-Analyzer, p50 was measured using an I.L. 237 Tonometer and 2.3-DPG using the UV-Boehringer-Biochemica method. $TcpO_2$ was monitored during the period of stasis using a Kontron Tc Microgas 7640, placing the transducer on the palmar side of the forearm.

Results

Looking at the results in Fig. 1 one observes a certain variability both in transcutaneous and in venous pO_2 between the individual cases. One sees also that transcutaneous pO_2 sometimes comes very close to the level arterial pO_2 would be expected to reach.

Venous stasis always provokes a decrease in pO_2 values, as shown by Fig. 2, where mean values are given. Mean base values of transcutaneous pO_2

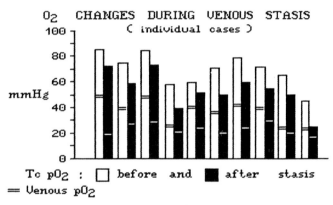

Fig. 1. Changes in transcutaneous pO_2 (tcpO$_2$) and venous pO_2 values registered in the 10 subjects before and after 30 min of venous stasis

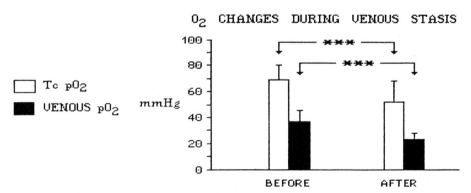

Fig. 2. Mean values of transcutaneous pO_2 (tcpO$_2$) and venous pO_2 registered in base conditions and after 30 min of venous stasis. Student's t-test for paired data. n=10, mean ±SD, *** = $p < 0.001$

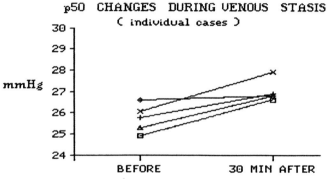

Fig. 3. Changes in p50 values registered in 5 subjects before and after 30 min of venous stasis

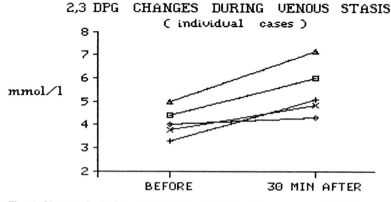

Fig. 4. Changes in the intraerythrocytary 2.3 Diphosphoglycerate (2.3 DPG) observed in 5 subjects before and after 30 min of venous stasis

being 70 mmHg, one could argue that using the transcutaneous probe we measured at a point presumably in the middle of the capillary, between the arterial and venous sides. Furthermore, reduction of tcpO$_2$ after stasis demonstrates that at this point variations in O$_2$ transfer at capillary level are signalled by the probe.

In venous blood, p50 increases during stasis (Fig. 3), making the slope of the Hb curve shift to the right. There is also an increase in 2.3-DPG (Fig. 4). Both these changes are signs of a reduced affinity between Hb and O$_2$.

Conclusion

Firstly these findings demonstrate that during venous stasis there is an increase in O$_2$ transfer from capillary to tissue, due to increase in hydrostatic pressure on the one hand and decreased affinity between hemoglobin and oxygen on the other.

Furthermore, from the methodological point of view, we can confirm that tcpO$_2$ reflects variations in the capillary blood due to gas exchange at the microcirculatory level.

References

1. Forconi S (1988) Regional ischemia and hyperviscosity. Clinical Hemorheology 8:321
2. Forconi S, Pieragalli D, Guerrini M, Galigani C, Monaci A, Domini L, Ralli L, De Franco V, Sani P, Di Perri T (1987) Hemorheological changes during venous stasis. In: Tsuchiya M, Asano M, Mishima Y, Oda M (eds) Microcirculation – an update. Excerpta Medica International Congress Series No 755, Elsevier Science Pbs., Amsterdam, Vol 2, p 709
3. Forconi S, Guerrini M, Laghi Pasini F, Cappelli R, Franchi M, Pieragalli D, Acciavatti A, Messa GL, Pasqui AL, Galigani C, Sani P, Frigerio C, Capecchi PL, Landini F, Domini L, Monaci A (1988) La stasi venosa come modello di studio dei rapporti tra endotelio e sangue a livello microcircolatorio. In: Pupita F, Ansuini R, Frausini G (eds) Microcircolazione. Abbott Pbs, Fano, p 47

Improved Reliability of tcpO$_2$ Measurements at 37°C by Use of Histograms

L. Caspary, A. Creutzig, K. Alexander

Introduction

The initial purpose of the tcpO$_2$ method was to record the arterial oxygen pressure. However, below a skin perfusion rate of 90 ml/100 ml tissue · min, the recorded signal is flow-dependent [4].

In recent years, tcpO$_2$ measurements have been increasingly applied to the assessment of flow in the skin, especially in patients with peripheral vascular disorders [3]. At a moderate hyperemisation temperature of 37°C, the regional capillary blood flow can be recorded [2], whereby, in contrast to measurements at 44°C, vasoregulatory processes are mostly preserved.

This is a great advantage of the application at 37°C regarding the possibility of recording vasomotional reactions to provocation tests and application of drugs. However, due to the great variability of skin perfusion, the signal at rest is poorly reproducible. Yet, it could be useful to obtain information on the microcirculatory state of the skin at rest, which can be expected to differ from the hyperemia state under an electrode heated to 44°C.

Since tcpO$_2$ at 37°C cannot be determined in a representative way by a single measurement, we recorded complete histograms of healthy subjects as well as of patients with peripheral vascular disease. Procedure and preliminary results are presented below.

Subjects and method

The measurements were performed in 5 healthy young men of 28 to 35 years age and with no detectable signs of vascular disorders or diabetes (Table 1).

Additionally, 6 patients of 42 to 68 years with proven peripheral arterial occlusive disease (PAOD) in various stages were investigated. 3 suffered from severe claudication stage IIb, the others from arterial ulcers. 1 patient with ulcer was diabetic. The ankle artery pressure of the patients ranged from 40 to 95 mmHg.

Clinical Oxygen Pressure Measurement II
A. M. Ehrly et al. (Eds.)
© Blackwell Ueberreuter Wissenschaft Berlin 1990

Table 1. Values of tcpO$_2$ at 37°C histograms from the forefoot of 5 healthy volunteers (and in 3 cases from the calf) as well as in 6 patients with PAOD stages IIb or IV

healthy persons	n	mean	S.D.	median
1	80	4.8	2.9	4.0
2	75	4.8	2.9	5.0
			.0	
3	66	4.4	2.9	4.0
3 (calf)	80	12.3	9.7	9.0
4	68	7.7	3.8	7.0
4 (calf)	68	9.4	7.2	8.0
5	74	6.4	3.3	7.0
patients stage IIb				
1	76	3.8	2.5	4.0
2	72	3.3	1.9	3.0
3	58	4.5	3.7	3.0
patients stage IV				
4	72	1.1	1.5	1.0
5	70	1.9	1.3	2.0
6 (diabetes)	68	5.2	2.4	5.0

All the participants had been asked not to smoke the day before. During the investigation the subjects lay on an examination bank at a room temperature of 21-23°C.

4 commercially available tcpO$_2$ electrodes (TCM-2, Radiometer, Copenhagen) identified as A, B, C & D, were calibrated at 37°C according to the manufacturer's instructions. The zero point was checked with a sodium dithionite solution. After thoroughly cleansing the skin, five rings of the original fixation kit, identified as 1, 2, 3, 4 & 5, were positioned on the epidermal region we wanted to examine, with as little space in between as possible. Most of the measurements were performed on the forefoot.

The electrodes were first inserted into rings 1-4. The values were recorded after 15-20 mins, when the skin had adapted to the electrodes and stable resting values been established. Then electrode A was moved to ring 5, B to ring 1 and so on. Ring 4, which remained empty, was tapped, so as to preserve the temperature. Once the skin under the fixation ring had warmed up, the equilibration time needed before a stable new baseline could be recorded shortened considerably, so that the rotation procedure could be repeated after about 5 mins. Thus it took 20-25 mins to complete a cycle in which each electrode had been in each location once. The procedure was continued until 3-4 cycles yielding 60-80 recorded values in all had been completed. These were then computed in the form of a histogram.

Differences between the histograms were tested using the Kolmogorov-Smirnov-test (KS-test).

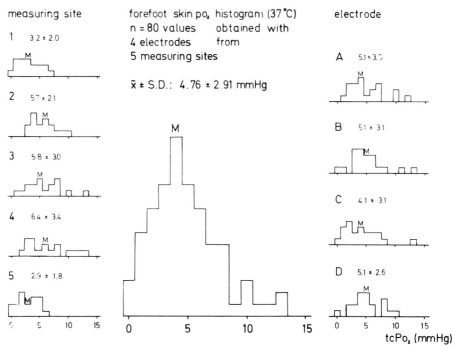

Fig. 1. Composition of the tcpO₂ at 37°C forefoot histogram of a healthy subject, sub-histograms of the 5 measuring sites and of the 4 electrodes

Results

Composition of the histogram

The influence of the measuring site as well as of the electrode applied is shown in Fig. 1, which represents the histogram of the forefoot of a healthy subject. The mean (and median) values of the sites 1 to 5 vary between 2.9 (3) and 6.4 (6) mmHg, whereas the variation between the electrodes A to D is only 1 mmHg. The other measurements behaved similarly, the variation between the measuring sites always being greater than that between the electrodes.

Reproducibility

In 1 healthy subject in the 3 patients in stage IIb measurements were repeated on four consecutive days. The mean and median values of the histograms thus obtained varied by 0.8 to 1.5 mmHg. The KS-test did not reveal significant intraindividual differences (Fig. 2).

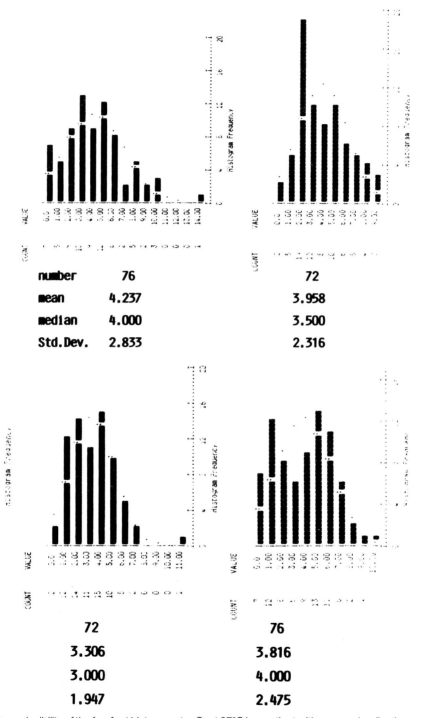

Fig. 2. Reproducibility of the forefoot histogram tcpO$_2$ at 37°C in a patient with severe claudication – measurements taken on 4 consecutive days

226   L. Caspary et al.

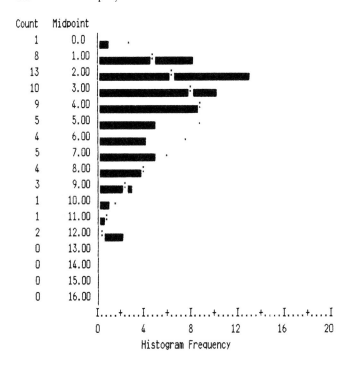

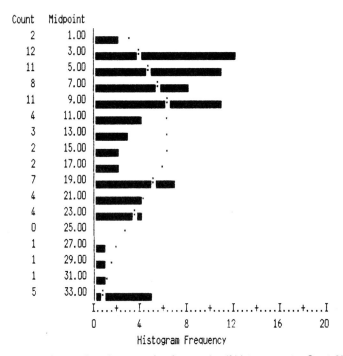

Fig. 3. Comparison between forefoot and calf histograms tcpO$_2$ at 37°C in a healthy subject

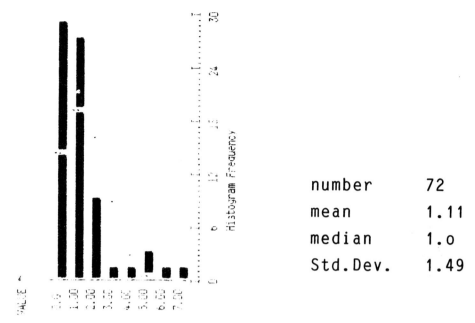

number   72

mean   1.11

median   1.0

Std.Dev.   1.49

Fig. 4. tcpO$_2$ at 37°C histogram from the forefoot of a patient with severe PAOD

Different skin regions

In 3 healthy subjects, the forefoot histogram was compared with that taken from the lower third of the calf. The mean and median values from the calf were higher in all cases. This was also the case when comparing the 5 sub-histograms from measuring sites 1-5 with the calf histogram. Fig. 3 gives an example showing that the results at the different sites can still be distinguished from the sum histogram of the calf.

Differences between patients and healthy subjects

In the patients, mean and median values of the forefoot histogram were lower than in the healthy subjects, although nearly normal values were recorded in 2 of the patients in stage IIb and in the diabetic patient in stage IV. In the other 3 patients, the histograms were markedly left-shifted (Fig. 4) and significantly differentiated by the KS-test.

Influence of other factors

In 1 healthy subject a histogram was taken with the foot in a dependent position. Then, after returning to the supine position, he was allowed to smoke several cigarettes while another histogram was being recorded.

228   L. Caspary et al.

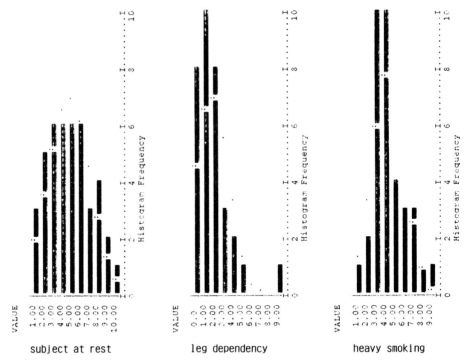

subject at rest   leg dependency   heavy smoking

Fig. 5. Forefoot tcpO$_2$ at 37°C of a healthy subject, reaction to leg dependency and heavy cigarette smoking

Leg dependency produced a significant reduction in mean and median tcpO$_2$ of 3 mmHg (p<0.05), whereas during smoking mean and median values fell non-significantly by about 1 mmHg (Fig. 5).

Discussion

The pO$_2$ histogram, obtained with surface or needle electrodes, is known to be a reliable tool for the assessment of tissue oxygen supply. A sum of at least 100 measured values is required [5]. In contrast to measurements at the skin surface, smaller platinum wires are used in the electrodes, and recordings of pO$_2$ can be performed under isothermic conditions at body temperature. Skin pO$_2$ measurements can only be obtained if external heat is applied, thus creating an artificial state of the skin.
Therefore, our histograms cannot be directly compared to tissue pO$_2$ histograms. Nevertheless, our recorded over-all histograms are more representative than single tcpO$_2$ measurements at 37°C. This was the case both in healthy subjects as well as in patients [1]. The fact that the values stemmed from five different sites does not devaluate the method: on the contrary, the reproducibility of the histogram is increased thanks to the

integration of a larger surface. The differences between the measuring sites only underline the inhomogeneity of dermal perfusion.

One great advantage of individual measurements taken at 37°C, namely the rapid assessment of perfusion reactions to different stimuli, must be abandoned. However, alterations in skin perfusion provoked by long lasting stimuli, can be revealed. Thus, the decrease in tcpO₂ under conditions of leg dependency proved to be long lasting.

Although the equilibration process is considerably accelerated once the skin has adapted to the electrode, the method is very time consuming. In all, the recording of one histogram takes 2 hours, which restricts the method to scientific experiments.

Our investigation shows that by rotating the tcpO₂ electrodes at 37°C, reproducible and reliable histograms can be obtained which are more representative of the microcirculatory system at rest. Further investigations, especially with multiwire electrodes in order to provide shorter measuring times, will be needed to give this method a place among the other applications of the tcpO₂ method.

References

1. Creutzig A, Dau D, Caspary L, Alexander K (1987) Transcutaneous oxygen pressure measured at two different electrode core temperatures in healthy volunteers and patients with arterial occlusive disease. Int J Microcirc Clin Exp 5:373
2. Ewald U, Rooth G, Tuvemo T (1981) Postischemic hyperemia studied with a transcutaneous oxygen electrode used at 33-37°C. Scand J Clin Lab Invest 41:641
3. Franzeck UK, Talke P, Bernstein EF, Golbranson FL, Fronek A: Transcutaneous pO₂ measurements in health and peripheral arterial occlusive disease. Surgery 91:156
4. Huch R, Huch A, Lübbers DW (1981) Transcutaneous pO₂. Thieme-Stratton Inc., New York, p 156
5. Lübbers DW, Baumgärtl H, Grunewald W (1975) Micromethods for monitoring local tissue oxygen supply and microcirculation. Bibl Anat 13:53

tcpO$_2$ Measurements in Patients with Chronic Venous Incompetence before and after Babcock Stripping

L. Caspary, A. Creutzig, H. v.d. Lieth, K. Alexander

Introduction

Venous incompetence leads to alterations in the skin circulation. These can be assessed on the microvascular level by means of laser Doppler fluxmetry, capillary microscopy and tcpO$_2$ measurements [1, 4]. In a former investigation we observed increased tcpO$_2$ (37°C) values at rest, a strong signal decrease upon leg dependency and an impaired reactive hyperemia on macroscopically indemned skin areas of the forefoot [1]. Babcock stripping of the saphena vein has proved to be effective with respect to skin varicosis and subjective well-being of patients suffering from incompetence of the saphena valve [6]. We investigated alterations in the skin microcirculation of a group of patients with primary varicosis, aiming to answer the following questions: What significant differences are observable compared to an age-matched group of healthy controls? What are the effects of surgical treatment?

Patients and methods

15 patients from our outpatient department, 11 women and 4 men of mean age 44 years, gave their informed consent to participate in this study. They suffered from venous incompetence grade II according to Widmer and had been designated for Babcock operation. Saphena insufficiency had been ascertained by Doppler investigation and phlebography films, which precluded any damage to the deep veins. Venous outflow, determined by strain gauge plethysmography, exceeded 80 ml/100 ml · min.

The measurements were performed before and 8 to 9 weeks after the operation which consisted in exairese of the saphena vein and in meticulous ligation of all incompetent perforator veins. By the time of the second investigation, the post-operative edema had completely disappeared and venous outflow values had fallen to the normal range. Doppler investigation did not reveal any reflux to superficial veins during Valsalva manoeuvre. Post-operative phlebography was not performed.

Clinical Oxygen Pressure Measurement II
A.M. Ehrly et al. (Eds.)
© Blackwell Ueberreuter Wissenschaft Berlin 1990

A group of 15 healthy subjects matched for age and sex served as controls. They had no history of varicosis and Doppler investigation revealed no reflux.

None of the subjects in either group suffered from diabetes. tcpO$_2$ was determined using 4 platinum electrodes (Radiometer, Copenhagen) which were first calibrated at 37°C. They were all fixed within a 5 by 5 cm field of the thoroughly cleansed foot dorsum. The subjects were in a comfortable supine position at a room temperature of 21-23°C and had not smoked on the day of the examination.

After 20 minutes stable measuring conditions were achieved and resting values recorded. Then the leg was passively elevated to about 40 cm above heart level for about 5 minutes and a second recording taken. After a further 15 minutes in the supine position the subjects were asked to stand for 5 minutes so as to record the leg dependency reaction.

After resting conditions had been re-established in the supine position, a five minute venous occlusion was performed at calf level by inflating a cuff to 40 mmHg and values recorded. After a further 15 minutes a supra-systolic cuff occlusion at the thigh level was performed and terminated after 3 minutes, the postischemic signal overshoot being recorded and followed up for 20 minutes.

Then the electrodes were recalibrated at 44°C and again inserted into the rings of the fixation kit. Once a stable value had been reached, the signal increase during 5 minutes of oxygen breathing was monitored.

Pre- and post-operative results were compared and analyzed using the paired t-test. For comparision with the controls, the Mann-Whitney-Wilcoxon test was used.

Results

Resting values

tcpO$_2$ values at 37°C were significantly higher in the group of patients than in the controls ($p < 0.05$). There were no differences between the pre- and post-operative values of the varicosis group. At 44°C no significant differences between any of the groups were observable (see Table 1).

Changes of position

Leg elevation led to a signal increase or decrease in both groups, whereby there was a small but not significant ($p = 0.104$) tendency towards signal increase in the patients' group. After the operation, this tendency disappeared.

Leg dependency produced a tcpO$_2$ (37°C) decrease in both groups, whereby the decrease was significantly more pronounced in the patients' group ($p < 0.05$). The difference between tcpO$_2$ during leg elevation and

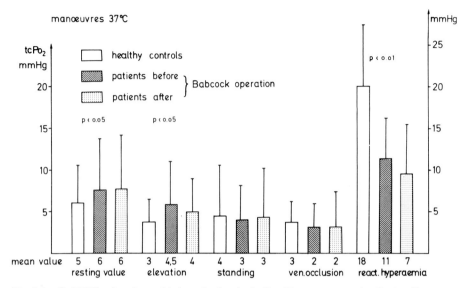

Fig. 1. tcpO$_2$ (37°C) values in mmHg from the forefoot of healthy persons and patients with venous incompetence; reactions to various stimuli

leg dependency was significantly higher in the patients' group (p<0.02). The operation did not alter this difference.

Occlusion

Upon venous occlusion, tcpO$_2$ fell to about 40-60 % of the initial value in all groups. The fall was more pronounced in the patients than in the controls, but the difference between the two groups was not significant.

Arterial occlusion produced a signal decrease to zero, which was delayed in some of the patients. After deflation of the cuff, a reactive hyperemia with a high signal overshoot was observed. The extent of the overshoot was significantly reduced in the patients' group both before and after the operation (p<0.01).

The various tcpO$_2$ values at 37°C are displayed in Fig. 1.

Oxygen inhalation

Breathing pure oxygen during resting significantly increased tcpO$_2$ (44°C) in both groups. The differences between controls and patients, both before and after the operation, were not significant (Table 1).

Table 1. tcpO$_2$ values from the forefoot of patients with venous incompetence and healthy controls in mmHg, mean values ± S.D., median values in brackets

	healthy persons	patients before stripping	patients after stripping
at rest 37°C	6.1 ± 4.5 (5.0)	7.6 ± 5.8 (6.0)	7.7 ± 6.3 (6.0)
44°C	51.3 ±14.9 (51)	56.0 ±10.2 (56)	55.3 ±14.0 (58)
oxygen 44°C breathing	198 ±41 (192)	193 ±32 (180)	200 ±38 (196)

Discussion

As was the case in a former investigation [1], measurement of tcpO$_2$ revealed alterations in the microcirculation of patients with chronic venous incompetence even on the macroscopically unchanged foot region. Compared to a group of healthy controls matched for age tcpO$_2$ at 37°C revealed significant differences consisting in higher resting values, a greater decrease upon leg dependency, a greater difference between leg elevation and leg dependency and a reduced reactive hyperemia reaction. These results can be partly explained by a chronic dilation of the skin capillaries due to increased venostatic pressure. In the supine position, the skin blood flow was shown to be increased [4].

In the dependent position, tcpO$_2$ at 37°C normally decreases as a result of the vasoconstrictor response [2]. In our patients, the increased venostatic pressure may additionally reduce the skin capillary flow.

During leg elevation, the skin blood flow will be rather facilitated in the presence of big varicose veins. Thus the increased signal difference between the two positions may indicate a lack of venostatic control.

Reactive hyperemia was markedly reduced in the patients' group with respect both to relative and absolute values. This phenomenon must have a functional explanation. It cannot be explained by a lack of flow capacity, since maximal hyperemia flow at 44°C was not reduced.

At 44°C no significant differences between patients and healthy subjects were observed. The increase of tcpO$_2$ during oxygen breathing was within the same range. Thus, the greater differences at 37°C cannot be explained by an assumed reduction in diffusion distance in the patients between capillaries and electrodes, since this should have been reflected by a stronger increase after oxygen breathing, which wasn't the case.

Although the Babcock operation had clearly improved the patients' clinical symptoms and led to normal venous capacity as determined by strain gauge plethysmography, 2 months after the operation the alterations in microcirculation were found to be as great as before.

One can speculate that the capillary disorders have been made permanent by the long duration of the disease. Other theories locate the ultimate cause of chronic venous incompetence in the postcapillary venular system [5]. As a third hypothesis one might consider a period of 8 weeks as insufficient to allow the alterations to resolve.

References

1. Creutzig A. Caspary L, Alexander K (1988) Disturbances of skin microcirculation in patients with chronic arterial occlusive disease and venous incompetence. Vasa 17:77
2. Creutzig A, Dau D, Caspary L, Alexander K (1987) Transcutaneous oxygen pressure measured at two different electrode core temperatures in healthy volunteers and patients with arterial occlusive disease. Int J Microcirc Clin Exp 5:373
3. Franzeck UK, Bollinger A, Huch R, Huch A (1984) Transcutaneous oxygen tension and capillary morphologic characteristics in patients with chronic venous incompetence. Circulation 70:806
4. Gowland Hopkins NF, Spinks TJ, Rhodes CG, Ramicar ASO, Jamieson CW (1983) Positron emission tomography in venous ulceration and liposclerosis: Study of regional tissue function. Brit Med J 286:333
5. Riede U, Staubesand J (1977) A unifying concept for the role of matrix vessels and lysosomes in the formal pathogenesis of diseases of connective tissue and blood vessels. Beitr Pathol 160:3
6. Myers TT (1957) Results and techniques of stripping operation for varicose veins. JAMA 163:87

Effects of Low Dose, Long Term Urokinase Therapy on tcpO$_2$ of Patients with Venous Ulcers

A. M. Ehrly, J. Schenk, U. Bromberger

Findings over the last decade indicate that venous ulcers cannot be explained by macrovascular disturbances only and that microvascular factors are also involved. Under the microscope, dilated capillaries and protein leakage can be observed [12]. A number of authors have found a reduction in transcutaneous oxygen pressure values in the vicinity of venous ulcers [3,13,17,18]. This finding was explained by Borzykowski and Krähenbühl [3], Bollinger and co-workers [2] and Franzeck [13] as being the result of microflow impairment due to a rarification of capillaries. Fagrell [12], Partsch [19] and Sindrup and co-workers [20] on the other hand actually found an increase in blood flow, and claimed oxygen diffusion problems were responsible. Browse and Burnand [4] described pericapillary fibrin cuffs in the skin surrounding venous ulcers which might be responsible for impairing diffusion of oxygen and nutrients. Other authors have reported the presence of microthrombi in the microcirculatory vessels close to or in the area surrounding venous ulcers [14,15,16,1].

Earlier studies done by our group yielded good therapeutic results using a low dose, long term urokinase therapy in patients with severe occlusive arterial disease [6] as well as in patients with severe therapy-resistant angina [9].

We have now performed a study in patients with postthrombic venous ulcers. The basic idea was to reduce the thickness of the extravascular fibrin wall or to dissolve microthrombi, factors which might impair oxygen diffusion into the surrounding tissue. This long term stimulation of fibrinolysis and fibrinogenolysis should also improve the flow properties of the blood [8], which would also lead to a more homogenous perfusion [5,7]. If this concept is valid, an increase in transcutaneous oxygen pressure and a clinical benefit could be expected.

Patients and methods

In an open study, 7 patients suffering from severe postthrombotic ulcers were investigated. Chronic arteriosclerosis was excluded by ankle pres-

Clinical Oxygen Pressure Measurement II
A.M. Ehrly et al. (Eds.)
© Blackwell Ueberreuter Wissenschaft Berlin 1990

sure measurements. These patients were hospitalized in the dermatology department of the university hospital and were being treated as usual with ointment, compression and so on. All patients had given their informed consent.

Urokinase (Ukidan®, Serono, Freiburg, FRG) was infused intravenously in daily doses of 500,000 I.E. or 1,000,000 I.U. The infusion lasted 60 min. Control parameters of thrombolytic therapy were plasma fibrinogen concentration and thrombin time. $tcpO_2$ and $tcpCO_2$ values 2 were measured next to the ulcers with an instrument from Radiometer, Copenhagen. The heating temperature of the electrode was 44°C; the patient was in a horizontal position. Healing progress of the ulcers was documented photographically and by planimetry, using a transparent plastic film placed directly on the ulcers.

Results

There was a continuous and significant increase in $tcpO_2$ values in the course of the four week, low dose Urokinase therapy. At the beginning of

Table 1. Low-dose, long-term urokinase therapy in patients with venous leg ulcers (n=7)

	Orig. values	after 1 week	after 2 weeks	after 3 weeks	after 4 weeks	after 3−6 months' therapy (n=3)
$tcpO_2$ (Torr)	11.14	23.85	32.71	38.00	32.00	42.33
$tcpCO_2$ (Torr)	54.28	48.85	44.00	48.71	49.25	34.33
ESR (mm/h)	25/55	13/33	12/31	9/22	12/29	
Hematocrit (%)	41.42	40.64	40.92	40.57	40.25	
Red cell count(x 10^6)	4.997	4.910	4.860	4.995	4.795	
Whole blood viscosity (H_2O = 1)	4.79	4.42	4.46	4.43	4.39	
Plasma viscosity (H_2O = 1)	1.79	1.74	1.72	1.73	1.73	
Erythrocyte aggregation ($\bar{x}$ α)	42.42	32.71	28.07	22.35	21.75	
Ankle pressure index	1.20	1.17	1.31	1.21	1.24	
Ulcer area (cm²)	19.05	15.80	14.13	11.86	5.27	

the therapy the average tcpO$_2$ values were 11,14 Torr and at the end 32,21 Torr ($p<0.01$). A reduction in the ulcer area as well as the disappearance of pains were observed concomitantly. In 2 out of 7 cases there was complete healing within the 4-week therapy. As expected, the hemorheological parameters improved (see Table 1). Side effects could not be registered. A more detailed description of this result has been published elsewhere [10,11].

Discussion

We suggest that a long term stimulation of fibrinolysis leads to a reduction of the thickness of the pericapillary fibrin wall due to an extraversation of urokinase and/or to a lysis of microvascular thrombi. The improvement of the flow properties of blood by Urokinase does not seem to play a dominant role, since similar studies on chronical occlusive arterial ulcers have not yielded increases in tcpO$_2$ values. The reduction in the area covered by the ulcer coincides (inversely) with the tcpO$_2$ results. However, further control studies are needed. The present results support the concept according to which disturbances in diffusion of oxygen and nutrients are the most important pathogenetic factor in venous leg ulcers. In addition, the results underline the significance of microvascular disturbances in the pathogenesis and pathophysiology of venous ulcers.

References

1. Bollinger, A. (1989): Evidence for microvascular thrombosis obtained by fluoresence videomicroscopy. *Int. Angiology* (in press).
2. Bollinger, A., Jäger, K., Geser, A., Sgier, F., Seglias, G. (1982): Transcapillary and interstitial diffusion of Na-Fluorescein in chronic venous insufficiency with white athrophy. *Int. J. Microcirc. Clin. Exp. 1:* 5
3. Borzykowski, M. and Krähenbühl, B. (1981): Mesure noninvasive de l'oxygénation cutanée en cas d'ulcères chroniques des membres intérieurs. *Schweiz. Med. Wschr. 111:* 1972
4. Browse, N.L., Burnand, K.G. (1982): The cause of venous ulceration. *Lancet I:* 243
5. Ehrly, A.M. (1980): New pathophysiological concept of ischemic diseases: microcirculatory blood maldistribution (MBM). *Bibl. Anatom. 20:* 456
6. Ehrly, A.M. (1986): Systemic low dose Urokinase therapy in patients with chronic arterial disease (stages III and IV): theoretical and practical considerations. In: *What is new in Angiology?* eds P. Maurer, H.M. Becker, H. Heidrich, C. Hoffmann, A. Kriessmann, H. Müller-Wiefel, C. Prätorius, Zuckschwerdt, Munich: p. 411.
7. Ehrly, A.M. (1980): Mikrozirkulatorische Blutverteilungsstörung (MBV) als pathophysiologisches Prinzip bei der chronischen arteriellen Verschlußerkrankung. In: *Mikrozirkulation und Blutrheologie, Therapie der peripheren arteriellen Verschlußkrankheit.* ed H. Müller-Wiefel, H. Witzstrock, Baden-Baden: p. 59-62.
8. Ehrly, A.M., Fuchs, H. (1987): Influence of Urokinase on the flow properties of blood. *Clin. Hemorheol. 7:* p. 665-669
9. Ehrly, A.M., Schenk, J. (1987): Systematische, niedrigdosierte Langzeit-Urokinasetherapie bei schwerster Angina pectoris -Grundlagen und erste Ergebnisse. In: *Fortschritte in der kardiovasculären Hämorheologie.* eds B.E. Strauer, A.M. Ehrly, M. Leschke. MWP-Press, Munich, p 35-38 and 1986: *Klin. Wschr. 64:* 1152

10. Ehrly, A.M., Schenk, J., Bromberger, U. (1988): Niedrigdosierte Urokinasetherapie bei Patienten mit Ulcus cruris. In: *Fortschritte in der Angiologie*. ed A. Kriessmann. *VASA Suppl. 23:* 283

11. Ehrly, A.M, Schenk, J., Bromberger, U. (1989): Mikrozirkulationsstörungen bei Ulcus cruris venosum: Niedrig dosierte systemische Langzeittherapie mit Urokinase. *Phlebol. u. Proktol. 18:* 166-168

12. Fagrell, B. (1979): Local microcirculation in chronic venous incompetence and leg ulcers. *Vasc. Surg. 13:* 217

13. Franzeck, U.K. (1983): Sauerstoffpartialdruck und Kapillarmorphologie bei Patienten mit chronischer venöser Insuffizienz (CVI). *Phlebol. u. Proktol. 12:* 149-160

14. Hasselbach, P., Vollenweider, U., Moneta, G., Bollinger, A. (1986): Microangiopathy in severe chronic venous insufficiency evaluated by fluorescence video-microscopy. *Phlebol. 1:* 159-169

15. Kulwin, M.H., Hines, E.A. (1950): Blood vessels of the skin in chronic venous insufficiency. *Arch. Dermatol. Syhphil. 63:* 293

16. Leu, H.J., Schneider, U.W. (1967): Epitheliale und kutan-vaskuläre Veränderungen beim postthrombotischen Ulkus, ihre prognostische Aussage und ihre Bedeutung für die Therapie. *Med. Welt 18:* 1024-28

17. Neumann, H.A.M., Berrety, P.J.M., v. Leuwen, M., v.d. Broek, M.J. (1983): Transcutaneous pO$_2$ measurement in chronic venous insufficiency syndrome. *Microvasc. Res. 26:* 262

18. Partsch, H. (1983): Transkutane Messung des Sauerstoffpartialdrucks bei trophischen Hautläsionen an der unteren Extremität. In *Probleme der Vor- und Nachsorge und der Narkoseführung bei invasiver angiologischer Diagnostik und Therapie*. eds. F. Nobbe and G. Rudofsky, pp. 209-214. Munich: Pflaum.

19. Partsch, H. (1984): Hyperaemic hypoxia in venous ulceration. *Br. J. Derm. 110:* 249-251

20. Sindrup, J.H., Avnstorp, Chr., Steenfos, H.H., Kristensen, J.K. (1987): Transcutaneous pO$_2$ and Laser Doppler blood flow measurements in 40 patients with venous leg ulcers. *Acta. Derm. Venereol. (Stockh.) 67:* 160-182

21. Sparkman, Th., Horwitz, O., Graham, J.H. (1964): Circulatory changes in the skin of patients with varicose ulcers as demonstrated by skin oxygen tension determinations and histological sections. *Circulation 29, Suppl. III:* 164

Transcutaneous pO_2 for Therapy Control in Mixed Connective Tissue Disease and Scleroderma

J. M. Steinacker, F. Nobbe

Mixed connective tissue disease (MCTD) is characterized by a combination of clinical symptoms similar to that of systemic lupus erythematosus, scleroderma, polymyositis and rheumatoid arthritis. The etiology of MCTD has not been clarified, but a number of immune aberrations have been found: high titers of nuclear ribonucleoprotein antigen, hypergrammaglobulinemia, suppressor T-cell defect, circulating immune complexes during active disease. There is a deposition of IgM and IgG within vascular walls and widespread lymphocytic and plasma cell infiltration of numerous tissues [5].

The primary event in scleroderma may be an endothelial cell injury in blood vessels ranging from small arteries to capillaries. The cause of this endothelial damage is not known. Hypergammaglobulinemia and antinuclear antibodies are frequent findings. The initial phase of sclerodermia is characterized by infiltration of the endothelium of small vessels, increased vascular permeability and edema, later followed by fibrosis [10].

Thromboangiitis obliterans (Buerger's disease) starts in the small arteries of the hands and feet. The initial inflammatory stage is later followed by arterial occlusion and fibrosis. In recent studies some abnormal immune responses were found in patients with Buerger's disease [9].

It is difficult to obtain a diagnosis in patients with small vessel disease because invasive and sensitive methods such as biopsies, arteriographies and immunological examinations are necessary. These methods mostly do not lend themselves to therapy control. Therefore, a non-invasive but sensitive method for measurement of tissue circulation would be helpful. Transcutaneous pO_2 is a method for measuring both arterial pO_2 and peripheral circulation [2, 3, 4, 6, 7]. The purpose of this study was to examine the possibilities of $tcpO_2$ measurements for therapy control in small vessel disease.

Method

We measured $tcpO_2$ in 10 patients with small vessel disease (mixed connective tissue disease [n=4], scleroderma [n=3], Buerger's disease [n=3]).

Clinical Oxygen Pressure Measurement II
A.M. Ehrly et al. (Eds.)
© Blackwell Ueberreuter Wissenschaft Berlin 1990

The diagnosis was made on the basis of case history, physical examination, laboratory, histological and immunological results. The lesions in the digital arteries were confirmed by arteriography.

Transcutaneous pO_2 was measured on the forearm, the hand and the finger of the patients before and during therapy. The electrode (Hellige Transoxode) was heated to 45°C and fixed with a self-adhesive ring. On the finger, the electrode was moulded in semi-elastic dental rubber, and reliable measurements were possible on the middle limb of the finger. The results were recorded after a heating period of 25 minutes during steady state of $tcpO_2$. At the same time p_aO_2 was determined in a capillary blood sample from the earlobe and a transcutaneous index $p_aO_2/tcpO_2$ was calculated [2, 6, 7]. Doppler pressure was recorded by a 8MHz unidirectional ultrasound probe by Doppler shift. A blood pressure cuff appropriate in size was attached around the limb (upper arm for brachial artery, forearm for ulnar and radial arteries, finger for digital arteries) and was inflated to suprasystolic levels. During the slow release of the cuff pressure the point of reoccurence of blood flow was taken as the systolic pressure in the artery [7, 10]. When necessary, the same procedure was applied to the lower limbs. Doppler pressure gradients were calculated as brachial-ankle pressure gradient (BAPD) and brachial-digital pressure gradient (BDPG). The Doppler index was calculated for each measurement as the ratio of local to brachial systolic blood pressure. Additionally, body plethysmography was performed in each patient.

Results

Fig. 1 shows values of a female patient of 45 years with MCTD. At first diagnosed as Raynaud's phenomenon, an angiography showed small forearm and lower leg arteries and stenosis in digital arteries. We decided first to try a hemorheological therapy with pentoxiphylline (Fig. 1, orhth) and during the next months the patient had no complaints.

Five months later, the patient came with a deep necrosis on the left big toe, small rat bite-like necrosis on some finger tips and blueish lips. First we carried out an isovolemic hemodilution and made infusions of dextrane and pentoxyphylline (Fig. 1, prhth), with only little improvement in all measured values. We found an increased blood sedimentation rate, antinuclear antibodies of speckle pattern, antibodies to microsomes and thyreoglobuline, slight hypergrammaglobulinemia, decreased renal clearance. The patient complained of athralgia and had swollen hands.

Both arterial pO_2 and peripheral $tcpO_2$ were decreased, pulmonary function was reduced (Fig. 1). These findings led to the diagnosis of MCTD, and we decided to make a trial with steroid therapy (Fig 1), which had significant effects on the patient's complaints, Doppler pressure, $tcpO_2$ and vital capacity. After reducing the dosis, clinical condition and values measured worsened initially, but after a second cycle, all values remained

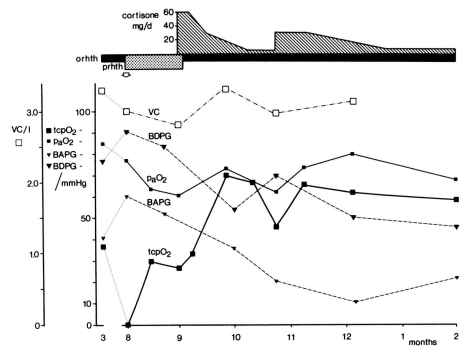

Fig 1. Transcutaneous pO₂ (tcpO₂), pₐO₂, brachial-digital Doppler pressure gradient BDPG, brachial-ankle Doppler pressure gradient BAPG and vital capacity VC during therapy in a 45 year old female patient with MCTD (orhth = oral rheological therapy, prhth = parenteral rheological therapy and hemodilution). For further explanation see text

nearly stable. The necrosis had healed and the patient was in fair condition.

In Fig. 2 tcpO₂ is plotted as a Box-and-Wisker-Plot for all patients for the forearm (2), the back of the hand (1), the finger (0) before (Fig. 2a) and during or after therapy (Fig. 2b). On the forearm tcpO₂ was 65.5 mmHg (s±11.3, n=26). The variance analysis showed significant differences in tcpO₂ depending on localization (p<0.0001) and a significant influence of therapy (p<0.05).

Transcutaneous index and Doppler index are plotted in Fig. 3 for all measured values. A hyperbolic dependency of tcpO₂ index on Doppler index can be seen, the correlation coefficient being 0.85.

Discussion

Transcutaneous pO₂ is non-invasive, objective and not dependent on the examiner, as is the case with Doppler methods [7, 10]. It is sensitive to cutaneous blood flow (CBF) and yields reliable data on the clinical con-

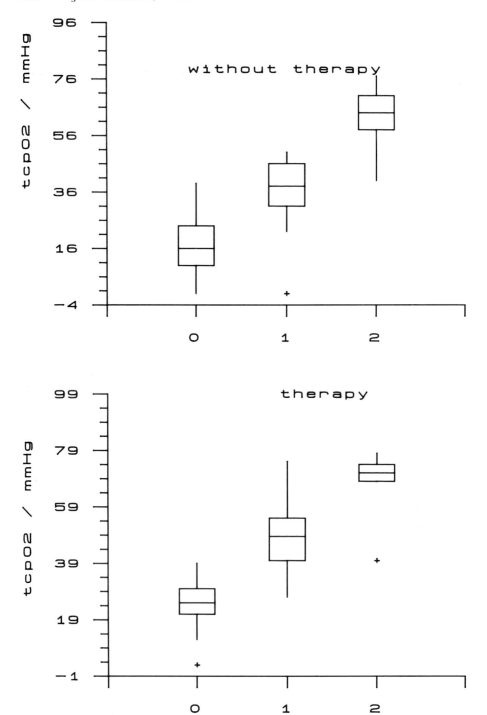

Fig 2. Transcutaneous pO$_2$ (tcpO$_2$) on the finger (0), the hand (1) and forearm (2) in 10 patients with small vessel disease before (left) and during or after therapy (right)

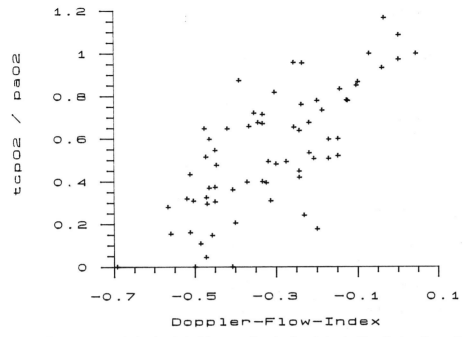

Fig 3. Transcutaneous index (tcpO₂/pₐO₂) versus Doppler-flow index in 10 patients with small vessel disease

dition of an immunologically induced small vessel disease as shown in Fig. 1. The therapy of immunologically induced vascular disease is a lengthy process [1, 5]. Sometimes therapeutical effects have to be "titrated" (Fig. 1). Transcutaneous pO₂ could be an important aid for the planning and evaluation of therapy in small vessel disease.

We had examined the blood flow dependency of tcpO₂ in another study [6, 8]. The heating power of the transcutaneous electrode and a Doppler flow signal showed a linear correlation to perfusion pressure and CBF. A hyperbolic dependence of transcutaneous pO₂ perfusion pressure and CBF was confirmed, such as has been proposed in the model of the circulatory hyperbola according to Lübbers and Huch [2, 3]. If there is high CBF under the electrode as is found in heat induced vasodilation at normal perfusion, tcpO₂ will reflect changes of pₐO₂ in the range of 70–100 % of normal perfusion pressure. If CBF is increasingly restricted, tcpO₂ will decrease and indicate changes in blood flow [2, 3, 6, 8]. The distal blood pressure gradient in the patients of this study with small vessel disease is demonstrated in Fig. 2 and is also of hyperbolic shape. These findings can be used in therapy control of vascular disorders. This was shown for arteriosclerosis obliterans [2, 4, 7]. This could also be the case in small vessel disease, where it is difficult to obtain any objective measurements of tissue blood flow and where the physician has to evaluate the therapy mostly on the basis of clinical findings.

References

1. Gilliland BC (1987) Progressive systemic sclerosis (diffuse scleroderma). In: Braunwald E et al. (eds) Harrison's principles of internal medicine, chap 264
2. Huch R, Huch A, Lübbers DW (1983) Transcutaneous pO_2. Thieme, Stuttgart
3. Lübbers DW, Grossmann U (1983) Gas exchange through human epidermis as a basis of $tcpO_2$ and $tcpCO_2$ measurements. In: Huch R, Huch A (eds) Continuous transcutaneous blood gas monitoring. M Deccer, Basel
4. Oghi S, Ito K, Mori T (1981) Quantitative evaluation of the skin circulation in ischemic legs by transcutaneous measurement of oxygen tension. Angiology 32:833
5. Sharp GC, Singsen BH (1984) Mixed connective tissue disease. In: McCarty DJ (ed) Arthritis and allied conditions. 10th ed., Lea & Febiger, chap 64
6. Steinacker JM, Spittelmeister W, Wodick RE (1987) Examinations on the blood flow dependence of $tcpO_2$ using the model of the "circulatory hyperbola". In: Huch A, Huch R, Rooth G (eds) Continuous transcutaneous monitoring. Adv Exp Med Biol, Plenum Press, New York, p 263
7. Steinacker JM, Brock F, Wodick RE, Nobbe F (1987) Control of the conservative therapy of arterial occlusive disease by means of transcutaneous pO_2 measurement. In: Ehrly AM, Hauss J, Huch R (eds) Clinical oxygen pressure measurement. Springer, Berlin, p 145
8. Steinacker JM, Spittelmeister W (1988) The dependence of transcutaneous pO_2 on cutaneous blood flow. J Appl Physiol 64:21
9. Steininger H (1985) Thrombangitis obliterans (Buerger's disease). Pathologe 6:204
10. Strandness DE, Summer DS (1975) Ultrasonic techniques in angiology. Huber, Bern

Transcutaneous pO$_2$-Measurement in Patients on Hemodialysis

N. Weindorf, U. Schultz-Ehrenburg, P. Altmeyer

Introduction

Chronic renal failure is known to induce disturbances in greater and smaller blood vessels. In 1977 Läppchen et al. found a higher incidence of Raynaud-phenomenon in comparison with controls (54 % versus 6 %). A higher calcification of the arteries in patients on dialysis (46 % versus 17 %) could be demonstrated by Renaud et al. (1985).

Previous ultrastructural studies performed by us on patients on dialysis revealed alterations in microcirculation such as multilamellar basement membranes and perivascular and pericollagenous deposits of an amyloid-like substance (Altmeyer et al. 1983). Further information could be obtained by immunostaining methods. Thus fibrinogen-positive deposits were found in the vessel walls, and beta$_2$-microglobulin deposits also in the surrounding tissue especially along the collagen fibers. These findings are of special importance because beta$_2$-microglobulin cannot be eliminated during hemodialysis, which may result in dialysis-specific amyloidosis (Ritz et al. 1988). These morphological changes can be expected to be accompanied or even preceeded by functional disturbances. In the present study we therefore examined the reactivity of cutaneous microcirculation to different stimulation tests using tcpO$_2$ measurements.

Patients and methods

We first performed a pilot test to determine the influence of the hemodialytic procedure itself. tcpO$_2$ was therefore measured in 3 patients before, during, and up to 1 hour after one dialytic treatment. We found no effect on the tcpO$_2$ values, providing blood pressure remained constant (Fig. 1).

We then performed a systematical functional study on a dialysis-free day with 13 patients on hemodialysis. The study included only patients without diabetes or longstanding hypertension. Their mean age was 46 years (ranging from 30 to 73 years), and they had been undergoing dialytic treatment for 0.5 to 14.5 years. Their mean hemoglobin value was 9.8 g%

Clinical Oxygen Pressure Measurement II
A. M. Ehrly et al. (Eds.)
© Blackwell Ueberreuter Wissenschaft Berlin 1990

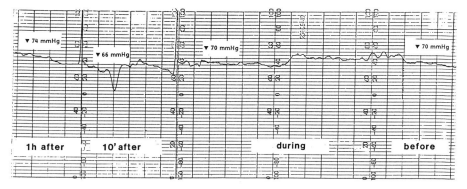

Fig. 1. Continuous tcpO₂ measurement before, during, 10 min and 1 h after one dialytic procedure; no change of the tcpO₂ values was observed

(ranging from 6.5 to 12.3 g%). The control group consisted of 15 healthy persons with a mean age of 48.3 years (ranging from 26 to 76 years). We used the apparatus of Radiometer, Copenhagen, with the Clark electrode E 5242. The electrode was heated to 37 °C and placed on the volar aspect of the forearm after stripping the horny layer 10 times. All subjects were studied in supine position at a room temperature of 24 – 28 °C. The following stimulation tests were applied:
– resting value (RV)
– postocclusive value (POV) after 4 min of ischemia using a sphygmo-manometer cuff
– rubefacient-induced value (RIV) after local application around the electrode of a commercially available ointment (Finalgon®, Thomae Company, FRG) containing nicotine acid butyl ester and nonylic acid vanillylamide
– 45 °C heating value (HV) after heating the electrode from 37 °C to 45 °C; this measurement was performed on the contralateral forearm because of the long-lasting hyperemia after application of the rubefacient.

Results

The results of all tcpO₂ measurements are shown in Table 1. Patients on hemodialysis displayed diminished tcpO₂ values for resting pO₂ and for all 3 stimulation tests, most clearly for the rubefacient-induced pO₂ value (patients 22.4 ±12.5 mmHg, controls 43.5 ±9.1. mmHg). As for the pO₂ increase, i.e. the difference between resting and stimulated pO₂ values, the rubefacient-induced hyperoxia for patients on hemodialysis was 19.1 ±13.0 mmHg, and for the controls 38.5 ±9.8 mmHg.

Table 1. Results of pO$_2$-measurement (x̄ ± SD in mmHg / kPa)

Stimulation test	Pat. on hemodialysis (n=13)	Controls (n=15)
Resting value (RV)	3.3 ± 4.0 / 0.4 ± 0.5	5.1 ± 4.1 / 0.7 ± 0.5
Postocclusive value (POV)	17.5 ± 5.4 / 2.3 ± 0.7	20.4 ± 8.6 / 2.7 ± 1.1
Rubefacient-induced value (RIV)	22.4 ± 12.5 / 3.0 ± 9.1	43.5 ± 9.1 / 5.8 ± 1.2
Heating value (HV)	97.1 ± 16.7 / 12.9 ± 2.2	102.0 ± 14.0 / 13.5 ± 1.9
Δ POV − RV	14.2 ± 4.7 / 1.9 ± 0.6	15.3 ± 4.5 / 2.0 ± 0.6
Δ RIV − RV	19.1 ± 13.0 / 2.5 ± 1.7	38.5 ± 9.8 / 5.1 ± 1.3
Δ HV − RV	93.3 ± 18.2 / 12.4 ± 2.4	97.0 ± 16.0 / 12.8 ± 2.1

Discussion

Patients on hemodialysis showed diminished tcpO$_2$ values for resting pO$_2$ and for all 3 stimulation tests. This is probably – to some extent at least – due to renal anemia diminishing all transcutaneously measured pO$_2$ values. Our patients too showed renal anemia with hemoglobin values from 6.5 to 12.3 g%. But besides anemia there must be other factors influencing the tcpO$_2$ values. For example, the curves on Fig. 2 represent a patient with a hemoglobin of 8.2 % and normal pO$_2$ values, whereas the curves on Fig. 3 represent a patient with a hemoglobin of 12.3 % but decreased rubefacient-induced and 45 °C heating values.

The 45 °C heating value gives information on the total capacity of the terminal vessels, because at this temperature the arterioles are maximally dilated. Therefore, a diminution of the 45 °C heating pO$_2$ can be regarded

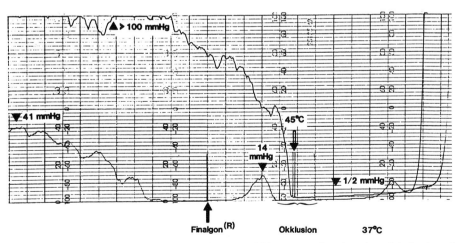

Fig. 2. tcpO$_2$ measurement on a male patient, aged 30 years and undergoing dialysis since 4 years; all tcpO$_2$ values are normal; simultaneous measurements on both arms

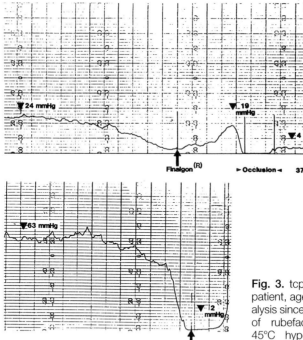

Fig. 3. tcpO$_2$ measurement on a female patient, aged 31 years and undergoing dialysis since 14.5 years; there is a decrease of rubefacient-induced hyperoxia and 45°C hyperoxia; successive measurements of both arms

as a sign of organic vessel wall changes. This is in good agreement with the morphological changes in patients on hemodialysis reported above.

The most striking result is the diminished rubefacient-induced hyperoxia which reaches only half the pO$_2$ value of the control group (22.4 ±12.5 mmHg versus 43.5 ±9.1 mmHg). This pO$_2$ value represents a pharmacological stimulation test which works by transcutaneous resorption and subsequent diffusion to the small vessels of the skin. Nicotonic acid as well as its various esters are widely used vasodilating agents. The mechanism of vasodilation is probably based on the release of prostaglandins, especially prostacyclin (Andersson et al. 1977). This is a typical endothelial cell function. Nonylic acid vanillylamide has vasodilating properties too. It probably works by stimulation of acetylcholine receptors of the endothelial cells (Crossland 1970). In a second step the endothelium-derived relaxing factor is released, leading to vasodilation (Furchgott and Zawadzki 1980). Thus, nicotinic acid butyl ester as well as nonylic acid vanillylamide induce actions which are mainly dependent on the endothelial cell function. Therefore, the rubefacient-induced pO$_2$ value can be regarded as an indicator of disturbances of the endothelial cell function. In comparison to diabetics, patients on hemodialyis show a different pattern of microangiopathy (Fig. 4). Diabetic patients displayed higher resting pO$_2$ values, probably as a result of reduced vasomotor tonus. They

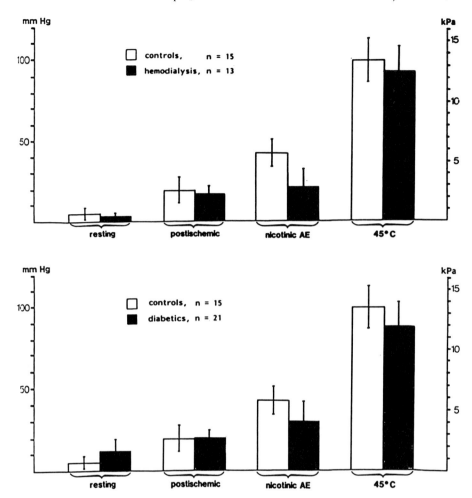

Fig. 4. Upper half: resting and stimulated pO$_2$ values in patients on hemodialysis and healthy controls. Lower half: resting and stimulated pO$_2$ values in in diabetics and the same control group as above

also had a lower total capacity, indicating that their organic vessel wall changes are more frequent resp. more severe than in patients on hemodialysis.

References

1. Altmeyer P, Kachel H-G, Runne U (1983) Mikroangiopathie, Bindegewebsveränderungen und amyloidartige Ablagerungen bei chronischer Niereninsuffizienz. Hautarzt 34:277
2. Andersson RGG, Aberg G, Brattsand R, Ericsson E, Lundholm L (1977) Studies on the mechanism of flush induced nicotine acid. Acta Pharmacol Toxicol 41:1

3. Crossland J (1970) Lewis' Pharmacology, Livingstone, Edinburgh
4. Furchgott RF, Zawadzki JV (1980) The obligatory role of endothelial cells in the relaxation of arterial smooth muscle by acetylcholine. Nature 288:373
5. Läppchen J, Ritz E, Koch A, Mörl H, Brommer J, Ossenkop Ch (1977) Raynaud-Phänomen bei Dialyse-Patienten. DMW 102:521
6. Renaud H, Attik H, Hervé M, Benelmouffok S, Galg C, Kambia B, Morrinière P, Fornier A (1985) Evaluation des facteurs favorisant la calcinose vasculaire des hémodialysés chroniques. Arch Mal Coeur 11:1696
7. Ritz E, Bommer J, Zeier M (1988) ß$_2$-Mikroglobulin-bedingte Amyloidose. DMW 113:190
8. Weindorf N, Schultz-Ehrenburg U, Altmeyer P (1987) Diagnostic assessment of diabetic microangiopathy by tcpO$_2$ stimulation tests. In: Huch A, Huch R, Rooth G (eds) Continuous transcutaneous monitoring. Plenum Publishing Corporation, New York

Influence of Erythropoietin on Transcutaneous Oxygen Pressure in Patients with Renal Anemia

A. Creutzig, L. Caspary

Introduction

Recombinant human erythropoietin (rh-EPO) therapy of chronic anemia due to end-stage renal disease may be complicated by the development of thrombosis and severe hypertension [1, 2, 3]. Acute elevation of hematocrit by transfusion in patients with renal anemia will be followed by a decrease in cardiac output and an increase in peripheral vascular resistance [4]. Up to now there is no knowledge about tissue oxygenation during rh-EPO therapy.

Patients and methods

We examined 14 patients (10 male and 4 female) with end-stage renal failure due to chronic glomerulonephritis (n=8), chronic interstitial nephritis (n=4) and primary malignant hypertension (n=2). Their median age was 48.5 years (ranging from 22 to 57 years). None suffered from diabetes mellitus or peripheral arterial occlusive disease. Seven patients were initially treated with antihypertensive drugs (beta-blockers and/or ACE inhibitors). After informed consent, they received rh-EPO intravenously three times weekly after dialysis (40-120 IU rh-EPO/kg body weight).

The following parameters were determined 12 – 20 h after the last dialysis: hemoglobin and hematocrit, blood pressure (Riva Rocci method), blood pressure in the tibial artery (Doppler method), and regional calf blood flow by strain gauge plethysmography (Periquant 3800, Gutmann, Eurasburg, FRG). The transcutaneous oxygen pressure (tcpO$_2$) was determined polarographically with commercially available electrodes (TCM 2, Radiometer, Copenhagen, Denmark) with a platinum wire of 25 µm in diameter covered by a polypropylen membrane. The patients were asked not to smoke for at least 12 hours before the examination, which took place in a well climatized room (22-23°C). They lay in a comfortable supine position for at least 30 mins before the measurements were started. First, tcpO$_2$ was measured with using 6 electrodes on both forefeet at an electrode core temperature of 37°C [5]. After 30 mins, resting values were

Clinical Oxygen Pressure Measurement II
A.M. Ehrly et al. (Eds.)
© Blackwell Ueberreuter Wissenschaft Berlin 1990

recorded. Then the patients were asked to stand for 5 mins to check for the orthostatic vasoconstrictor response. Then they moved back to the supine position. After recalibration the electrodes were run with a core temperature of 44°C. The whole procedure was repeated one week later, so that in all 12 tcpO$_2$ readings were obtained in every patient, which could then be averaged.

The patients were examined before rh-EPO treatment, 10-12 weeks and 22-24 weeks after beginning of treatment. For comparison, tcpO$_2$ values for 18 healthy subjects of median age 29 years (ranging from 21 to 49 years) are given.

Mean blood pressure was calculated as MAP = diastolic blood pressure + 1/3 (systolic – diastolic blood pressure) and peripheral vascular resistance as MAP/calf blood flow (mmHg/ml/min/100 ml tissue).

Results

Hemoglobin increased significantly within the first 10-12 weeks of rh-EPO therapy, and remained constant during the second period of 12 weeks. Correspondingly, hematocrit was elevated by about 50 % (see Table 1). Antihypertensive treatment had to be reinforced in 5 patients during the study. Under these conditions there were no significant changes in systolic, diastolic and tibial artery pressure (Table 1).

Table 1. Values given as x̄ ±SD; ** p<0.01; *** p<0.005; paired t-test

	prior to therapy		after 10–12 weeks therapy	after 22–24 weeks therapy
hemoglobin (g/dl)	6.7 ±1.0	***	10.4 ±1.4	10.4 ±1.1
hematocrit (%)	20.0 ±2.8	***	31.3 ±3.1	29.9 ±3.2
RR systolic (mmHg)	120 ±23		125 ±14	116 ±19
RR diastolic (mmHg)	75 ±15		80 ±13	77 ±13
tibial ankle pressure (mmHg)	163 ±26		157 ±21	153 ±25
regional calf blood flow (ml/100ml tissue)	4.5 ±2.1		3.2 ±1.5	2.5 ±0.9
peripheral vascular resistance (mmHg ml/min/100ml tissue)	15.6 ±5.5	***	31.0 ±21.3	35.4 ±14.1

Regional calf blood flow was significantly impaired by about 45 % during the observation period. Accordingly, the calculated peripheral vascular resistance more than doubled (Table 1).

Prior to therapy, tcpO$_2$ (37°C and 44°C) was significantly diminished compared to healthy volunteers. During treatment tcpO$_2$ (37°C) more than doubled and reached values within the normal range. tcpO$_2$ (44°C) increased by about 25 %, but nevertheless remained very significantly below that of healthy persons (Table 2).

Table 2. Transcutaneous oxygen pressure (tcpO$_2$) before and during rh-EPO treatment and in comparison to healthy volunteers. Values in mmHg, given as x̄ ±SD and medians; ** p<0.01; *** p<0.005; U-test

	healthy volunteers	prior to therapy	after 10–12 wks therapy	after 22–24 wks therapy
tcpO$_2$ (37°C)	5.6 ± 4.3 4.0 **	3.6 ± 3.8 2.0 ***	8.3 ± 6.9 6.0	7.9 ± 6.5 6.0
tcpO$_2$ (44°C)	62.8 ±10.9 62.0 ***	33.8 ±18.7 33.5 ***	42.2 ±15.8 43.5	42.9 ±16.2 44.0

During standing, an increase in tcpO$_2$ occurred significantly more often in patients than in probands (p<0.01, Chi-Square test). This was true for all measurements before and during rh-EPO therapy.

All parameters were again analysed in order to answer the question whether there existed detectable differences between the patients who needed reinforced antihypertensive treatment (n=5) and those who had a stable blood pressure during rh-EPO treatment (n=9). None of the parameters could discriminate between the two groups.

Discussion

Our investigation showed that despite a remarkable increase in peripheral vascular resistance skin oxygenation could be improved to a large extent by rh-EPO treatment. The increase in peripheral vascular resistance has already been described by Neff et al [4], who observed 6 patients with chronic renal failure during transfusion with packed blood cells up to a normal hematocrit level. One important contributing factor is the increase in whole blood viscosity due to the increase in total red cell mass. However, for a hematocrit below 30 %, which was present in our patients, the influence on whole blood viscosity was shown to be small [6]. Another influencing mechanism is the fact that improvement in tissue oxygenation increases vascular tone. It could be shown that hypoxia leads to vasodilatation, which is probably locally regulated by vasoactive mediators and is reversible after restoration of normal oxygen supply [7, 8].

Measurements of tcpO$_2$ revealed severe disturbances of skin microcirculation in these patients. TcpO$_2$, which is mainly influenced by skin capillary perfusion, was markedly diminished. In addition, hyperemia microcirculatory flow (tcpO$_2$ 44°C) was also reduced. Partial correction of anemia leads to normal tcpO$_2$ values at 37°C, whereas tcpO$_2$ at 44°C remains reduced compared to non-anemic persons. The increase in tcpO$_2$ at 37°C was much more pronounced than the increase in hematocrit. So we presume that there is a real improvement in skin microcirculation: probably a maldistribution of skin blood flow, which is described for muscle perfusion in patients with renal anemia and for muscle and skin perfusion in patients with peripheral arterial occlusive disease, is influenced favorably [9, 11]. There was a high incidence of pathological response to orthostasis in our patients. Standing normally leads to a vasoconstriction which can be monitored as a decrease in tcpO$_2$ (37°C) at the forefoot level [5, 12]. The frequent tcpO$_2$ increase in patients with renal anemia, which to our knowledge has for the first time been described in this study, may be regarded as a conseqence of bad tissue oxygenation. Remarkably, the incidence of this pathological reaction did not decrease in the course of treatment. We can speculate that this phenomenon in patients with renal anemia is not regulated by the level of tissue oxygenation but by metabolic mediators.

Measurement of tissue pO$_2$ could be one method to determine the optimal hematocrit in rh-EPO therapy. From experimental studies with hemodilution we know that from the rheological point of view a hematocrit of 30 % would be preferable [6]. This is the reason why we aimed at this value in our study. Probably repeated tcpO$_2$ determinations in the course of rh-EPO therapy could help find the optimal individual hematocrit.

Acknowledgements. We gratefully acknowledge the excellent cooperation with Dr. B. Nonnast-Daniel and Prof. Dr. J. Bahlmann (Dept. of Nephrology, MHH). We are indebted to Mrs. I. Kiegeland and Mrs G. Krause for their technical assistance and to Mrs. C. Glasser for preparing the manuscript.

References

1. Winearls CG, Oliver DO, Pippard MJ, Reid C, Downing MR, Cores PM (1986) Effects of human erythropoietin derived from recombinant DNA on the anemia of patients maintained by chronic haemodialysis. Lancet 1175
2. Eschbach JW, Joan MD, Egrie C, Downing MR, Browne JK, Adamson JW (1987) Correction of anemia of end-stage renal disease with recombinant human erythropoietin. New Engl J Med 316:73
3. Samtleben W, Baldamus CA, Bommer J, Fassbinder W, Nonnast-Daniel B, Gurland HJ (1988) Blood pressure changes during treatment with recombinant human erythropoietin. In: Koch KM, Kühn K, Nonnast-Daniel B (eds) Treatment of renal anemia with recombinant human erythropoietin. Karger, Basel, p 114
4. Neff MS, Kim KE, Persoff M, Onesti G, Schwartz C (1971) Hemodynamics of uremic anemia. Circulation 43:876

5. Creutzig A, Dau D, Caspary L, Alexander K (1987) Transcutaneous oxygen pressure measured at two different electrode core temperatures in healthy volunteers and patients with arterial occlusive disease. Int J Microcirc Clin Exp 5:373
6. Messmer K, Sunder-Plassmann L, Klövekorn WP, Holper K (1972) Circulatory significance of hemodilution: Rheological changes and limitations. Adv Microcirc 4:1
7. Duling BR, Berne RM (1970) Longitudinal gradients in periarteriolar oxygen tension: A possible mechanism for the participation of oxygen in local regulation of blood flow. Circulation Res 27:669
8. Duling BR, Pittmann RN (1975) Oxygen tension: Dependent or independent variable in local control of blood flow? Fed Proc 34:2012
9. Saborowski F, Kessler M, Höper J, Greitschus F, Rath K, Dickmans HA, Thiele KG (1983) Skeletal muscle oxygen pressure in patients with chronic renal insufficiency. In: Ehrly AM (ed) Determination of tissue oxygen pressure in patients. Pergamon, Oxford, p 79
10. Creutzig A, Wrabetz W, Lux M, Alexander K (1985) Muscle tissue oxygen pressure in patients with arterial occlusive disease. Microvasc Res 29:350
11. Creutzig A, Caspary L, Alexander K (1988) Disturbances of skin microcirculation in patients with chronic arterial occlusive disease and venous incompetence. Vasa 17:77
12. Eickhoff J, Henriksen O (1985) Local regulation of subcutaneous forefoot blood flow during orthostatic changes in normal subjects, in sympathetically denerved patients and in patients with occlusive arterial disease. Cardiovasc Res 19:219

On the Differences between Muscle pO_2 Measurements Obtained with Hypodermic Needle Probes and with Multiwire Surface Probes

W. Fleckenstein, A. Schäffler, R. Heinrich, C. Petersen, M. Günderoth-Palmowski, G. Nollert

Part 1: Differences between Tissue pO_2 and Tissue Surface pO_2 Observed in Dog Gracilis Muscle

Introduction

Reviewing available data, pO_2 histograms from the inner parts of tissues do not agree with those from tissue surfaces even when measured under equal experimental or clinical conditions (Schäffler 1987). Authors using multiwire pO_2 probes, according to Kessler and Grunewald (1969), observed only in a few cases low pO_2 values from muscle surfaces under physiological conditions. In contrast, within the muscle tissue, pO_2 values below 5 mmHg were frequently recorded when applying needle probes (according to Baumgärtl and Lübbers 1973, Ehrly and Schroeder 1977, Fleckenstein 1982, Kunze 1966, Silver 1965, Whalen et al. 1967). If available myoglobin oxygen saturation data are taken into account (Gayeski 1981; Gayeski et al. 1985), low pO_2 values also are to be expected under physiological conditions in resting gracilis muscle of dog.

In order to obtain information about the relation between muscle pO_2 values and the pO_2 values on its surface, we registered pO_2 histograms from gracilis muscles of beagle dogs simultaneously with needle probes and surface probes.

Materials and methods

The eight beagle dogs under examination (b.w. 10.41 ± 1.4 kg), were initially anaesthetized using 3 mg/kg Methohexitale and intubated. Narcosis was maintained by N_2O, Fentanyl ($15\ \mu g\ kg^{-1}h^{-1}$) and Pancuronium ($0.1\ mg\ kg^{-1}h^{-1}$). Rectal temperature was regulated at $36.9 \pm 0.4°C$ by a thermoregulated operating table. Endtidal pCO_2, acid/base, glucose and electrolyte values were controlled and kept at physiological levels. Loss of fluid was measured and substituted.

Before preparations, the volume of the shaved hind legs (distal of a plane given by ischiadic tuber, trochanter major and anterior inferior iliac spine)

Clinical Oxygen Pressure Measurement II
A.M. Ehrly et al. (Eds.)

was determined according to the Archimedian principle. Femoral artery and vein were cannulated and connected to pressure transducers; arterial flow in femoral artery was measured by an electromagnetic flow probe; O_2 content was determined in blood samples from femoral artery and vein. Thus the O_2 uptake of the hind limb could be determined and referred to the volume of hind limb tissue.

The animals were ventilated during the first three hours of the experiment with a gas mixture of 75% N_2O and 25% O_2 (phase 1). During the subsequent period of two hours, the fraction of inspired oxygen (FiO_2) was increased to 0.4 (phase 2), followed by a period of two hours at an FiO_2 of 0.9 (phase 3). The arterial pO_2 values during phase 1 were at 118 ± 14 mmHg, during phase 2 at 228 ± 20 mmHg and during phase 3 at 468 ± 39 mmHg. In four of the eight experiments, room temperature was regulated (at 50% relative air humidity) in order to keep the skin temperature 1-2 mm below the surface and at a distance of 2 cm from the gracilis muscle at a constant value of 29 ± 0.83 °C ("cold-skin-experiments"); during the other four experiments, the skin temperature in the same position was kept at 34 ± 0.94°C ("warm-skin-experiments") also by climatising the air of the room (relative humidity 50%). During the warm and the cold experiments, rectal temperature was kept nearly at the same level (37.1 ± 0.34°C). The mean muscle temperature, measured from the muscle surface during the cold experiments (34.2 ± 0.47°C), was only 0.6 ± 0.35°C below the mean temperature during the warm experiments; temperatures were measured simultaneously with muscle pO_2.

In Fig.1, the situs of the simultaneous pO_2 histogram determination is schematically shown. In order to dissect the free gracilis muscle, the skin of the inner thigh was incised to a length of 8 cm. For each series of 3 subsequent pO_2 histogram determinations with the surface probe, a muscle area of 2 – 4 cm² was freshly prepared; fascia, epimysial and peri-

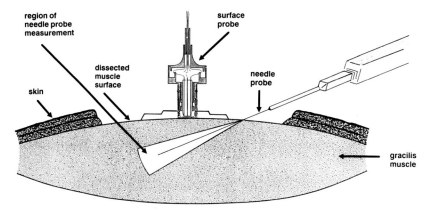

Fig. 1. Situs of simultaneous pO_2 histogram determination, schematically: gracilis muscle with a multiwire surface pO_2 probe (of the MDO type) and an inserted hypodermic needle probe. Before and during the measurements the edges of the wound were adapted by a reversible continued suture (not shown)

mysial connective tissue layers were removed under microscopic control; any bleeding or irritation of the muscle surface was avoided. After positioning of the surface probe (suspended on a micromanipulator) the edges of the wound were adapted by a reversible continued suture. Thus the suture could be easily opened in order to displace the probe, or slackly closed in order to protect the muscle surface against drying and cooling before and during the measurements of muscle temperature and pO_2. Most of the time during the experiments the suture was kept closed.

The hypodermic needle pO_2 probe was inserted into the muscle through the scision of the skin at a flat angle (of 10°-20°) to the long axis of the muscle fibres. The distance between tissue, from which pO_2 values were taken by the needle probe, and the surface probe, was kept shorter than 1.5 cm. The determination of one pair of histograms, comprising a histogram from the surface (with at least 100 single pO_2 values) and a histogram from the inner of the muscle (with at least 200 single pO_2 values), took 20 minutes. After each pair of histograms the O_2 content in blood samples from femoral artery and vein were determined. During each of the phases – each lasting at least 2 hrs – at constant FiO_2 at least 4 pairs of simultaneous histograms were taken.

After the final phase (3) of the experiments, a flat strip (2 cm x 2 cm x 0.3 cm) of the muscle tissue which was last in contact with the surface probe was rapidly excised and fixated. During these procedures the muscle strip was kept expanded to its in-situ length. The methods of preparation, fixation and histological examination were equivalent to those reported by Schramm et al. elsewhere (in this book).

The surface probe measurements were carried out with the "M.I.T. -pO_2 Meß-System" (mfg. by Bruins Instruments, Puchheim, FRG) and with an 8-wire multiwire polarographic surface probe of the Clark-type, known as "MDO probe" (mfg. by Eschweiler u. Co., Kiel, FRG). For the pO_2 measurements with needle probes, a "KIMOC® Gewebe pO_2-Histograph" was applied (mfg. by GMS, Gesellschaft für Medizinische Sondentechnik, Kiel-Mielkendorf, FRG) using polarographic, fast responding hypodermic needle pO_2 probes. Surface and needle probes were calibrated in an unstirred physiological saline solution, saturated with air or N_2 (99.996%) repectively. All tissue pO_2 data were corrected for the temperature differences between muscle tissue and the calibration solution. Temperatures of the skin, of the gracilis muscle and of the rectum were determined by thermocouples.

Results

On the left side of Fig.2, all pO_2 data (regardless of skin temperature) obtained within the tissue by needle probe are pooled from all dogs in histograms. Data from each of the three experimental phases are pooled in three separate histograms; on the right side, the correspondingly pooled pO_2 data of simultaneous surface measurements are shown. In

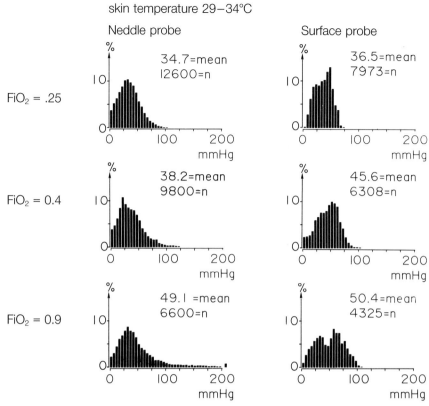

skin temperature 29–34°C

Neddle probe

Surface probe

FiO₂ = .25   34.7=mean   12600=n   36.5=mean   7973=n

FiO₂ = 0.4   38.2=mean   9800=n   45.6=mean   6308=n

FiO₂ = 0.9   49.1 =mean   6600=n   50.4=mean   4325=n

Fig. 2. Pooled histograms of pO₂ data which were simultaneously obtained from gracilis muscle of 8 dogs at different fractions of inspired oxygen (FiO₂). Data from the warm and cold skin experiments are pooled together. Upper row: ventilation with 25% O₂; middle row: ventilation with 40% O₂; lower row: ventilation with 90% O₂. Histograms of the left column were obtained by hypodermic needle probes, histograms of the right column by surface multiwire probes

both methods, an increase of the mean tissue pO₂ was observed when arterial pO₂ was increased. The mean values of the 145 pairs of simultaneously determined single histograms were significantly correlated (Mann-Whitney-U-test with z-transformation). At first glance, mean pO₂ values from tissue and from tissue surface seemed to be in the same range; means of histograms obtained by needle probes are slightly lower in Fig.2. However, the correspondence of mean pO₂ values obtained by the two methods is missing if pO₂ data are pooled taking into account the temperature of skin (Figs. 3, 4).

In order to show the effect of skin temperature on pO₂ within and on the surface of the muscle (at almost unchanged muscle temperature; see methods), all pO₂ data from the "warm-skin-experiments" (34°C) are pooled and compared to corresponding data from the "cold-skin-experiments" (29°C) (Fig. 3). Obviously the mean pO₂ values obtained by needle probes

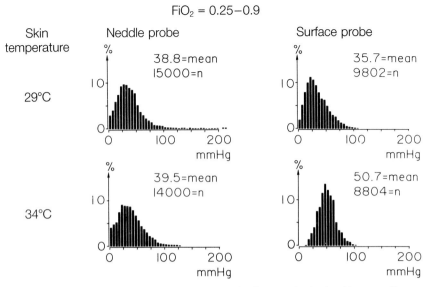

Fig. 3. Pooled histograms of pO₂ data which were simultaneously obtained from gracilis muscle of two groups of dogs, each of the groups with different temperatures of skin but nearly equal temperatures of rectum and muscle. Data obtained during phases of different levels of arterial pO₂ are pooled together. Upper row: temperature of the skin of the inner thigh laid at 29°C (data from 4 dogs); lower row: skin temperature was 34°C (data from 4 dogs). Histograms of the left column were obtained by hypodermic needle probes, histograms of the right column by surface multiwire probes

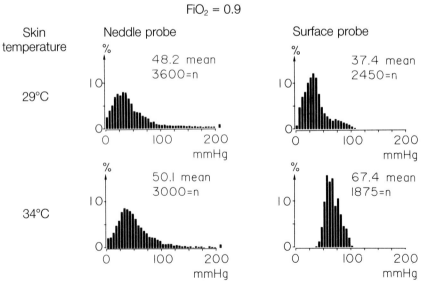

Fig. 4. Histograms calculated in an equal manner as in Fig.3; however, only pO₂ data obtained during arterial hyperoxia are pooled in these histograms

were only minimally influenced by skin temperature. In contrast, the mean pO_2 values from the muscle surface were significantly correlated to skin temperature although muscle surface temperature was practically at the same level during cold and warm skin experiments. Surprisingly, the mean surface pO_2 distribution was more elevated by the increase in skin temperature from 29 to 34°C (see Fig.3, right column) than by an increase in arterial pO_2 from 118 mmHg to 468 mmHg (see Fig.2, right column). In Fig.4 the effect of skin temperature on mean pO_2 within and on top of the muscle is shown during the third experimental phase (at an FiO_2 of 0.9). As can be seen (by a comparison of Figs. 2, 3, 4), during the cold-skin-experiments the mean pO_2 of muscle surface was almost unchanged despite of the dramatic change in mean arterial pO_2 value. In contrast to this, during the warm-skin-experiments, the mean surface pO_2 was highly dependent on the arterial pO_2. In Fig.4 it can once more be seen that the mean pO_2 of the inner parts of the muscle is practically independent of skin temperature.

During the warm-skin-experiments, the mean femoral flow was increased by 18.2% in comparison to the cold-skin-experiments; also, the mean values in femoral O_2 delivery (+3.9%), the hind limb O_2 uptake (+12.3%), the hind limb O_2 extraction (+4.2%) and the femoral arteriovenous difference in O_2 content (+6.6%) were slightly higher during the warm-skin-experiments. The mean vascular resistance of hind limbs was reduced by 15.7% during the warm-skin-experiments. The mean values of femoral perfusion pressure, acid/base status and blood gases were independent of the skin temperature.

The scatter of the single pO_2 values around the mean value in each of the individual histograms was formally described by means of the standard deviation of the pO_2 values. Mean values and the standard deviations of the so determined scatters are shown in Fig.5. In Fig.5 arterial pO_2 values

Fig. 5. Mean values of the standard deviations of the single pO_2 histograms determined during each of the experimental phases; 145 pairs of simultaneously obtained single histograms are evaluated. Left side: data obtained by surface probe; right side: data obtained by needle probes

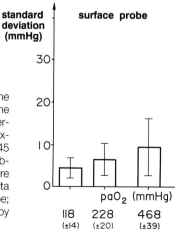
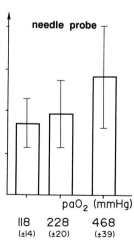

and methods of pO_2 measurement are regarded. As can be seen from the figure, the (above-defined) scatter of pO_2 values was markedly (by a factor of up to 4) higher in the pO_2 measurements performed by needle probes. The difference of the scatter is more evident at high arterial pO_2 values. The higher scatter of histograms determined within the muscle can also be seen clearly, comparing the pooled pO_2 histograms from the warm-skin-experiments (Fig.4, lower row). On the surface no values above 105 mmHg or below 40 mmHg were registered although mean arterial pO_2 was at 468 mmHg (Fig.4). In the pooled histograms of Fig.2 the method-dependent scatter-differences cannot clearly be seen because in Fig.2, pO_2 data are pooled regardless of the skin temperature.

In Table 1 numerical data of the histograms from Fig.2 are listed. Only 1.1% of the surface pO_2 values were below 5 mmHg. In contrast, within the muscle 3.5% of values were below 5 mmHg. That difference was qualitatively observed during each of the three experimental phases and most evident in warm skin experiments.

Table 1. Numerical data of histograms that are shown in Fig. 2

	needle probe				surface probe			
FiO$_2$	n	mean mmHg	SD mmHg	rel. frequ. <5 mmHg	n	mean mmHg	SD mmHg	rel. frequ. <5 mmHg
0.25	12600	34.7	17.1	3.7 %	7973	36.5	4.7	0.2 %
0.40	9800	38.2	19.2	3.8 %	6308	45.6	6.6	2.3 %
0.90	6600	49.1	24.6	2.4 %	4325	50.4	9.5	0.9 %
0.25...0.9	29000	39.2	20.4	3.5 %	18606	42.8	6.4	1.1 %

n: number of local pO_2 measurements; mean: mean of local pO_2 values; SD: mean of scatters (standard deviations) of single histograms which are comprised in the pooled histogram; rel. frequ. <5 mmHg: relative frequency of pO_2 values below 5 mmHg

Sixteen histological sections of muscle surfaces which had been (not longer than 30 min before fixation) in contact with the surface probe were examined. In Fig.6 typical sections and a control section are shown. The connective tissue layers on the surface had thicknesses between 10 and 180 µm (mean: 82 ± 32 µm). In all areas of probes' contact necrotic muscle fibres were seen in the uppermost muscle cell layer. In the area of contact interstitial edema and dilated capilliaries were seen within some upper cell layers. In most preparations erythrocytes and granulocytes were detected in extravascular positions within the superficial cell layers.

Discussion

The results of pO_2 measurements from surfaces and inner parts of dog gracilis muscle do not agree. The most important aspect of this discre-

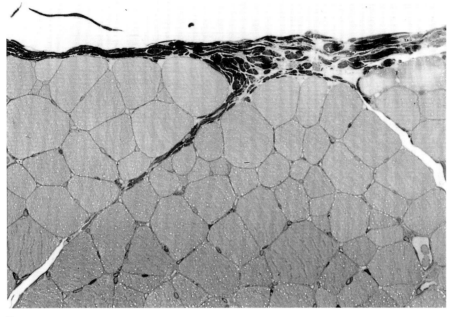

a

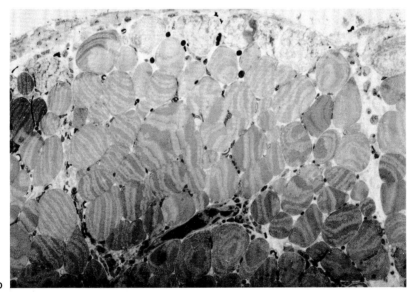

b

Fig. 6a-c. Sections of dog gracilis muscle surfaces (stained according to Richardson): **a)** muscle surface that had no contact with a surface probe, fixated 30 min after removal of fascia and epimysial and perimysial connective tissue. Due to the relief of muscle bundles, the thickness of the superficially left connective tissue layer is locally varied up to a factor of 5. **b)** and **c)**: muscle surfaces fixated 30 min after start of a continued contact between a measuring multiwire surface probe and the tissue. Tissue damage can be derived from dilation of vessels, cell immigration, interstitial edema and fibre necrosis in the uppermost cell layer(s)

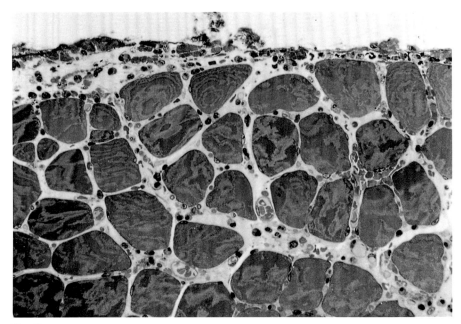

Fig. 6c

pancy is the marked influence of the skin temperature on the mean surface pO_2 value. Changes of skin temperature by 5°C, at almost constant temperature of muscle and muscle surface, have more influence on the mean surface pO_2 than switching the O_2 content of inspired gas from 25% to 90%. In contrast, skin temperature changes between 29°C and 34°C have practically no influence on the mean pO_2 within the muscle.

The measurements were performed by two independent teams; each of the teams had been practicing "their" method on muscle tissue for 5 years. So a lack of technical skill in the application of the compared methods can be excluded as a reason for the observed discrepancies.

Our results show that the mean pO_2 values obtained by the two methods could only lead to comparable data if the thermal conditions during the surface measurements were well defined and correlated to skin temperature effects. These effects may possibly be manifested to a different degree in other species and muscles. In practice, it seems to be unrealistic that thermal conditions of clinical surface measurements can be sufficiently standardised in order to allow a direct comparison between the absolute mean values obtained in different examinations. The wide range of muscle surface pO_2 values reported by different groups examining comparable clinical situations (Schäffler 1987), could be partly explained by differences in thermal conditions.

The histological examination of muscle surfaces which were fixated (at in-situ lengths) not later than 30 min after contact with the surface probe showed interstitial edema, dilated capillaries and microvessels as well as damaged muscle fibres in the superficial cell layers. First signs of an inflammatory reaction could be seen. It can certainly be doubted whether the regulation of local blood flow corresponds to physiological conditions within the tissue area that has contact to the surface probe. Particularly the dilation of capillaries suggests that, near the surface probe, the capillary flow rates are not regulated to the local demand and in accordance with the normal blood flow regulation within the tissue. This hypothesis is supported by the observation that the 18% increase in femoral flow attending the skin temperature elevation leads (at FiO$_2$ of 0.9) to an increase in mean surface pO$_2$ reading by 80%, whereas the muscle pO$_2$ was increased by only 4%.

The histological finding of an interstitial edema leads us to the assumption that the distribution of the local O$_2$ diffusion coefficients within the surface layer attached to the probe does not correspond to physiological conditions. The histological finding of single fibre necrosis within the superficial cell layer inevitably leads to the assumption that the spacial pattern of O$_2$ uptake is also disturbed under the surface probe. It is reasonable to assume that the O$_2$ uptake of severely damaged fibres is reduced. If so, the pO$_2$ gradients as observed physiologically within the muscle tissue are levelled out at that surface, and mean O$_2$ consumption within that muscle surface is reduced. Any tissue pO$_2$ distribution is determined by the local balances of local O$_2$ delivery and local O$_2$ consumption values; hence an unphysiological pattern of local O$_2$ consumption and local perfusion leads to artificial pO$_2$ distributions. If the mean O$_2$ uptake of tissue surface is reduced, the mean surface pO$_2$ is increased. According to this hypothesis it could also be explained that the mean pO$_2$ value at the surface, attached to the multiwire probe, is more elevated than the mean pO$_2$ value within the tissue at higher femoral flow rates .

If the histological findings are not taken into account, the pO$_2$ increase, due to elevation of skin temperature, could be explained by a thermoreflectory hyperemia within superficial muscle layers; however, no experimental evidence has been reported showing differences in the regulation of perfusion between the surface and inner parts of muscle in the course of thermoregulation.

Comparison of the widths of the scatter of pO$_2$ values around the mean values obtained by surface and needle measurements shows marked differences (Figs. 3–5, Table 1). High and low values in the histograms of surface measurements are missing. It is hard to explain why an arterial hyperoxia of 468 mmHg should not lead to at least a few high pO$_2$ values of over 105 mmHg at the muscle surface (as they are observed within the tissue). On the other hand, the frequency of low pO$_2$ values was also significantly reduced at the surface, even when mean pO$_2$ values (in cold-skin-experiments) at the surface were below mean values within the muscle. Most studies on pO$_2$ distributions with microneedle probes show a wide range of distribution of pO$_2$ values, e.g. from below 1 mmHg to 110 mmHg in the tibialis anterior muscle of healthy volunteers (Kunze 1969[a]).

pO_2 values below 10 mmHg were frequently measured in most experimental studies on skeletal muscle with pO_2 needle probes (e.g. Ehrly and Schroeder 1977, Kunze 1966, Kunze 1969[a], Kunze 1969[b], Schroeder et al. 1976, Whalen et al. 1976) as well as with O_2 microtonometers (Piiper 1985). Sunder-Plasmann (1981) stated that the pO_2 histogram of most organs reveals a considerable frequency of pO_2 values in the range of $0-5$ mmHg. Lübbers (1981) reported that when using microneedle probes very low pO_2 values are frequently obtained from tissue showing no signs of impairment of the O_2 supply. Low pO_2 data as measured by needle probes are in agreement with results of spectrophotometric measurements of myoglobin oxygen saturation in dog gracilis muscle (Gayeski 1981, Gayeski et al. 1985). Hence, pO_2 values below 5 mmHg are to be expected under our experimental conditions in resting gracilis muscle of dog.

From the available evidence and from our data, we can conclude that surface probe measurements lead to pO_2 distributions which do not show the correct frequency of the low tissue pO_2 values. This "systematic error" of surface pO_2 measurement can be explained at the low value edge of the distributions by the histologically observed fibre necrosis, coupled with a reduction in O_2 consumption in the damaged superficial cell layer.

However, none of the histological findings discussed so far can explain the absence of extreme values at the high end (the right tail) in surface pO_2 distributions. High pO_2 values near the arterial pO_2 are to be expected in the adjacency of the arterial end of capillaries (e.g. Grunewald and Sowa 1977). In this and in another study (Fleckenstein and Petersen, this book), carried out with pO_2 needle probes in the femoral quadriceps muscle of man and in the gracilis muscle of dog, it was shown that the highest pO_2 values of a tissue pO_2 histogram are sensitive to arterial hyperoxia; at a mean arterial pO_2 of 470 mmHg, 1% out of 6600 pO_2 values recorded by needle probes from dog gracilis muscle was found to lie above 200 mmHg. Authors of surface probe measurements emphasize that a muscle surface must be prepared in such a manner that no bleeding or damaging of the muscle surface occurs (Hauss et al. 1982). In order to achieve this it is necessary to leave some connective tissue on the fibres; in our examination, the thickness of this layer varied between 10 and 180 μm (mean 82 μm); the scatter of the local thicknesses of remaining connective tissue is dependent on the "microroughness" of the superficial relief of the muscle fibres (see Fig.6a). Authors using the surface probe method showed that the capture radius of pO_2 measurement around the single pO_2 measuring wire ends (of the surface probe) is at approx. 25 μm. If so, the surface probe measures the pO_2 distribution within the connective tissue layer which lies between the muscle tissue and the probes' membrane. The O_2 uptake and the capillarisation of connective tissue lie far below that of muscle. So, this layer can be regarded as a diffusion barrier with negligible O_2 uptake; therefore, we call this diffusion membrane the "inert layer". The 2-dimensional pO_2 distribution, which is located directly on the surface of the muscle fibres, is "projected" into this inert layer by diffusion.

Since O_2 diffusion is a 3-dimensional process this "projection" within the inert layer not only leads to O_2 diffusion directed perpendicularly to the muscle surface but also horizontally. So the extremely high and low pO_2 values at the muscle cell surfaces that are adjacent to the inert layer can be levelled out by horizontal diffusion within the inert layer. This hypothe-this can plausibly explain the absence of high and also of low pO_2 values in pO_2 histograms obtained by multiwire surface probes. In part 2 of this paper mathematic modelling is performed in order to examine the quan-titative influence of the thickness of an inert layer, and of the pO_2 gradients located directly at the muscle cell surfaces, on pO_2 histograms obtained by surface probes.

Conclusions

Mean values of simultaneous pO_2 measurements performed by needle probe and by surface multiwire probes (MDO-probes) do not lead to the same absolute values.

In contrast to needle pO_2 measurements, the mean values and distribu-tions of surface pO_2 measurements are markedly influenced by changes in the temperature of the skin even if the temperature of the muscle surface is nearly constant.

Histological findings from the contact area between surface probes and muscle tissue suggest that surface histograms do no represent tissue pO_2 distributions of a physiologically regulated microcirculation; the local pat-terns of O_2 diffusion conductivity, O_2 consumption and O_2 delivery values within the superficial tissue layer are most probably severely disturbed. The strong dependency of mean pO_2 values obtained by surface probes on skin temperature and femoral flow rates can be explained by that tissue damage at the site of measurement.

In pO_2 histograms taken from muscle surfaces, the relative frequencies of high and low pO_2 values are markedly underestimated; it is hypothesised that this error is a systematic one; that artifact could be caused by O_2 diffusion in a horizontal direction within a thin connective tissue layer located between the muscle cell surface and the probes' membrane.

For references see part 2 of the study.

On the Differences between Muscle pO$_2$ Measurements Obtained with Hypodermic Needle Probes and with Multiwire Surface Probes

W. Fleckenstein, A. Schäffler, R. Heinrich, G. Nollert

Part 2: A Systematic Diffusion Error of the Multiwire Surface pO$_2$ Probe when Applied on Tissue

Introduction

Muscle pO$_2$ measurements with multiwire surface probes are carried out on surgically exposed muscle surfaces; in order to avoid bleeding or damage of muscle surfaces, which are well known to be adverse to surface measurements, a thin layer of connective tissue must be left on the muscle fibres.

In Part 1 of the study it was shown that the frequencies of high and low pO$_2$ values of muscle tissue are underestimated if the tissue pO$_2$ distribution is determined by a multiwire surface probe. It was suggested that this error is due to an O$_2$ diffusion process within a superficial layer of tissue; this layer lies between the uppermost layer of oxygen metabolizing muscle fibres and the probes' membrane and was called "inert layer". Our hypothesis was that oxygen within the inert layer – in contrast to muscle tissue – is virtually not consumed and that the tissue volume from which pO$_2$ measurements are taken by the surface probe is restricted to the inert layer. The radius of pO$_2$ catchments of the surface probes electrodes lies at 25 μm, and the mean thickness of the low O$_2$ consuming connective tissue layer exceeds that catchment radius manifold. Therefore both prerequisites of our hypothesis seem to be fulfilled.

Necrosis of muscle fibres, observed under the surface probe on top of the muscle, leads to the assumption that the "inert" layer of low O$_2$ consumption can be even thicker than the uppermost connective tissue layer.

In this study, O$_2$ diffusion within an inert layer is calculated by modelling. The influence of the thickness of the inert layer on the pO$_2$ distribution that is "projected" from the metabolically active muscle cells into the pO$_2$ catchment area of the surface probe is evaluated. The model enables us to estimate direction and amount of O$_2$ diffusion within the inert layer at steady state conditions of diffusion. Calculations are carried out regarding thicknesses of the inert layer between 12.5 and 200 μm. In order to estimate the contribution of the oxidative metabolic activity of tissue to the error of surface pO$_2$ measurements, mean tissue pO$_2$ gradients of 4.3 mmHg/40 μm, of 7.7 mmHg/40 μm and of 12.6 mmHg/40 μm are ex-

Clinical Oxygen Pressure Measurement II
A. M. Ehrly et al. (Eds.)
© Blackwell Ueberreuter Wissenschaft Berlin 1990

amined. Modelling is made assuming tissue normoxia as well as tissue hypoxia.

Methods

In Fig. 1, the tissue model is outlined. O_2 diffusion from a border plane – the uppermost O_2 metabolizing muscle cell layer – into the inert tissue layer was calculated. For simplification it was assumed that no O_2 metabolism is present within the inert layer; additionally, the O_2 diffusion coefficient and the O_2 solubility were assumed to be homogeneous within it. The border plane consisted of narrow strips of high pO_2 (O_2 sources) alternating with broader strips of lower pO_2 (O_2 sinks). O_2 sources represented capillary properties whereas O_2 sinks represented properties of O_2 consuming muscle cells lying between the capillaries. The pO_2 field of the border plane qualitatively represented a pO_2 field which could be obtained on a surface of intersection of Krogh' cylinders cut in half, and arranged side by side (see Fig. 1). The mean distance between capillaries was assumed to be 80 μm (Kunze 1969 [a]).

According to the spectrum of pO_2 values in Krogh' cylinders, pO_2 values of the border plane were assumed to lie under normoxic conditions in the range of 1 mmHg to 97 mmHg (mean pO_2 of 36 mmHg). In order to calculate hypoxic conditions as well, a pO_2 distribution between 0.5 mmHg and 63 mmHg was also assumed (mean pO_2 of 18 mmHg); the hypoxic distribution was explained by a reduction of systemic O_2 delivery through bleeding (Fleckenstein et al. 1986). Taking available values for O_2 diffusion conductivity (Grunewald and Sowa 1977; Kunze 1968 [a]) and O_2 consumption of resting skeletal muscle (Stainsby and Lambert 1979), mean pO_2 gradients between pO_2 sources and neighbouring pO_2 sinks were calculated to be 4.3 ± 3.4 mmHg over a distance of 40 μm. However, a few measurements of pO_2 gradients in anterior tibialis muscle of man obtained by doublebarreled pO_2 microelectrodes revealed mean gra-

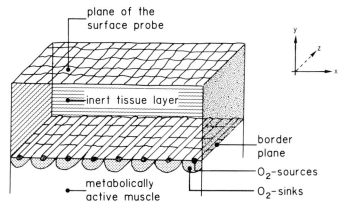

Fig. 1. Outline of the muscle surface model

dients between 12.2 ± 8.1 mmHg/60 µm and 21.6 ± 13.6 mmHg/50 µm (Kunze 1966, Kunze 1969 [a], Kunze 1969 [b]). For this reason we also modelled higher mean pO_2 gradients of 7.7 ± 6.4 mmHg and 12.5 ± 7.7 mmHg over a distance of 40 µm in order to examine the influence of the oxidative metabolic rate of muscle tissue on the error of surface probes.

A model of network diffusion was applied; thus, numerical methods for the calculation of local pO_2 and O_2 transport within the inert layer could be used. This method of simulating diffusion by the modelling of networks was first applied by Niesel and Thews (1959) and by Hutten (1973). Theoretical and experimental prerequisites regarding the applicability of the model to our question, regarding the assumed values of O_2 consumption and transport, and regarding the applied methods of mathematical transformations and calculations, have been given elsewhere (Schäffler 1987).

The calculation procedures were performed with the network analysis program SPICE (Simulation Programm with Integrated Surface Emphasis, Hoefer 1986) which is also suitable for simulating microcirculation (Mickulecky 1980).

Results

In Fig. 2, calculated pO_2 distributions within, and on top, of the inert layer are shown. The profiles and the histograms of the lower rows (in diagram 2A and 2B) represent the assumed conditions directly on the surface of O_2 consuming muscle fibres. These assumed distributions represent normoxic conditions at tissue pO_2 values between 1 mmHg and 97 mmHg (mean tissue pO_2 of 36 mmHg), at a mean of pO_2 gradients of 7.7 ± 6.4 mmHg/40 µm at the muscle cell surfaces. Under the given boundary conditions of calculation, no pO_2 values higher than 85 mmHg occur on the surface of an inert layer as thin as 50 µm, and values below 5 mmHg are reduced in relative frequency (Fig. 2A). On the surface of an inert layer of 200 µm, neither values below 10 mmHg nor values higher than 65 mmHg occur (Fig. 2B), although pO_2 values in the range between 1 mmHg and 97 mmHg exist at the tissue surface. In Table 1 numerical data from calculations of Fig. 2B are given. It can be seen that the pO_2 distribution on the surface of an inert layer of 50 µm in thickness is not exactly equal to the distribution that is present 50 µm above the muscle cell surface within an inert layer of 200 µm in thickness; the difference can be explained by the boundary conditions at the surface of the 50 µm inert layer. However, the results are qualitatively in agreement. Therefore, the other diagrams shown (Figs. 3–5) are calculated only for inert layers of 200 µm in thickness, and corresponding results for thinner inert layers can be derived approximately from the intermediate pO_2 profiles.

In Fig. 3 and Table 1, results from the calculations equivalent to Fig. 2b are shown assuming a lower muscle O_2 consumption resulting in lower mean

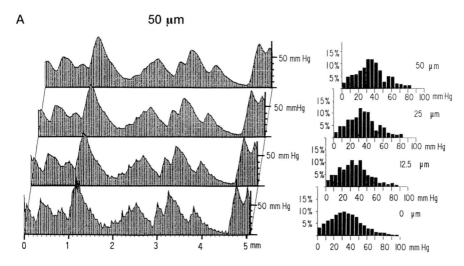

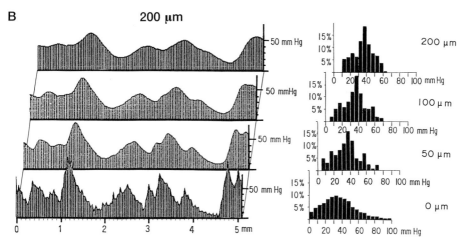

Fig. 2. Results of network simulations of pO₂ distributions within and on the surface of inert tissue layers; diagram 2A: inert layer has a thickness of 50 μm; diagram 2B: inert layer has a thickness of 200 μm. In each diagram pO₂ profiles are shown on the left side. Bottom profiles of each of the diagrams: assumed pO₂ profiles along a line directly adjacent to the oxygen metabolizing muscle cells (conditions: mean of pO₂ gradients is 7.7 ± 6.4 mmHg/40 μm; tissue pO₂ values lie between 1 mmHg and 97 mmHg with a mean of 36 mmHg). Top profiles of each of the diagrams: calculated pO₂ profile along a line which is located on top of the inert layer in shortest distance and in parallel to the line from which the bottom pO₂ profile is taken. In each of the diagrams 2 intermediate (calculated) pO₂ profiles, located within the respective inert layers, are shown. On the right side in each of the diagrams the pO₂ histograms which result from the respective pO₂ profiles at varied distances to the muscle cell surfaces are shown; bottom histograms: directly on the muscle cells; top histograms: on top of the inert layers

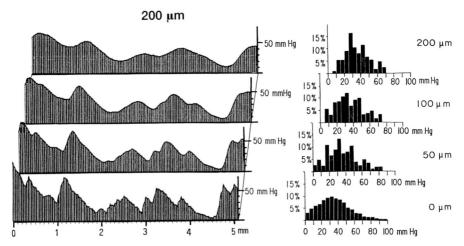

Fig. 3. Results of network simulation of pO₂ distributions within and on top of an inert tissue layer of a thickness of 200 μm. In contrast to Fig. 2, a lower tissue oxygen consumption is assumed resulting in a mean value of pO₂ gradients on the muscle cells of 4.3 ± 3.4 mmHg/40 μm. See legend of Fig. 2 and text for details

Table 1. Numerical data of calculations of Fig. 2B, 3, 4 and 5

mean (SD) of pO2 gardients directly on muscular tissue: 7.7 (±6.4) mmHg / 40 μm					
distance to muscle cells	scatter of histogram	rel. frequency of pO2 < 5 mmHg	number of missing pO2 classes at high / low end of histogram		see histogram in Fig. Nr.
μm	SD	%	low classes	high classes	
0	18.8	3.1			2 B
12.5	18.4	2.7	0	1	
25	18.0	2.5	0	2	
50	17.3	2.4	0	3	2 B
100	15.8	0.0	1	5	2 B
200	13.5	0.0	2	7	2 B

mean (SD) of pO2 gardients directly on muscular tissue: 4.3 (±3.4) mmHg / 40 μm					
distance to muscle cells	scatter of histogram	rel. frequency of pO2 < 5 mmHg	number of missing pO2 classes at high / low end of histogram		see histogram in Fig. Nr.
μm	SD	%	low classes	high classes	
0	18.8	3.1			3
12.5	18.7	3.1	0	1	
25	18.1	2.9	0	2	
50	17.1	2.7	0	3	3
100	15.9	0.0	1	5	3
200	14.1	0.0	1	6	3

Table 1. (continued)

mean (SD) of pO2 gardients directly on muscular tissue: 12.5 (±7.7) mmHg / 40 μm					
distance to muscle cells	scatter of histogram	rel. frequency of pO2 < 5 mmHg	number of missing pO₂ classes at high / low end of histogram		see histogram in Fig. Nr.
			low classes	high classes	
μm	SD	%			
0	18.8	3.1			4
12.5	18.7	1.2	0	1	
25	18.6	0.0	1	3	
50	18.5	0.0	1	4	4
100	16.4	0.0	2	6	4
200	12.2	0.0	3	8	4

mean (SD) of pO2 gardients directly on muscular tissue: 3.6 (±3.5) mmHg / 40 μm					
distance to muscle cells	scatter of histogram	rel. frequency of pO2 < 5 mmHg	number of missing pO₂ classes at high / low end of histogram		see histogram in Fig. Nr.
			low classes	high classes	
μm	SD	%			
0	11.3	12.2			5
12.5	11.1	11.0	0	1	
25	11.0	10.2	0	1	
50	10.7	9.4	0	2	5
100	10.0	7.5	0	3	5
200	8.2	2.7	0	5	5

pO₂ gradients directly on the muscle tissue of 4.3 ± 3.4 mmHg/40 μm. In Fig. 4 and Tab. 1 corresponding results are given for higher muscle O₂ consumption values resulting in a mean pO₂ gradient of 12.5 ± 7.7 mmHg directly on the muscle tissue. As can be seen from Fig. 3 and 4 as well as from numerical data of Tab. 1, the high and low pO₂ values are missing on the surface of the inert layer, particularly when metabolic activity of tissue is increased.

In Fig. 5, a hypoxic pO₂ distribution on the surface of muscle fibres is assumed. The histogram has a shape which was determined by needle probes from a dog gracilis muscle in the process of bleeding (blood loss 4% of b. w.). A mean value of muscular pO₂ gradients of 3.6 ± 3.5 mmHg/40 μm and a range of tissue pO₂ between 0.5 mmHg and 63 mmHg were assumed. Especially under these conditions, the marked effect of O₂ diffusion within the inert layer on the reduction of the relative frequency of low pO₂ values can be clearly seen. The left shifted form of the tissue pO₂ histogram, within the inert layer, is transferred into a more symmetrical form; see Tab. 1 for numerical data.

200 µm

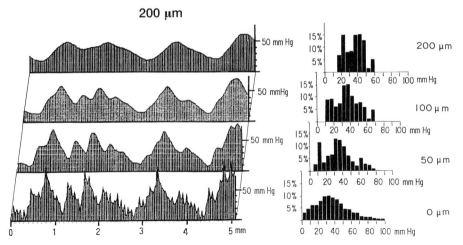

Fig. 4. Results of network simulation of pO$_2$ distributions within and on top of an inert tissue layer of a thickness of 200 µm. In contrast to Fig. 2, a higher tissue oxygen consumption is assumed resulting in a mean value of pO$_2$ gradients on the muscle cells of 12.5 ± 7.7 mmHg/40 µm. See legend of Fig. 2 and text for details

200 µm

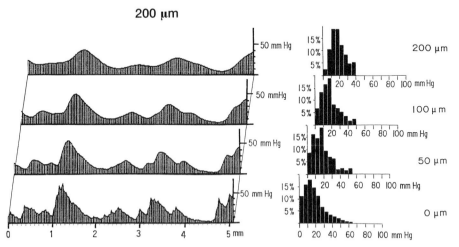

Fig. 5. Results of network simulation of pO$_2$ distributions within and on top of an inert tissue layer of a thickness of 200 µm. In contrast to Fig. 2, tissue hypoxia and a lower tissue oxygen consumption are assumed resulting in a mean tissue pO$_2$ value of 18 mmHg (scatter of single pO$_2$ values between 0.5 mmHg and 63 mmHg) and a mean value of pO$_2$ gradients of 3.6 ± 3.5 mmHg/40 µm. See legend of Fig. 2 and text for details

Discussion

The comparison of pO$_2$ values obtained by pO$_2$ surface probes and by pO$_2$ needle probes showed that surface probes delivered other mean pO$_2$ values and a narrower distribution of pO$_2$ values (see part 1 of this study). This second part of the study was primarily directed towards finding an explanation for the smaller scatter of the measured surface histograms. This smaller scatter is unlikely to represent the prevailing conditions within the tissue since considerable pO$_2$ gradients are to be expected on the surface of O$_2$-consuming and adequately perfused tissue. The histological examinations lead us to assume that the horizontally directed component of O$_2$ diffusion within a connective tissue (and/or a necrotic cell) layer, located between the surface probe's wires and the metabolically active tissue could plausibly explain the small scatter in pO$_2$ distributions measured on muscle surfaces. In our tissue model we calculated the O$_2$ diffusion (under steady state conditions of diffusion) within a non-oxygen-consuming and isotropic inert tissue layer which is located between the muscle surface and the membrane of the surface probe. The values of the parameters of calculation were taken from available experimental data.

It was shown by mathematical modelling that under all of the given boundary conditions, layers of 25 to 200 μm in thickness cause considerable changes in the resulting pO$_2$ histograms. The more O$_2$ is metabolized in the tissue, the more both high and low pO$_2$ values in surface histograms are underestimated. If pO$_2$ gradients, as measured by Kunze (1966; 1969 [a]; 1969 [b]) within tibialis anterior muscle of man (up to mean values of 21.6 ± 13.6 mmHg/50 μm), are assumed to be present also on muscle surfaces, then the disturbing influence of the inert tissue layer on surface probe pO$_2$ readings is even worse than shown in the worst case of our model calculations (maximal modelled mean of pO$_2$ gradients was 12.5 ± 7.7 mmHg/40 μm).

Our modelling also shows that tissue hypoxia under conditions of disturbed O$_2$ supply to the muscle, is drastically underestimated if histograms are taken on the surface of the inert layer:

We explain the underestimation of low and high tissue pO$_2$ values in histograms measured from tissue surfaces by the horizontal component of O$_2$ diffusion within an inert layer. However, this diffusion error of surface probes when applied to muscle cannot be avoided since, even under microscopic control of preparation, the inert connective tissue layer cannot be removed completely without damaging tissue. We assume that not only the connective tissue layer, but also necrotic cells on top of the muscle must be regarded as inert layer (see part 1 of the study). So, radical removal of connective tissue will lead to an increase of this other kind of inert layer.

Under practical experimental or clinical conditions, the amount of superficial cell necrosis and the thickness of the connective tissue layer are unknown. Hence, the extent of underestimation of high and low pO$_2$

values in surface pO_2 histograms cannot be estimated. The duration of the contact between probe and tissue is an important factor in tissue damage (Schramm et al., this book), and the duration of MDO probe measuring procedures is not standarized. So, it must be assumed that surface pO_2 data obtained under equivalent clinical conditions differ considerably.

Conclusions

The horizontal component of O_2 diffusion within the thin connective tissue layer which is left on the surface of a muscle leads to a marked underestimation of high and low pO_2 values in pO_2 histograms obtained by a multiwire surface probe. As shown in part 1 of the study, a connective tissue layer of a thickness between 10 and 180 μm (mean 82 μm) could not be removed in the preparation of the muscle surface, or else local bleeding or damage to the muscle tissue occurred. Due to the "micro-roughness" of the superficial relief of muscle bundles, the thickness of the connective tissue layer that must be left on the muscle, varies considerably.

If fibres on the surface of the muscle are damaged, high and low pO_2 values will be additionally underestimated. However, fibre necrosis is a common finding on muscle surfaces that have been in contact with a surface probe. Since the thickness of the connective tissue and necrotic cell layer is unknown in available studies, it must be assumed that surface pO_2 data obtained under equivalent clinical condition differ considerably for methodical reasons.

Hypoxic tissue pO_2 values can be almost completely absent in the surface histogram; hence, it is difficult to interpret surface pO_2 histograms obtained under conditions of disturbed tissue O_2 supply, e. g. during shock syndromes.

References

1. Baumgärtl H, Leichweiss HP, Lübbers DW, Weiss C, Huland H (1972) The oxygen supply of the dog kidney: measurements of intrarenal pO_2. Microvasc. Res. 4: 247–257
2. Baumgärtl H, Lübbers DW (1973) Platinum needle electrode for polarographic measurement of oxygen and hydrogen. In: Kessler M, Bruley DT, Lübbers DW, Silver IA, Strauss J (eds) Oxygen supply. Urban & Schwarzenberg, München, 130–136
3. Bruley DF (1973) Mathematical considerations for oxygen transport to tissue. Adv Exp Med Biol 37a: 749–759
4. Ehrly AM, Schroeder W (1977) Oxygen pressure in ischemic muscle tissue of patients with chronic occlusive arterial diseases. Angiology 28: 101–108
5. Feifel B (1986) Allgemeine Analyseverfahren für lineare Netzwerke. In: Feifel B, Trautwein A (eds) Formelsammlung Elektrotechnik I, Fachhochschule Aalen, 21–22
6. Fleckenstein W (1982) In vivo measurements of pO_2 histograms using a hypodermic needle electrode system. Pflügers Arch 392: R209
7. Fleckenstein W (1985) Ein neues Gewebe-pO_2-Meßverfahren zum Nachweis von Mikrozirkulationsstörungen. Med Diss Lübeck

8. Fleckenstein W, Kersting T, Schäffler A, Heinrich R, Reinhart K, Weiss C (1986) The effects of hemodilution and bleeding on muscular pO₂ in the dog. In: Ehrly AM, Haus J, Huch R (eds) Clinical oxygen pressure measurement. Springer, Heidelberg, 208–215

9. Fleckenstein W (1987) Die Entwicklung der Feinnadel-Gewebe-pO₂-Histographie zum klinisch eingesetzten Diagnoseverfahren. In: Präsident der FU Berlin (ed) 2. Forum Medizintechnik. Verlag Forschungsvermittlung, Berlin, 92–105

10. Fleckenstein W, Petersen C (this book) On the effects of arterial hyperoxia on muscle oxygen supply of man and dog.

11. Gayeski TEJ (1981) A cryogenic microspectrophotometric method for measuring myoglobin oxygen saturation in subcellular volumes; application to resting dog gracilis muscle. PhD thesis Univ Rochester

12. Gayeski TEJ Connet RJ, Honig CR (1985) O₂ transport in the rest-work transition illustrates new function of myoglobin. Am J Physiol 248: H914–H921

13. Grunewald WA, Sowa W (1977) Capillary structures and O₂-supply to tissue. Rev Physiol Bioch Pharmacol, 77: 150–209

14. Hauss J, Schönleben K, Spiegel U (1982) Therapiekontrolle durch Überwachung des Gewebe pO₂. Aktuelle Probleme in der Angiologie. Verlag Huber, Bern (CH) 41

15. Hoefer E, Nielinger H (1986) SPICE – Analyseprogramm für elektronische Schaltungen. Springer, Berlin

16. Hutten H (1973) Some special problems concerning the oxygen supply to tissue as studied by an anologue computer. In: Kessler M, Bruley DT, Lübbers DW, Silver IA, Strauss J (eds) Oxygen supply. Urban & Schwarzenberg, München, 25–30

17. Kessler M, Grunewald W (1969) Possibilities of measuring oxygen pressure fields in tissue by multiwire platinum electrodes. Progr Resp Res. 3: 147–152

18. Kessler M (1981) Grundlegende Prinzipien der Sauerstoffversorgung des Gewebes. In: Mirkozirkulation and arterielle Verschlußkrankheiten. Karger, Basel, 45–58

19. Kunze K (1966) Die lokale kontinuierliche Sauerstoffdruckmessung in der menschlichen Muskulatur. Pflügers Arch 292: 151–160

20. Kunze K (1969 [a]) Das Sauerstoffdruckfeld im normalen und pathologisch veränderten Muskel. Springer, Berlin

21. Kunze K (1969 [b]) Significance of oxygen pressure field measurements in human muscle, with special remarks on pO₂ micro-needle electrodes. Progr Resp Res 3: 153–157

22. Lübbers DW (1981) Grundlagen und Bedeutung der lokalen Sauerstoffdruckmessung und des pO₂-Histogramms für die Beurteilung der Organe und des Organismus. In: Ehrly AM (ed) Messung des Gewebesauerstoffdruckes bei Patienten. Witzstrock, Baden-Baden, 11–21

23. Meuer HJ (this book) Local oxygen consumption of blood perfused skeletal muscle determined with oxygen microelectrodes under stop flow conditions.

24. Mickulecky DC (1980) The use of a circuit simulation program (SPICE 2) to model microcirculation. In: Schneck DJ (ed) Biofluid mechanics, 2: 327–345

25. Niesel W, Thews G (1959) Ein elektrisches Analogverfahren zur Lösung physiologischer Diffusionsprobleme. Pflügers Arch 269: 282–305

26. Piiper J (1985) Blood flow distribution in dog gastrocnemius muscle at rest and during stimulation. J Appl Physiol 58: 2068–2074

27. Schäffler A (1987) Methodenkritische Untersuchung über Unterschiede der Muskel-Gewebe-pO₂-Daten von Nadelsonden und Oberflächensonden. Med Diss Lübeck

28. Schramm U, Fleckenstein W, Weber C (this book) Morphological assessment of skeletal muscle injury caused by pO₂ measurements with hypodermic needle probes.

29. Silver IA (1965) Some observations on the cerebral cortex with an ultramicro membrane-covered oxygen electrode. Med Electron Biol Engng 3: 377–387

30. Stainsby WN, Lambert CR, 1979 (1979) Determinants of oxygen uptake in skeletal muscle. Am J Physiol 206: 125–151

31. Sunder-Plassmann L (1981) Quantitative assessment of microvascular integrity by tissue oxymetry in patients. In: Effros RM (ed) Microcirculation. Academic Press, New York 267–280
32. Whalen WJ, Riley J, Nair P (1967) A microelectrode for measuring intracellular pO_2. Appl J Physiol 23: 798–801
33. Whalen WJ, Burek D, Thuning C, Kanoy BE, Duran WN (1976) Tissue pO_2, VO_2, venous pO_2 and perfusion pressure in resting dog gracilis muscle perfused at constant flow. Adv Exp Med Biol 75: 639–655

Verification of the Tissue Oxygen Distribution in the Carotid Body

H. Acker

Introduction

Since de Castro's [1929] and Heyman's [1930] fundamental findings, the carotid body is considered to be a peripheral chemoreceptor which transduces changes in arterial pO_2 and arterial pCO_2 or pH into nervous signals. These signals predominantly regulate ventilation via the respiratory center and thus help to normalize the arterial blood gases. But other organs like heart and kidney [Acker and O'Regan, 1983] can also be influenced by the nervous signal of the carotid body. With regard to the pO_2 chemoreception the specific stimulus for this process is to be found in the oxygen pressure distribution of the carotid body tissue.

The oxygen pressure distribution in a tissue is mainly determined by the following parameters:

1. The microcirculation in the tissue and an adequate capillary network
2. The arterial pO_2 and the oxygen transport capacity of the blood
3. The local oxygen consumption.

In order to characterize the oxygen supply to the carotid body direct tissue pO_2 measurements have been performed by two groups with the aid of microelectrodes. Acker et al. [1971] and Weigelt et al. [1980] measured the tissue pO_2 in the cat and rabbit carotid body. The tissue pO_2 displayed in form of a histogram was found to range between 0 to 100 Torr with a mean value of about 20 Torr for the cat and 10 for the rabbit carotid body (Fig. 1). Whalen et al. [1981] found mean pO_2 values of 40 to 50 Torr and top values of up to 100 Torr in the cat carotid body. These findings were unexpected since the carotid body possesses a high venous pO_2 with a small arteriovenous O_2 difference and a high total flow of about $2000ml/(100g*min)$ [Purves, 1970]. To find an explanation for this discrepancy several parameters and their interconnections influencing the oxygen supply of an organ were investigated.

Clinical Oxygen Pressure Measurement II
A.M. Ehrly et al. (Eds.)
© Blackwell Ueberreuter Wissenschaft Berlin 1990

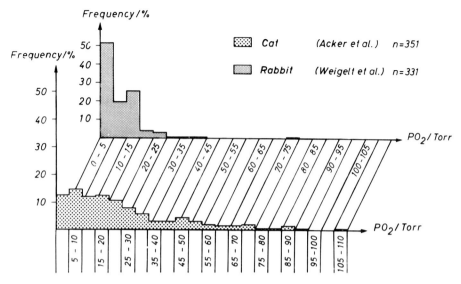

Fig. 1. Tissue pO₂ histograms of the cat and rabbit carotid body

Microcirculation and capillary network

The carotid body possesses a high total blood flow of about 2000 ml/(100g·min) [Daly et al., 1954]. Direct determination of the blood flow inside the organ with the aid of hydrogen clearance curves measured with microneedle electrodes [Keller and Lübbers, 1972] exhibits flow values between 600 and 3000 ml/(100g·min), depending on the location inside the tissue, at a blood pressure of about 100 mmHg. However, Degner and Acker [1986] were able to calculate local flow velocities from histologically reconstructed capillaries of the cat carotid body comparable to values known for capillaries in other organs. For this purpose various segments of vessels whose length from one ramification to the other and whose radius as well as the viscosity of the blood streaming through had been individually calculated were substituted by a single resistance value R according to the law of Hagen Poiseuille

$$R=(8{*}\eta{*}l)/(\pi{*}r^4)=p/I=p/(v{*}\pi r^2) \text{ (Equation 1)}$$

where η=viscosity, v=velocity of the streaming blood, l=length of the vessel, r=radius of the vessel, I=flow, p=blood pressure difference between the beginning and the end part of the vessel and p/I=R (law of Ohm). The network of resistance can be reduced stepwise into one resistance value for parallel resistances and one value for resistances in series. Resistances connected in a triangular set-up are substituted with the aid of:

$R=(R_2*R_3)/(R_1+R_2+R_3)$ (Equation 2)

where R_1,R_2,R_3 are individual resistances and R is the total substituted resistance. Assuming a given arteriovenous blood pressure difference and a given viscosity value for the flowing blood (hematocrit), a velocity of the streaming blood for each part of the vessels is computable stepwise according to Eqs. 1 and 2. This calculation leads to the flow velocity values given in Table 1 if our morphometrical data of capillaries in cat carotid body are taken into account.

Table 1. Calculated flow velocities in the carotid body; v=flow velocity, avbp diff.=arteriovenous blood pressure difference

v=0.02 cm/s 60%	v=0.05 cm/s 29%	v=0.5 cm/s 16%	viscosity mNS/m² 3	avbp diff. Torr 100

It can be seen that in 60% of the vessels a flow velocity of 0.02 cm/s is computable. This value is comparable to values known from capillaries in other organs.

Direct measurements of the flow velocities in the carotid body have been carried out by Hilsmann et al. [1987]. They used double pH_2-microelectrodes with one H_2 generating and one pH_2 measuring electrode. By determining the pH_2 in the carotid body tissue under perfused and non-perfused conditions the prevailing flow velocity could be determined with the aid of the following equation:

$v = 2D/(r-x)*\ln p_o/p_v$ (Equation 3)

where **v**=flow velocity, D=diffusion coefficient, r=known distance between the electrode tips, x=measuring angle of 90°, p_v and p_o=measured pH_2 values with and without blood perfusion respectively. At a perfusion pressure of 120 mmHg a mean value of about 0.014 cm/s could be measured, which tallied very well with the calculated values in Table 1. Taking the whole carotid volume as a reference volume this value yields a local blood flow of about 84 ml/(100g*min). The discrepancy with the blood flow values as published by Keller and Lübbers [1972] might be due to the difference in the measuring distance covered by the pH_2-microelectrodes. The small measuring distance of the double electrodes of about 100 μm provides the necessary spatial resolution for distinguishing between the flow within the particular tissue and the shunt flow of the vessels of the carotid body.

The vascular structure of the carotid body permits normal flow velocities parallel to the high flow velocities through arteriovenous anastomoses or vessels of different length [Seidl, 1976]. This structure seems to act as a stationary controller of the flow heterogeneity, since pO_2 changes only have an influence on the local flow velocity except under conditions of hypotension or ischemia.

The functional importance of a low flow system in the carotid body may be derived from the location of the organ near the common carotid artery with its high flow velocity and perfusion pressure. With the aid of the described vascular structure the organ reduces this high flow and perfusion pressure to avoid edema in the immediately adjoining cell area of the carotid body. A mean local flow velocity of about 0.014 cm/s under normal physiological conditions permits pO_2 changes in the carotid body as fast as in other organs during arterial pO_2 variations.

Arterial pO_2 and hematocrit

Hypoxia and hyperoxia in the arterial blood leads to a prompt response of the carotid body tissue pO_2 histogram with a left or right shift of the mean value. Assuming the chemoreceptor possesses a certain pO_2 threshold at which the chemoreceptive process is started, the variations of the pO_2 histogram determine the number of activated chemoreceptive units. Several authors tried to rule out the importance of the local hematocrit on chemoreceptor activity [Chiodi et al., 1941; Duke et al., 1952; Lahiri et al., 1981]. It has been demonstrated that most carotid body chemoreceptor fibers do not respond to a moderate decrease in O_2 content of the arterial blood, but that aortic chemoreceptors do. For the carotid body Acker and Lübbers [1977] offered the explanation that the organ is perfused with blood of low hematocrit as a result of plasma skimming. This would mean that the physically dissolved O_2 in the plasma is on the one hand sufficient to supply the organ with oxygen and on the other hand able to establish a close relationship between oxygen pressure and chemoreceptor activity without being disturbed by hematocrit or, to be more precise, by oxygen solubility changes of the local blood flow.

Oxygen consumption

The absolute level of oxygen consumption under control conditions depends on the kind of oxygen supply. The blood perfused carotid body reveals oxygen consumption values of about 0.12 µl O_2/min [O'Regan, 1979; Purves, 1970], whereas the saline perfused carotid body or the non-perfused carotid body in vivo and in vitro with an oxygen supply from the outside shows oxygen consumption values of about 0.021 µl O_2/min [for review see Eyzaguirre et al., 1983]. Nearly all groups found a clear pO_2 dependence of the oxygen consumption since decreasing the pO_2 lowers oxygen consumption.

Summary

All these results, together with the total number of glomoids in one carotid body counted as the number of specific cell aggregates assumed to be

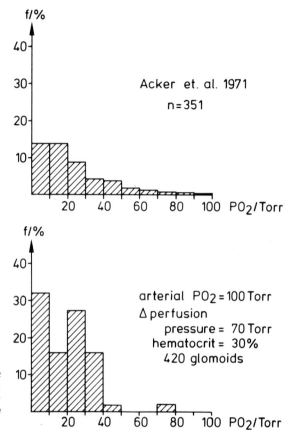

Fig. 2. Top: Measured tissue pO₂ histogram of the cat carotid body. Bottom: Recalculated pO₂ histogram taking into consideration the listed parameters

equally distributed along the whole length of vessels, were combined in a mathematical model as described by Metzger [1969] to recalculate the published pO₂ histograms of the carotid body. Fig. 2 shows as a result of these calculations that the left-shifted pO₂ histogram of the cat carotid body can be recalculated on the basis of the flow velocity distribution as shown in Table 1 and the parameters as mentioned in Fig. 2. A reduction of the mean capillary length of 40% would shift the pO₂ distribution to the right with a mean value between 40 and 50 Torr resembling then more the pO₂ histogram as described by Whalen et al. [1981]. Variations either of the oxygen consumption by a factor of 10, or the blood viscosity by a factor of 3, or the flow velocity by 67% result in a change of the median pO₂ of about 5 Torr only.

Fig. 2 shows that it is possible to verify measured pO₂ histograms with the aid of a mathematical model of physiological parameters determining the oxygen supply of an organ. This verification is important to understand the development of the pO₂ histogram in each individual organ as well as to give an assessment of the accuracy of pO₂ microneedle measurements in tissue.

References

1. Acker H, Lübbers DW, Purves MJ (1971) Local oxygen tension field in the glomus caroticum of the cat and its change at changing arterial pO_2. Pflügers Arch 329:136
2. Acker H, Lübbers DW (1977) Oxygen transport capacity of the capillary blood within the carotid body. Pflügers Arch 366:241
3. Acker H, O'Regan RG (eds) (1983) Physiology of the peripheral arterial chemoreceptors. Elsevier, Amsterdam
4. Chiodi H, Dill DB, Consolazio F, Horvath SM (1941): Respiratory and circulatory responses to acute CO poisoning. Am J Physiol 134:683
5. Daly M, Lambertsen CJ, Schweitzer A (1954) Observations on the volume of blood flow and oxygen utilization of the carotid body in the cat. J Physiol 125:67
6. De Castro F (1929) Über die Struktur und Innervation des Glomus Caroticum beim Menschen und bei Säugetieren. Anatomisch-experimentelle Untersuchungen. Z Anat Entw-gesch 89:250
7. Degner F, Acker H (1986) Mathematical analysis of tissue pO_2 distribution in the cat carotid body. Pflügers Arch 407:305
8. Duke HN, Green JH, Neil E (1952) Carotid chemoreceptor impulse activity during inhalation of carbon monoxide mixtures. J Physiol 118:520
9. Eyzaguirre C, Fitzgerald RS, Lahiri S, Zapata P (1983) Arterial Chemoreceptors. In: Handbook of Physiology – The Cardiovascular System. Shepherd JT, Abboud FM (eds) Bethesda, Am Physiol Soc, p 557
10. Heymans C, Bouchaert JJ, Dautrebrande L (1930) Sinus carotidien et réflexes respiratoires, II. Influences respiratoires, réflexes de l'acidose, de l'alcalose, de l'anhydride carbonique, de l'ion hydrogène et de l'anoxémie. Sinus carotidiens et échanges respiratoires dans les poumons et au delà des poumons. Arch Int Pharmacodyn Theer 39:400
11. Hilsmann J, Degner F, Acker H (1987) Local flow velocities in the cat carotid body. Pflügers Arch 410:204
12. Keller HP, Lübbers DW (1972) Flow measurements in the carotid body of the cat by hydrogen clearance method. Pflügers Arch 336:217
13. Lahiri S, Mulligan E, Nishino T, Mokashi A, Davies RO (1981) Relative responses of aortic body and carotid body chemoreceptors to carboxyhemoglobinemia. J Appl Physiol 50:580
14. Metzger H (1969) Distribution of oxygen partial pressure in a two dimensional tissue supplied by capillary meshes and concurrent and countercurrent systems. Math Biosci 5:143
15. O'Regan RG (1979) Responses of the chemoreceptors of the carotid body perfused with cell-free solutions. Int J Med Sci 148:78
16. Purves MJ (1970) The effect of hypoxia, hypercapnia and hypotension upon carotid body blood flow and oxygen consumption in the cat. J Physiol 209:395
17. Seidl E (1976) On the variability of form and vascularisation of the cat carotid body. Anat Embryol 149:79
18. Weigelt H, Seidl E, Acker H, Lübbers DW (1980) Distribution of oxygen partial pressure in the carotid body region and in the carotid body (rabbit). Pflügers Arch 388:137
19. Whalen WJ, Nair P, Sidebotham T, Spande J, Lacerna M (1981) Cat carotid body: Oxygen consumption and other parameters. J Appl Physiol 50:129

On the Effects of Arterial Hyperoxia on Muscle Oxygen Supply of Man and Dog

W. Fleckenstein, C. Petersen

Introduction

Arterial hyperoxia leads to a reduction of cardiac output and an increase in peripheral vascular resistance (Bergovsky and Bertun 1966; Chapler et al. 1984; Bachofen et al. 1971; Duling 1972). Hence, muscle perfusion can be decreased during arterial hyperoxia. In previous studies we observed an aggravation of local hypoxia in muscle tissue of patients suffering from syndromes of hypercirculation whilst respiring a gas mixture containing 40% O_2 (Fleckenstein 1985; Fleckenstein et al. 1985); in some cases even the mean muscular tissue pO_2 value was decreased when arterial pO_2 was increased. We explained this "paradox" effect by a constriction of arteriolar resistance vessels induced by arterial hyperoxia. In healthy human volunteers subjected to the same procedure, the mean muscular pO_2 value was increased and relative frequency values in left classes of pO_2 histograms were reduced (Fleckenstein et al. 1985). In critically ill patients Lund et al. (1980[b]), and also in healthy volunteers Lund et al. (1980[a]), observed a development of local tissue hypoxia when a gas mixture containing 80% O_2 was administered; in the latter study, only one histogram was taken from each of the individuals shortly after starting the arterial hyperoxia. The authors explained their observations by a redistribution of bloodflow within the microcirculation.

In an introductory study we examined pO_2 distributions of the femoral quadriceps muscle from 6 critically ill patients undergoing arterial hyperoxia. Their arterial pO_2 values varied from 321 mm Hg to 609 mm Hg in consequence of 100% O_2 breathing. The arterial hyperoxia was administered within a time span of 60 minutes. In order to examine the changes of the muscle pO_2 distributions in course of time, 3 histograms were taken from each of the patients during arterial hyperoxia. For comparison, before arterial hyperoxia, one histogram, and Swan Ganz catheter data were determined. As can be seen from the data of all patients pooled in histograms (Fig. 1), before arterial hyperoxia was started a physiological pO_2 distribution was observed at a mean arterial pO_2 of 118 mm Hg; 10 minutes after start of arterial hyperoxia the mean muscular pO_2 was increased and the frequency of low pO_2 values was decreased. Surprisingly

Clinical Oxygen Pressure Measurement II
A.M. Ehrly et al. (Eds.)
© Blackwell Ueberreuter Wissenschaft Berlin 1990

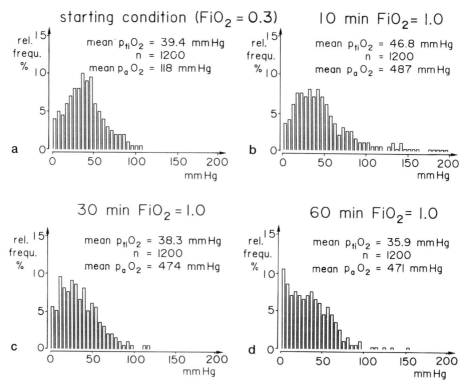

Fig. 1a–d. Histograms of pooled pO_2 data obtained from quadriceps femoral muscle of 6 patients: **a)** respired gas contains 30% O_2; **b)** 10 min after start of respiring 100% O_2; **c)** 30 min after start of respiring 100% O_2; **d)** 60 min after start of respiring 100% O_2. $p_{ti}O_2$: Mean muscular pO_2; FiO_2: Fraction of inspired oxygen; p_aO_2: mean arterial pO_2; n: Number of local muscular pO_2 values

however, after 60 minutes of arterial hyperoxia, mean tissue pO_2 decreased and the histogram was dramatically shifted to the left. The cardiac output, determined 15 and 30 minutes after onset of the arterial hyperoxia, was reduced on mean by 6%. Mean systemic vascular resistance was increased by 19%. The mean total body oxygen consumption was decreased by 12% at an increased mean oxygen delivery (+2.5%). Hence, the decrease of pO_2 within peripheral tissue, due to arterial hyperoxia, could not be explained by a reduction of total body oxygen delivery in consequence of a reduction of cardiac output. Additionally, the results of the introductory study clearly demonstrated that hyperoxemia-studies from peripheral tissue of man only lead to evaluable results if the oxygen effects are referred to their course in time.

In order to study systematically the effects of prolonged arterial hyperoxia on the peripheral oxygen supply, we examined pO_2 distributions and femoral oxygen delivery values in the hind limb of dogs. Our question was whether arterial hyperoxia of 2 hrs induces a reduction of peripheral blood flow which could possibly explain disturbances in peripheral oxygen supply.

Materials and methods

Experiments were carried out on 10 pure-bred beagle dogs with a mean body weight of 10.0 kg. The dogs were intubated and artificially ventilated with gas mixtures containing different fractions of O_2 and N_2O. Eucapnic conditions were kept accurately. Fentanyl was continuously infused (15 µg/kg*h). Muscle relaxation was induced by Pancuronium (0.08 mg/kg*h). Before preparations, the volume of the shaved hind legs (distal of a plane given by ischiadic tuber, trochanter major and anterior inferior iliac spine) was determined according to the Archimedian principle. Femoral vessels were then surgically exposed. The femoral artery of one leg and the vein of the other were cannulated and connected to a pressure transducer. The femoral blood flow in the non-cannulated femoral artery was measured by means of a perivascular electromagnetic flow transducer. Blood gases and acid/base status were determined from blood samples drawn from femoral artery and vein; hemoglobin concentration was determined spectrophotometrically and hemoglobin O_2-saturation was calculated according to Cain and Rossig (1976). So, the O_2 delivery and uptake of the hind limb could be determined and referred to the volume of hind limb tissue. Rectal temperature was kept constant at 37°C by a thermoregulated operating table.

Tissue pO_2-measurements from the gracilis muscle were performed by hypodermic needle probes of the fast responding type which were driven forward in steps (device KIMOC®, mgf. Ges. Med. Sondentechnik, Kiel-Mielkendorf, FRG). Methodical aspects have been described elsewhere (Fleckenstein 1982; Fleckenstein and Weiss 1982; Fleckenstein and Weiss 1984; Fleckenstein 1985; Weiss and Fleckenstein 1986).

Three gas mixtures of N_2O and O_2 were administered, each of them during a period of 2 hrs; during the first period, the fractional volume of O_2 was 25%, subsequently 40% and finally 90%. During each of the periods, 6 pO_2 histograms, each of them comprising 200 local pO_2 values, were taken from the gracilis muscle.

Results

During the first period of ventilation with 25% oxygen, the pO_2 histograms were shaped physiologically as demonstrated in Fig. 2a; the mean arterial pO_2 value lay at 117 ± 11 mm Hg and the mean muscle pO_2 value at 33 ± 6.4 mm Hg. When the dogs were ventilated with 40% O_2, the mean arterial pO_2 was 230 ± 18 mm Hg; at 90% O_2 ventilation, the arterial pO_2 rose to 470 ± 40 mm Hg. The pooled tissue pO_2 values under hyperoxe-

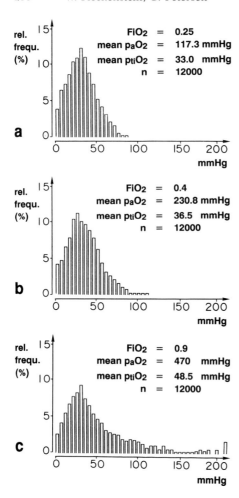

Fig. 2. Histograms of pooled pO_2 data obtained from gracilis muscle of 10 dogs during different ventilation periods of 2 hrs duration: **a)** ventilation with 25% O_2; **b)** ventilation with 40% O_2; **c)** ventilation with 90% O_2. Abbreviations see Fig. 1

mic conditions are shown in Fig. 2b and 2c. Compared with the first period (at 25% O_2 ventilation) during the arterial hyperoxia, mean tissue pO_2 was increased by 10.6% (at 40% O_2 ventilation) and by 47.2% (at 90% O_2 ventilation); during 90% O_2 ventilation, single highest muscle pO_2 values were observed at 250 mm Hg. In contrast to the patients, the mean muscle pO_2 values and the relative frequencies of low and high pO_2 values in the dogs remained nearly unchanged during the 2 hrs of arterial hyperoxia. The mean values of heart rate and blood pressure were significantly reduced during both phases of arterial hyperoxia. As shown in Fig. 3, during arterial hyperoxia the mean femoral oxygen delivery was decreased significantly and by the same percentage as the mean femoral blood flow (-26%). The mean oxygen consumption of the hind limb remained constant (at 0.21 ± 0.07 ml O_2/100 ml hind limb * min); consequently the mean femoral oxygen extraction ratio was increased significantly during arterial hyperoxia.

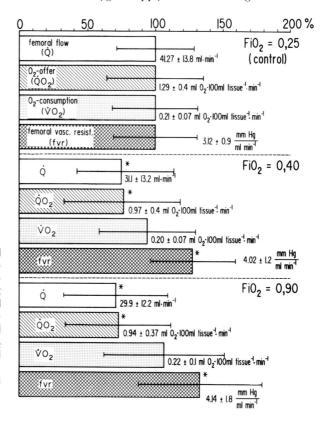

Fig. 3. Parameters of femoral oxygen transport and consumption; mean values obtained from 10 dogs at different levels of arterial pO_2. $\dot{Q}$: Femoral flow; $\dot{Q}O_2$: Femoral oxygen delivery, referred to the hind limb volume; $\dot{V}O_2$: Hind limb O_2 uptake, referred to the hind limb volume; fvr: Femoral vascular resistance; FiO_2: Fraction of inspired oxygen

significant change:
* = p < 0.001   n = 60
(Wilcoxon matched pairs
signed rank test)

Comparing the effects of arterial hyperoxia on the muscle pO_2 of individual dogs, two different "types" of changes in pO_2 distributions were observed: In 4 of the 10 dogs the mean muscular pO_2 was not significantly increased at both levels of arterial hyperoxia. Pooled pO_2 data of these dogs were less scattered at each of the 3 levels of arterial pO_2. At arterial hyperoxia the mean femoral flow was reduced by 35% in these 4 dogs which had no significant increase in mean muscular pO_2, whereas the corresponding flow reduction lay at only 22% in the other 6 dogs. In contrast to the findings in patients, during arterial hyperoxia, the relative frequency of muscle pO_2 values below 15 mm Hg in dogs was neither significantly increased nor reduced; the latter finding was made at elevated arterial pO_2 values in the dogs with increased as well as in the dogs with nearly unchanged mean muscular pO_2 values.

Discussion

Arterial hyperoxia of 230 mm Hg/pO_2 and 470 mm Hg/pO_2 led to a significant decrease in the femoral oxygen delivery; its relative decrease lay within the range of reduction of the femoral flow that was observed in other studies (Bachofen et al. 1971; Wilson and Stainsby 1978). The reduction of peripheral flow can be explained by an increase in vascular resistance and vagotonia (Bergovsky and Bertun 1966; Chapler et al. 1984; Daly and Bondurat 1962; Duling 1972; Duling 1973; Duling 1974; Duling and Klitzman 1980; Eggers et al. 1962; Gyton et al. 1965; Lambertsen 1978, Lübbers et al. 1978; Whalen and Saltzman 1965).

The oxygen content of arterial blood was not increased significantly by switching arterial pO_2 from 117 mm Hg to 230 mm Hg and 470 mm Hg respectively, since hemoglobin was already nearly saturated at 118 mm Hg. Additionally, at arterial hyperoxia the small increase in oxygen content of arterial blood, due to physically dissolved oxygen, was compensated by a small decrease in blood hemoglobin concentration as a consequence of withdrawal of blood samples. Hence, during arterial hyperoxia, the mean femoral oxygen delivery was decreased by the same percentages as the mean femoral flow.

In most pO_2 histograms recorded from the dogs a "physiological" distribution was observed; neither increases in relative frequencies at low pO_2 values nor pathological leftshifts nor wide scattered maldistributions were observed in the histograms of the dogs. Comparing the histograms of dog and man obtained during arterial hyperoxia, the latter findings show a distinct contrast: in patients the histograms were extremely leftshifted by 60-minutes-lasting arterial hyperoxia, whereas in 6 of the 10 dogs mean tissue pO_2 and, in all dogs, the relative frequency of high values up to 250 mm Hg, were markedly increased. At arterial hyperoxia, these high tissue pO_2 values are to be expected in the immediate adjacency of the arterial end of capillaries (Grunewald and Sowa 1977). These high pO_2 values lying near the arterial pO_2 values indicate perfused capillaries. Hence, it can be assumed that in consequence of arterial hyperoxia, the amount of reduction in tissue perfusion is negatively correlated to the mean tissue pO_2 value and to the relative frequency of high values of tissue pO_2 distributions. Indeed, during arterial hyperoxia less high pO_2 values and no increase of mean muscular pO_2 were seen when the mean femoral flow was strongly reduced by 35% (in 4 dogs); in the other 6 dogs, the hyperoxemic flow reduction was 22%. The hypothesis of a negative correlation between the hyperoxemic peripheral flow reduction and the tissue pO_2 values also fits an observation of Koop et al. (1981); during arterial hyperoxia, the authors observed less impairment of peripheral O_2 supply in patients with high cardiac output levels. It can be assumed that, due to a constriction of resistance vessels, the numbers and perfusion rates of functional nutritive capillaries are reduced during arterial hyperoxia. Hence, the microcirculatory and diffusive conditions of tissue oxygen supply are impaired during arterial hyperoxia; a detailed discussion has been given elsewhere (Petersen 1988).

However, in spite of a significant reduction in femoral flow in dogs during arterial hyperoxia, no increase in relative frequencies of low gracilis muscle pO_2 values was observed in them. This finding might be due to the slightness of the dogs' muscular O_2 consumption in consequence of muscular relaxation by Pancuronium. In patients, their higher yet normal level of muscular oxygen uptake may have led to the observed dramatic impairment of tissue O_2 supply after 60 minutes of 100% O_2 respiration; the delay between the start of the arterial hyperoxia and the impairment of muscle oxygen supply remains as yet unexplained. Our results clearly demonstrate that prolonged "Oxygen-Therapy" procedures can lead to a severe impairment of tissue oxygen supply.

References

1. Bachofen, M., Gage, A., Bachofen, H.: Vascular response to changes in blood oxygen tension under various blood flow rates. Am. J. Physiol. 220, 1786-1792 (1971)
2. Bergofsky, E.H., Bertun, P.: Response of regional circulation to hyperoxia. J. Appl. Physiol. 21, 567-572 (1966)
3. Cain, S.M., Rossig, R.G.: A nomogram relating pO_2, pH, temperature and hemoglobin saturation in the dog. J. Appl. Physiol. 21, 195-201 (1966)
4. Chapler, C.K., Cain, S.M., Stainsby, W.N. (1984): The effect of hyperoxia on oxygen uptake during acute anemia. Can. J. Physiol. Pharmacol. 62, 809-814 (1984)
5. Daly, W.J., Bondurat, S.: Effects of oxygen breathing on the heart rate, blood pressure, and cardiac index of normal men: resting, with reactive hyperemia, and after atropine. J. Clin. Invest. 41, 35-48 (1962)
6. Duling, B.R.: Microvascular responses to alterations in oxygen tension. Circ. Res. 31, 481-489 (1972)
7. Duling, B.R.: Microvascular diameter changes during local blood flow regulation: Independence of changes in pO_2. Adv. Exp. Med. Biol. 37a, 591-95 (1973)
8. Duling, B.R.: Oxygen sensititity of vascular smooth muscle. II: In vivo studies. Am. I. Physiol. 227, 42-49 (1974)
9. Duling, B.R., Klitzman, B.: Local control of microvascular function: role in tissue oxygen supply. Ann. Rev. Physiol. 42, 373-82 (1980)
10. Eggers, G.W.N., Paley, H.W., Leonard, J.J., Warren, J.V.: Hemodynamic responses to oxygen breathing in man. J. Appl. Physiol. 17, 75-79 (1962)
11. Fleckenstein, W.: In vivo measurements of pO_2 histograms using a hypodermic needle electrode system. Pflügers Arch, 392, R209 (1982)
12. Fleckenstein, W., Weiss, C.: Evaluation of pO_2 histograms using hypodermic needle electrodes. Proc. world congress on Med. Phys. Biomed. Eng. Kinzel Göttingen, 7.14. (1982)
13. Fleckenstein, W.: Ein neues Gewebe-pO_2-Meßverfahren zum Nachweis von Mikrozirkulationsstörungen. Med. Diss. Lübeck (1985)
14. Fleckenstein, W., Weiss, C.: A comparison of pO_2 histograms from rabbit hind limb muscles obtained by simultaneous measurements with hypodermic needle probes and with surface probes. Adv. Exp. Med. Biol. 169, 447-445 (1984)
15. Fleckenstein, W., Heinrich, R., Grauer, W., Schomerus, H., Dölle, W., Weiss, C.: Rapid local regulations of muscular pO_2 fields in patients suffering from cirrhosis of the liver. Adv. Exp. Med. Biol. 180, 687-694 (1985)
16. Grunewald, W.A., Sowa, W.: Capillary structures and O_2-supply to tissue. Rev. Physiol. Biochem. Pharmacol. 77, 149-209 (1977)
17. Guyton, A.C.: Walker, J.R.: Carier, O.: Relationship of tissue oxygen tension to autoregulation. Proc. Int. Conf. Hyperbaric Med. (1965)
18. Koop, K.H., Kieser, M., Sinagowitz, E.: Muscle pO_2 measurements in critically ill patients and its correlation to cardiac output and arterial pO_2. In: Monitoring of vital parameters during extracorporeal circulation. Karger, Basel (1981)
19. Lambertsen, C.J.: Effects of hyperoxia on organs and their tissues in: E.D. Robbin (ed.): Extrapulmonary manifestations of respiratory diseases. Marcel Dekker Inc., N.Y., Basel 8. (1978).

20. Lübbers, D.W.,Skolansiska, K., Haubig, K., Wodick, R.: pO_2 and microflow histograms of the beating heart in response to changes in arterial pO_2. Basic Res. Cardiol. 73, 307-319 (1978)

21. Lund, N., Jorfeldt, L., Lewis, D.H.: Skeletal muscle oxygen pressure fields in healthy human volunteers. Acta. Anaesthesiol. Scand. 24, 272-278 (1980(a))

22. Lund, N., Jorfeldt, L., Lewis, D.H., Ödmann, S.: Skeletal muscle oxygen pressure fields in artificially ventilated, critically ill patients. Acta. Anaesth. Scand. 24, 347-353 (1980(b))

23. Petersen, C.: Die Auswirkungen arterieller Hyperoxie auf die Sauerstoffversorgung des Skelettmuskels. Med. Diss. Lübeck (1988)

24. Weiss, Ch., Fleckenstein, W.: Local tissue pO_2 measured with "thick" needle probes. Funktionsanalyse biologischer Systeme 5, 155-166 (1986)

25. Wilson, B.A., Stainsby, W.N.: Effects of O_2 breathing on RQ, blood flow, and developed tension in in-situ dog muscle. Med. Sci. Sports Exerc. 10, 167-170 (1978)

26. Whalen, R.E., Saltzman, D.H., Holloway, jr., H.D., McIntosh, H.D.: Cardiovascular and blood gas response to hyperbaric oxygenation. Am. J. Cardiol. 15, 638-646 (1965)

The Effect of Normovolemic Hemodilution on Skeletal Muscle pO$_2$ in a New Animal Model of Chronic Arterial Occlusive Disease

U. Martin, E. Böhm, D. Gärtner, N. Würtz, K. Strein

An animal experimental model of chronic peripheral arterial occlusive disease (PAOD) should resemble as far as possible the typical pathophysiological situation in occlusive diseases. A combination of vascular disorders, hemodynamically effective vascular occlusion and disturbed flow properties of the blood is desirable. A rat model is presented below which includes this combination of disorders. The distribution of muscle tissue pO$_2$ is used as a parameter for the in vivo assessment of microcirculatory perfusion. As the model was developed especially in order to investigate the action of drugs on impaired microcirculation, we wanted to test it to see whether normovolemic hemodilution under these conditions led to changes in the distribution of muscular tissue pO$_2$.

Materials and Methods

The investigations were carried out on nine normotensive Wiga rats aged 6 months and 34 spontaneously hypertensive Wistar rats (SHR) (SHR/N/Ibm/BM) aged 12 months. The animals were all male and weighed on average 390 g. The hypertensive rats received, with the exception of a hypertensive control group, free access during the 5-week feeding period to the usual sniff standard food which had been enriched with 1.5% cholesterol (Merck, Darmstadt, Article No. 3670) and 0.5% cholic acid (Merck, Darmstadt). On day 0 of the feeding period 250 units horseradish peroxidase (HRP, BM No. 413 470) in 0.2 ml NaCl solution supplemented with 0.2 ml complete Freund's adjuvant (No. 0638-59, DIFCO Laboratories, Detroit, Michigan, USA) in a suspension solution were injected subplantarily into the hind paws (half the total amount per paw). Reimmunisation with 125 units HRP intracutaneously into the abdominal skin was carried out 28 days later. On day 32, 50 units HRP were administered i.v. as a booster. Measurements were carried out on day 36 [1, 2].

The normotensive and hypertensive controls received normal food and were not injected. Ligature of the right femoral artery was carried out in the hemodilution and control animals on day 29.

Clinical Oxygen Pressure Measurement II
A.M. Ehrly et al. (Eds.)
© Blackwell Ueberreuter Wissenschaft Berlin 1990

After premedication with 0.05 mg atropine (atropine sulphate Braun)/kg BW s.c., anesthesia was induced by inhalation with enfluran (Ethrane®) and was maintained with 1.5 mg piritramide (Dipidolor®)/kg BW/h and with 1 mg pancuronium (Pancuronium Organon®)/kg BW/h. The animals were tracheotomised and ventilated with an O_2:N_2O mixture of ratio 0.21:0.79. Blood pressure and heart rate were recorded via a carotid catheter which also permitted the collection of blood for measurement of blood gases, fibrinogen, cholesterol and erythrocyte aggregation.

In the hemodilution experiments, 4.5 ml 10% hydroxy ethyl starch (HAES-steril® 10%) with a molecular weight of 200,000 was infused for 30 min intravenously and at the same time 4 ml blood were removed continuously from the carotid artery. In the control group 1 ml of the solvent was infused i.v. for 10 min. Both groups were treated with 300 IU heparin/kg BW.

The tissue partial oxygen pressure was determined polarographically with multiple wire surface electrodes (L. Eschweiler, Kiel, FRG) on the exposed surface of the anterior tibial muscle of both legs. The position of the electrodes was repeatedly altered by slight twisting until 104 individual measurements were obtained. Histograms were produced and the arithmetic means calculated [3, 4]. Cholesterol in the serum was determined using BM Monotest®, Cholesterol and fibrinogen with BM Test Combination No. 524 484 (Boehringer, Mannheim, FRG). The erythrocyte aggregation index was measured in a Myrenne erythrocyte aggregometer (Myrenne, Roetgen, FRG). At the end of the experiment the femoral vein was punctured and the blood removed was examined in a lactate analyzer (Model 23 L, Yellow Springs Instruments Inc., Ohio, USA).

In the first part of the investigations, a group of normotensive rats (n = 9), a group of SHR (n = 7) and a group of SHR (n = 9) which had been fed and inoculated were compared. In the second part, only the SHR of the cholesterol-fed groups with inoculation were examined and in addition the right femoral artery was chronically ligated. In nine of these animals hemodilution was carried out and in a further nine solvent was injected.

The means and standard deviations were calculated for the individual parameters. Statistical comparison of two independent samples was carried out by the U-test according to Wilcoxon, Mann and Whitney. Paired observations were compared with the Wilcoxon Test for paired differences.

Results

The partial oxygen pressure on the surface of the anterior tibial muscle of normotensive rats was 28.3 ±6.6 torr on the left and 28.7 ±8.4 torr on the right. SHR without inoculation and feeding showed in contrast a tissue pO$_2$ on the left of 20.9 ±5.8 torr and on the right of 19.9 ±8 torr. After five weeks' feeding with cholesterol and 3-fold inoculation, the SHR showed a tissue pO$_2$ of 11.3 ±5.6 torr on the left and 10.5 ±6.7 torr on the right. The difference from the two control groups was statistically significant. After the cholesterol diet, an increased serum cholesterol content of 205.4 ±35.8 mg% was found in comparison with 75.4 ±11.6 mg% in the normotensive controls. Measurement of plasma fibrinogen showed 206 ±22.4 mg% in the normal group and 307 ±22.1 mg% in the cholesterol-fed group. The index of erythrocyte aggregation was 16.1 ±2.1 in the feeding group compared with 9.4 ±1.0 in the normotensive control group. The lactate level in the femoral venous blood of the feed group was 3.2 ±0.7 mmol/l compared with 0.95 ±0.3 mmol/l in the normotensive controls. Statistically significant differences from the normotensive controls were found for all four parameters.

Pilot histological examination of the muscle tissue revealed plaque-like intima proliferations of small arteries (< 100 µm) with partial perivascular cell infiltration, which can be regarded as an expression of early arteriosclerotic lesions.

In the second part of the investigations, the muscle tissue pO$_2$ rose to a statistically significant degree after completion of normovolemic hemodilution in the ligated leg from 5.7 ±6.5 torr to 14.9 ±9.3 torr. Injection of solvent in the control group led to a slight non-significant rise in tissue pO$_2$ from 2.2 ±3.1 torr to 5.8 ±5.6 torr. Whilst tissue pO$_2$ did not show any statistically significant difference in comparison with the two groups before the therapeutic measures, there was a statistically significant higher tissue pO$_2$ in comparison with controls after hemodilution.

Packed cell volume was reduced to a statistically significant degree from 46 ±1.4 % to 36 ±1.4 % by the blood exchange procedure, whilst it remained unchanged in the control group. The heart rate increased significantly from 342 ±23 beats/min to 384 ±26 beats/min after hemodilution, whilst it remained unchanged in the controls.

Discussion

The investigations were carried out in an animal experimental model of chronic arterial occlusive disease that is desirable from the pathophysiological point of view. The model facilitates hemorrheological investigation by combining an induced disorder of hemodynamics with an induced metabolic disorder. Artificial femoral artery occlusion [5] in isolation simulates the conditions in chronic PAOD patients to only a limited degree. According to Seiffge, the occlusion even leads to a 14 % improvement in erythrocyte deformability [6].

The single subplantar administration of complete Freund's adjuvant produces a chronic inflammation. The adjuvant arthritis model [7] leads to alteration of the physicochemical condition of the blood. A marked rise in fibrinogen, alpha$_2$-macroglobulin and later of gamma-globulin is accompanied by increased plasma viscosity and increased apparent blood viscosity at low and high shear forces. Furthermore, erythrocyte filterability is reduced and the degree of erythrocyte aggregation is increased. Thrombus formation in the mesenteric microcirculation, as investigated with laser technique, is increased in the arthritic rat [8]. Leucocyte adhesiveness is also increased, as shown by the intravital microscopic examination. Platelet aggregation also occurs to an increased degree in the early phase of the disease [9].

Vascular disorders were obtained by provoking early arteriosclerotic lesions. This was achieved by immunising spontaneously hypertensive rats [1]) with horseradish peroxidase and feeding them with a cholesterol-rich diet [2].

These model forms were combined in the animal model under investigation. This provided a relevant test situation for hemorrheologically active therapeutic measures. The measurement of muscle tissue pO_2 permits the direct assessment of the functional state of the terminal circulation [11].

This model showed that muscular microcirculation in older SHRs that had been kept for five weeks on a cholesterol-rich diet and been immunised three times was clearly impaired in comparison with equally old control SHRs and normal rats. The animal model also exhibited hemorrheological changes relating to chronic AOD. Reduced perfusion pressure in the limb was achieved by additional experimental ligature of the artery. In the presence of these massive disorders of blood distribution in the microcirculation normovolemic hemodilution leads to an improvement of tissue supply, which is seen as a rise in tissue pO_2. On the basis of these results, this animal model appears to be suitable for pharmacological investigations, but this must be shown in further studies.

References

1. Horsch AK, Kuhlmann WD, Bleyl U, Salomon JC (1978) Early atherosclerotic lesions in rat aorta. Res Exp Med (Berl) 173:251
2. Horsch AK, Jost-Vu E, Hofmann W, Clopath O, Staubesand J (1986) Der Einfluß von Sulfinpyrazon auf die Entstehung arteriosklerotischer Frühläsionen bei der Ratte. Herz/Kreisl. 18:397
3. Kessler M, Höper J, Krumme BA (1976) Monitoring of tissue perfusion and cellular function. Anaesthesiology 45:184
4. Lübbers DW (1969) The meaning of the tissue oxygen distribution curve and its measurement by means of Pt electrodes. Prog Resp Res 3, Karger, Basel, p 112
5. Messmer K, Fujita Y, Forst H, Weissm Th, Brückner UB (1984) Reversal of skeletal muscle hypoxia in chronic arterial occlusive disease. Microcirc Clin Exp 3:372
6. Seiffge D (1984) Veränderungen hämorheologischer Parameter bei verschiedenen Tierkrankheiten. In: Kiesewetter H, Ehrly AM, Jung F (eds) Hämorheologische Meßmethoden. Münchner Wissenschaftliche Publikationen, München, p. 74
7. Seiffge D, Kremer E (1983) Haemorheological long-term study of adjuvant arthritic disease in rats. Clinical Haemorheology 3:469
8. Görög P, Kovacs B (1976) Thrombus formation, hemostasis, adhesiveness of leucocytes and morphological abnormalities in the microcirculation of adjuvant arthritic rats. Agents and Actions 6/5:607
9. Lassmann HB, Kirby RE, Norick WJ (1974) Alterations in platelet aggregation associated with adjuvant arthritis in rats. Pharmac Res Comm 6:493

10. Limas C, Westrum B, Limas CJ (1980) The evolution of vascular changes in the spontaneously hypertensive rat. Am J Pathol 98:357
11. Ehrly AM, Schroeder W (1979) Zur Pathophysiologie der chronischen arteriellen Verschlußerkrankung. Herz/Kreisl 11:275

Circadian pO$_2$ Oscillations in Skeletal Muscle of Rats

**M. Günderoth-Palmowski, R. Heinrich, P. Palmowski, S. Dette,
W. Daiss, H. Schomerus**

Introduction

The influence of the 24 hour day-night cycle on physiological processes is
gaining more and more importance in medical research. The majority of
physiological oscillations have been found to depend on the circadian
rhythm (Wever, 1979). It is now known that the mammalian organism is a
multioscillator system composed of oscillations of different period length.
They are synchronized one by the other, or by an external "Zeitgeber"
(synchronizer) (Hoffmann, 1972; Wever, 1977).
In rats many circadian oscillations e.g. locomotor activity, food and water
intake (Borbely, 1978), body temperature, heart rate, and blood pressure
(Meinrath, 1979) have been investigated. It is still unknown whether circadian oscillations are present in the rats' terminal vascular bed, because
no suitable evaluation method has been available up to now. For the
present, the measurement of tissue pO$_2$ has been found to be a valid
parameter of microcirculation (Lübbers, 1981).
The aim of this study was to evaluate whether there are circadian oscillations of tissue pO$_2$ in skeletal muscles in rats.

Methods

10 female Sprague Dawley rats were kept under constant conditions
throughout the whole experiment:
– natural day-night changes
– air humidity 42 %
– room temperature 22 – 23 °C
– free access to food and water.

The measurement of tissue pO$_2$ of skeletal muscle was carried out at an
animal age of 90 days (mean body weight 252.9 ±7.0 g). pO$_2$ histograms
were taken from m. rectus abdominis under constant ether anesthesia
with a multiwire surface electrode according to Kessler and Lübbers
(1966).

Clinical Oxygen Pressure Measurement II
A. M. Ehrly et al. (Eds.)
© Blackwell Ueberreuter Wissenschaft Berlin 1990

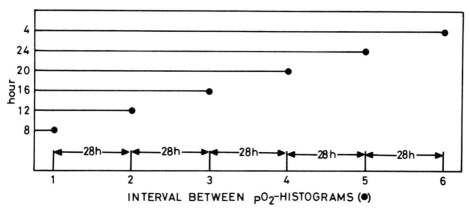

Fig. 1. Schedule of pO₂ measurement

In order to avoid a "Zeitgeber" effect of the measuring procedure, the animals were divided into pairs and the first pO₂-histogram of each pair was taken at a different time of the day, e.g. the first pair started at 8 o'clock, the second at 12 o'clock, etc. Each pair was measured 6 times at intervals of 28 hours. See Fig. 1 for the experimental schedule.

At the end of the experiment a circadian course for each animal and one for the whole group was calculated.

To test the statistical significance of the pO₂ differences at 4, 8, 16, and 20 hours of the mean circadian course a Student's t-test was evaluated.

For the sake of better visual representation of the circadian course, the time axis of the curves were reduplicated, and in this way a pO₂ course over a 48 hour period was obtained.

Results

Fig. 2 shows the circadian course of mean muscle pO₂ for all rats. The course was characterized by an amplitude of 14 mmHg ($p<0.005$) and a period length of approximately 24 hours. Thus the mean pO₂ course resembled a sinus oscillation.

Fig. 3 shows the individual pO₂ curves. The lowest pO₂ values occurred between 12 and 20 hours. After that, the pO₂ increased and the highest values occured at night. Only one animal showed an approximately sine oscillation, whereas the other rats had a double-peaked curve.

Discussion

Measurements of circadian oscillations have to be made very carefully without disturbing the individuals examined. Otherwise, the test itself operates as a "Zeitgeber" influencing the measured oscillation.

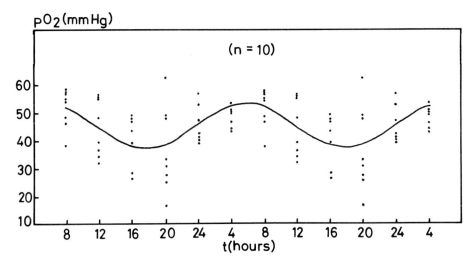

Fig. 2. Circadian course of mean muscle pO_2 of 10 rats

The effect of the pO_2 measurements themselves on the circadian cycle cannot be estimated. It is highly probable that the measuring procedure does cause some considerable disturbance to the rat organism and its circadian rhythm. Therefore, with regard to circadian oscillations of muscle-pO_2, these results can only be considered as preliminary. However, the similarity of the individual pO_2 curves inspite of different starting times of the measurements shows that the measurement procedure does not influence the circadian course of muscle pO_2 as much as might have been expected. Otherwise, we should have found identical muscle pO_2 curves correlating with the *first measurement* and not with the *time of day*. In fact, no matter at what time the measuring procedure was started, all individual pO_2-curves displayed high pO_2 values at night and low values in the afternoon.

The day and night cycle has indeed proved to be a dominant synchronizer for the sleeping and waking rhythm of practically all animal species that have been investigated (Borbely, 1978). Taking into account that laboratory rats are active at night, the increase in skeletal muscle pO_2 could be due to elevated locomotor activity. On the other hand the low pO_2 values during daytime relate to a relaxing period with decreased locomotor activity. The circadian cycle is a phylogenetical adaptation to the environmental time structure. The internal copy of this time structure helps the individuals to adjust themselves to the expected variations of the environment. As Benessiano et al. (1983) have shown, heart rate and body temperature of rats increase immediately at the beginning of the night period so as to prepare the organism for its active period.

In contrast to heart rate and body temperature, muscle pO_2 increased slowly, and the first maximum was reached some time after the beginning

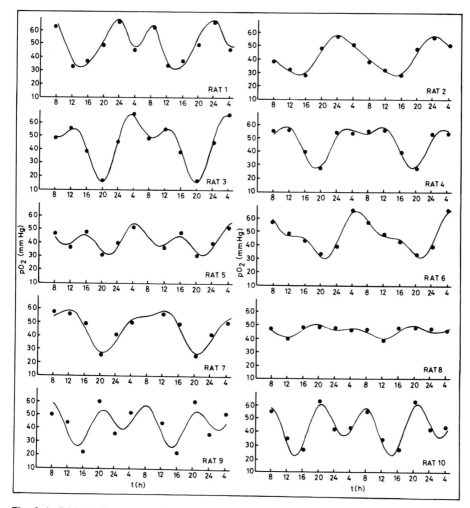

Fig. 3. Individual pO₂-courses of 10 rats

of the night period. It can be assumed that this increase was controlled by locomotor activity.

The circadian course of mean muscle pO_2 of all rats showed a sinus oscillation with high values at night and in the morning and low values in the afternoon. Thus the pO_2-oscillation was similar to the circadian rhythms of heart rate, body temperature and locomotor activity (Meinrath et al., 1978). However, in relation to the beginning of the night period and the beginning of locomotor activity, the high pO_2 values appeared delayed. Therefore, the findings of this study show that circadian muscle pO_2 oscillations are determined mainly by circadian locomotor activity and not by other oscillations.

Acknowledgements. This study was supported by the Deutsche Forschungs-gemeinschaft (HE 1293/1-2)

References

1. Benessiano J, Levy B, Samuel JL, Leclercq JF, Safar M, Saumont R (1983) Circadian changes in heart rate in unanaesthetized normotensive and spontaneously hypertensive rats. Pflügers Arch 397:70
2. Borbely AA, Neuhaus HU (1978) Daily pattern of sleep, motor activity and feeding in the rat. Effects of regular and gradually extended photoperiods. J Comp Physiol 124:1
3. Hoffmann K (1972) Zur Synchronisation biologischer Rhythmen. Ver Dtsch Zool Ges 18:266
4. Kessler M, Lübbers DW (1966) Aufbau und Anwendungsmöglichkeiten verschiedener pO$_2$-Elektroden. Pflügers Arch Ges Physiol 291:82
5. Lübbers DW (1981) Grundlagen und Bedeutung der lokalen Sauerstoffdruckmessung und des pO$_2$-Histogramms für die Beurteilung der Sauerstoffversorgung der Organe und des Organismus. In: Ehrly AM (ed) Messung des Gewebesauerstoffdruckes bei Patienten. Witzstrock, Baden Baden
6. Meinrath M, D'Amato MR (1979) Interrelationships among heart rate, activity, and body temperature in the rat. Physiol Behav 22:491
7. Wever R (1977) Quantitative studies of the interaction between different circadian oscillators within the human multioscillator system. The Publishing House, Il Ponte Milan, 1977
8. Wever R (1979) The circadian system of man. Springer, Berlin

Local Oxygen Consumption of Blood-Perfused Skeletal Muscle Determined with Oxygen Microelectrodes under Stop-Flow Conditions

H. J. Meuer

Abstract

The oxygen consumption rate, $\dot{V}O_2$, of blood perfused skeletal muscles was determined from the measured decrease of tissue pO_2 during stop-flow. By simulating stop-flow conditions using the Krogh tissue cylinder model an equation was derived which describes the influence of a definite value of pO_2 decrease and other parameters, such as hemoglobin and myoglobin concentration, on the oxygen consumption rate.
The method was applied to the blood-perfused rat gracilis muscle. The tissue pO_2 during stop-flow was measured in concurrent and countercurrent perfused tissue areas by oxygen microelectrodes. Additionally, the density of perfused capillaries and the percentage of fibers with high oxidative activity was determined. In the concurrent tissue type we found a mean density of perfused capillaries of 561 mm^{-2} and a mean fraction of oxidative fibers identified by strong SDH staining of 15.8%. For the countercurrent tissue type the respective values were higher (748 mm^{-2} and 25.5%) suggesting a higher oxygen consumption rate. This was confirmed by the results of the $\dot{V}O_2$ determinations. The mean values were 0.85 in concurrent and 0.97 ml $O_2/110$g x min in countercurrent perfused tissue areas. The sources of errors are discussed.

Introduction

The Fick principle is commonly used for determining the oxygen consumption rate, $\dot{V}O_2$, of living tissue. However, since the results of the measurements represent mean values of a large tissue portion or a whole organ, the method is not suitable for detecting local variations in $\dot{V}O_2$ which are to be expected in skeletal muscles composed of muscle fibers of different metabolic types.

Higher spatial resolution of consumption rate measurements can be achieved by the stop-flow principle. The basic idea is that the decrease in tissue pO_2 following a sudden stop of perfusion depends on the magnitude of the oxygen consumption rate. If the pO_2 decrease is measured by

Clinical Oxygen Pressure Measurement II
A.M. Ehrly et al. (Eds.)
© Blackwell Ueberreuter Wissenschaft Berlin 1990

oxygen microelectrodes, local values of the consumption rate can be obtained. Leniger-Follert and Lübbers (1973) used this principle for determining myoglobin concentrations in the hemoglobin-free perfused heart muscle of the guinea-pig.

The aim of the present study was to develop a method suitable for determining the local oxygen consumption rate of skeletal muscle tissue. The method should allow measurements under physiological conditions and not require hemoglobin-free perfusion or perfusion at an unphysiologically high pO_2, since a high tissue pO_2 may interfere with oxygen delivery and uptake.

In blood-perfused tissue the oxygen demand during stop-flow is not only met by the physically dissolved oxygen fraction, but also by oxygen bound to hemoglobin and myoglobin. Consequently, since the relationship between pO_2 and the concentration of oxygen bound to hemoglobin and myoglobin is non-linear, the decrease of the tissue pO_2 will not be constant in time, even if the consumption rate does not change (Fig. 1). This makes it difficult to extract information about the consumption rate from a measured pO_2 time course.

By simulating stop-flow conditions in a tissue cylinder we found a measurable quantity reflecting the oxygen consumption rate, and derived an equation describing the relationship between both parameters. The applicability of this equation is demonstrated by experiments.

Tissue model

Stop-flow conditions were simulated using Krogh's model of tissue cylinder. It was assumed that the tissue oxygen consumption rate does not change with time and is the same for every tissue location. Diffusion in axial direction was neglected (long cylinder with small radius). Hemoglobin and myoglobin were considered to be homogeneously distributed in the capillary and the tissue, respectively.

The diffusion of oxygen in respiring tissue is described by the equation (Hill, 1929):

$$dC/dt = D \text{ div grad } C - \dot{V}O_2 \tag{1}$$

where C is the oxygen concentration, D is the diffusion coefficient, $\dot{V}O_2$ is the oxygen consumption rate, and t is time. For the Krogh cylinder (no axial diffusion, radial symmetry) equ. 1 can be reduced to

$$dC/dt = D (d^2C/dr^2 + 1/r \, dC/dr) - \dot{V}O_2 \tag{2}$$

where r is the radius.

In the capillary the relationship between oxygen concentration, C_C, and partial pressure, P_C, is given by the oxygen hemoglobin dissociation curve (physically dissolved oxygen in the capillary is neglected). This curve is approximated by the well-known Hill equation

$$C_c = H \, C_{Hb} \, P_c{}^n/(P_c{}^n + P_{50Hb}{}^n) \tag{3}$$

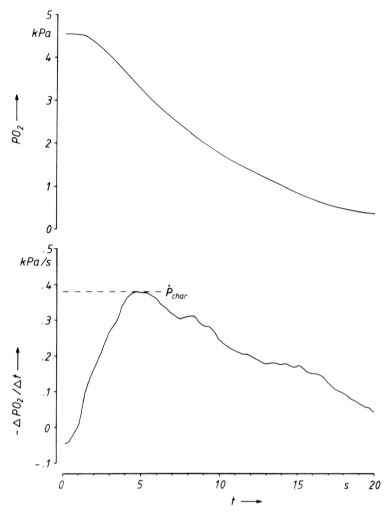

Fig. 1. Typical pO₂ time course (upper panel) measured in the resting rat gracilis muscle by an oxygen microelectrode under stop-flow conditions. The corresponding pO₂ slope is plotted in the lower panel

where P_{50Hb} is the half-saturation pressure of hemoglobin, C_{Hb} is the hemoglobin concentration in the capillary, H is the Hüfner number (maximum O₂ capacity [ml O₂] of 1 gm Hb), and n is the Hill exponent.

In the tissue, oxygen is physically dissolved and bound to myoglobin. Therefore, the relationship between oxygen concentration, C_t, and partial pressure, P_t, in the tissue,

$$C_t = S_t\,P_t + H\,C_{Mb}\,P_t/(P_t + P_{50Mb}) \tag{4}$$

consists of two components: the physically dissolved oxygen, which is proportional to the partial pressure (S_t = solubility coefficient for oxygen in tissue), and the chemically bound oxygen represented by a first order reaction term (C_{Mb} = myoglobin concentration, P_{50Mb} = half-saturation pressure for myoglobin).

Boundary conditions have to be met at the capillary/tissue interface

$$P_c = P_t(R_1) \tag{5}$$

where capillary pO_2, P_c, is equal to tissue pO_2 (R_1 = capillary radius), and also at the border of the tissue cylinder,

$$dC/dr = 0, \text{ for } r = R_2 \tag{6}$$

where no oxygen flux exists (R_2 = cylinder radius).

The initial condition is given by the steady-state solution of equ. 2 (Krogh, 1929):

$$C(r) = C(R_1) + [(r^2 - R_1^2)/2 - R_2^2 \ln(r/R_1)] \dot{V}O_2/2D \tag{7}$$

After transforming the differential equations to difference equations, estimates of the time dependent pO_2 field in the tissue during stop-flow were calculated by numerical iteration using the over-relaxation method (Björck and Dahlquist, 1972).

An example for the calculated pO_2 time course and corresponding pO_2 decrease is shown in Fig. 2. One can see that soon after the begin of stop-flow the pO_2 decrease reaches a maximum value. It can be demonstrated that this value is the same at every location within the tissue

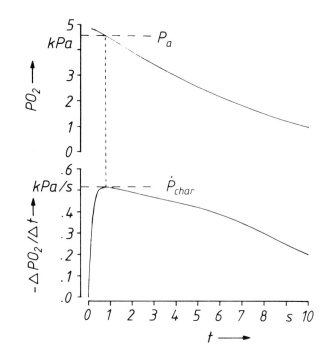

Fig. 2. Calculated time courses of pO_2 and corresponding pO_2 slope in a tissue cylinder under stop-flow conditions. The following parameters were used for the calculation: capillary radius R_1 = 1.5 µm, cylinder radius R_2 = 32 µm, hemoglobin concentration C_{Hb} = 75 g/l, myoglobin concentration C_{Mb} = 2 mg/g, and oxygen consumption rate $\dot{V}O_2$ = 1 ml O_2 /(100g min) (STPD conditions). These values approximate the situation of the resting rat gracilis muscle

cylinder. Therefore, we call this parameter the characteristic pO₂ decrease, $\dot{P}_{char}$.

In order to investigate the dependency of the characteristic pO₂ decrease on the oxygen consumption rate, different supply conditions were simulated by varying the values of the parameters influencing tissue oxygen supply, such as capillary density, capillary hematocrit, and myoglobin concentration. The values used for these calculations are listed in Table 1.

Table 1. Numerical values for constants and parametric ranges used for simulating stop-flow in the tissue cylinder. Gas volumes are given in STPD

Quantity, Unit	Value	Reference
D, 10^{-5} cm²/s	1.7	Thews (1960)
S_t, 10^{-4} ml O₂/(g kPa)	2.35	Altman & Dittmer (1971)
$\dot{V}O_2$, ml O₂/(100g min)	0.5–6	
R_1, µm	1.5–4	
R_2, µm	12.0–50	
C_{Hb}, g/l	37.0–112	
P_{50Hb}, kPa	4.0–5.3	
n	3.22	Bork et al. (1975)
C_{Mb}, mg/g	0–6	
P_{50Mb}, kPa	0.43	Theorell (1934)

From the results of these simulations an equation was derived describing the relationship between the oxygen consumption rate and the characteristic pO₂ decrease:

$$\dot{V}O_2 = (S_t + m_{Mb} \, H \, C_{Mb} + m_{Hb} \, H \, C_{Hb} / F^*) \, \dot{P}_{char} \qquad (8)$$

where

$$m_{Mb} = P_{50Mb}/(P_a + P_{50Mb})^2 \qquad (9)$$
$$F^* = (R_2/R_1)^2 - 1 = 1/(CD \, R_1^2 \, \pi) - 1 \qquad (10)$$

Equ. 8 shows that the oxygen consumption rate $\dot{V}O_2$ is proportional to the characteristic pO₂ decrease, $\dot{P}_{char}$. The proportional factor consists of three terms, each representing one of the oxygen pools covering the oxygen demand during stop-flow: physically dissolved oxygen, oxygen bound to myoglobin, and oxygen bound to hemoglobin (from left to right). m_{Mb} and m_{Hb} are the respective slopes of the oxygen myoglobin and oxygen hemoglobin dissociation curves at a partial pressure P_a which corresponds to $\dot{P}_{char}$ (see Fig. 2). m_{Mb} can easily be calculated from the dissociation curve (equ. 9).

F^* is the ratio of tissue to capillary cross-sectional area (equ. 10). The cylinder cross-section area can either be expressed by the cylinder radius, R_2, or by the capillary density, CD, assuming that $R_2^2 \, \pi = 1/CD$. The influences of F^*, C_{Hb}, and C_{Mb} on the proportional factor between oxygen consumption and characteristic pO₂ decrease are shown in Figure 3.

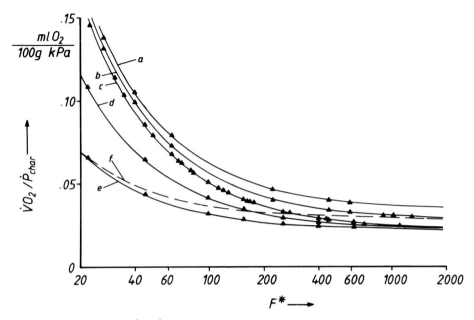

Fig. 3. Proportional factor $\dot{V}O_2/\dot{P}_{char}$ vs. F* calculated from equ. 8 (solid lines) for $P_a = 4.5$ kPa and different hemoglobin and myoglobin concentrations. a: $C_{Hb} = 112$ g/l, $C_{Mb} = 4$ mg/g; b: 112.2; c: 112.0; d: 75.0; e: 37.0; f: 37.2. Curve f probably applies to resting skeletal muscle best. Symbols represent control values obtained from the tissue model

Experimental Methods

Local oxygen consumption was determined in the anterior portion of the resting rat gracilis muscle. The animals (female Han-Wistar, 160 to 220 g body weight) were anesthetized with thiobutabarbital (0.1 g/kg b. w.). Central blood pressure, expiratory carbon dioxide fraction and body temperature were monitored continuously.

The gracilis muscle was isolated similar to the method described by Henrich and Hecke (1978) and mounted to a freezing device illustrated in Fig. 4. Blood supply was provided only by branches of the femoral artery and vein.

Tissue pO_2 was measured by recessed-tip oxygen microelectrodes with a tip diameter of 3 to 5 µm. Details of the construction and the performance have been described elsewhere (Meuer and Baumann, 1988).

After recording the pO_2 time course during stop-flow the muscles were shock-frozen and stored in liquid nitrogen until subsequent treatments.

Serial cryostat sections (20 µm) were cut from the same tissue portion in which the pO_2 decrease had been measured. Some of the slices were stained for succinic dehydrogenase (SDH) using the method of Dubowitz and Brooke (1973) with slight modifications. In these slices the relative

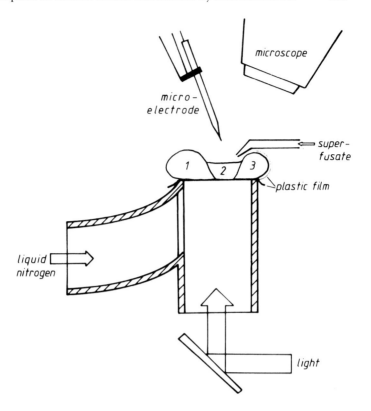

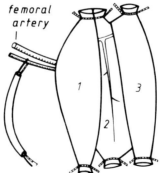

Fig. 4. Schematic drawing of the experimental set-up. The isolated muscles (1: posterior gracilis muscle; 2: anterior gracilis muscle; 3: major adductor muscle) were mounted to the top of a metal tube. To protect tissue from drying and cooling, the muscles were wrapped in plastic film and superfused by physiological salt solution at 36°C, equilibrated with 95% N_2 and 5% CO_2. Stop-flow was achieved by pulling the femoral artery into a small flexible tubule. For shock-freezing, liquid nitrogen was forced through the lateral connection of the metal tube

cross-sectional area of those muscle fibers displaying strong staining was determined. The other sections were stained for capillary endothelia by the ATPase reaction after pre-incubation at pH 4.3 (Sillau and Banchero, 1977) and used for determining the number of perfused capillaries per cross-sectional area, CD. Only those capillaries which showed an inner diameter of more than 3 μm at least once in a continuous series of five sections were counted.

Samples of venous blood were taken for determining the oxygen hemoglobin dissociation curve at standard pH (required for calculating m_{Hb}), the hematocrit and the hemoglobin concentration using standard methods.

Results

For $\dot{V}O_2$ determinations tissue areas were selected in which capillaries ran parallel to the muscle fibers and no major vessels were visible. In these areas one can distinguish between two different types of perfusion pattern: the concurrent type, where adjacent capillaries are perfused in parallel direction, and the countercurrent type, where red blood cells in adjacent capillaries move in opposite directions. We assumed that these differences in blood supply indicate different aerobic metabolic rates. This was supported by morphometric examination of the tissue: In the countercurrent type we found a significantly ($p < 0.01$) higher density of perfused capillaries and a significantly higher percentage of fibers with high oxidative activity identified by strong SDH staining (Table 2). Since the object of the experiments was to demonstrate whether the method is suitable for detecting local differences in the oxygen uptake rate, we determined and compared $\dot{V}O_2$ in both types of tissue.

Table 2. Density of perfused capillaries, CD, percentage of oxidative fibers, OF, identified by strong SDH staining, and estimates of the oxygen consumption rate, $\dot{V}O_2$, determined from tissue pO_2 decrease during stop-flow in concurrent and countercurrent perfused tissue areas. $\dot{V}O_2$ was calculated from the characteristic pO_2 decrease using equ. 8. The numerical values of the parameters required for this calculation are listed in Table 3. Values are means ± SD, gas volumes are given in STPD. ** = $p < 0.01$

Quantity, Unit	Concurrent	Countercurrent
CD, mm^{-2}	561 ±81	748 ±135**
OF, %	15.8 ±5.6	25.5 ±6.1**
$\dot{V}O_2$, ml O$_2$/(100g min)	0.85 ±0.21	0.97 ±0.36

In Table 2 the mean values of a total of 72 determinations of the local $\dot{V}O_2$ are given. The values are different for $p < 0.1$. The results correspond well to the data reported by Honig et al. (1971), who determined the oxygen consumption rate of the whole rat gracilis muscle at rest by the Fick principle and found a mean value of 0.95 ± 0.44 ml O$_2$/(100 g x min).

Discussion

The principal item of the method is equ. 8, derived from a tissue model and describing the relationship between the oxygen consumption rate and the characteristic pO$_2$ decrease. When using this equation one has to consider several sources of error which arise in part from the assumptions made for the model and also from the errors in the numerical values of the required parameters.

For the simulations it was assumed that the oxygen consumption rate is not affected by stop-flow. This is, of course, no longer true when the tissue pO$_2$ reaches values near zero. But, since the characteristic pO$_2$ decrease appears a few seconds after the begin of stop-flow while the tissue pO$_2$ is still high, it is unlikely that the consumption rate should change in the meantime.

In contrast to the model, the tissue volume which is supplied by a single capillary is not a cylinder, but irregularly shaped. Consequently, the steady state pO$_2$ field in living tissue differs from the pO$_2$ field in the cylinder. However, it is not the absolute pO$_2$ value which is evaluated, but the pO$_2$ slope over time. The computed curve for the pO$_2$ decrease shows that from about one second after the onset of stop-flow the pO$_2$ slope is the same at any distance from the capillary surface in spite of different pO$_2$ values and different spatial pO$_2$ gradients. This supports the assumption that the characteristic pO$_2$ decrease in a non-cylindrical tissue unit does not differ basically from the characteristic pO$_2$ decrease obtained in a tissue cylinder of the same cross-sectional area. For the same reason it is also unlikely that diffusion in axial direction which was suppressed in the model will considerably alter the results.

These considerations apply to tissues with the following morphological properties: the capillaries run straight and parallel, and the length of the cylinder is distinctly greater than the cylinder radius. These preconditions are satisfactorily fulfilled by skeletal muscle tissue at rest where the cylinder radius is roughly 50 µm and the cylinder length 500 µm.

Concerning the experimental requirements, a perfect stop-flow condition is essential for $\dot{V}O_2$ determinations. If the perfusion is not interrupted completely or not within about one second, the maximum pO$_2$ decrease will be lower than the true characteristic pO$_2$ decrease. The resulting error which cannot be estimated in any way affects the numerical value of the oxygen consumption rate at full magnitude, whereas an error in one of the other parameters of equ. 8 influences the result only in part.

Figure 3 shows that the influence of the myoglobin concentration on the $\dot{V}O_2$ evaluation should not be underestimated. Raising the myoglobin concentration from 0 to 2 mg/g at F* = 200 (ratio of tissue to capillary cross-sectional area), influences $\dot{V}O_2/\dot{P}_{char}$ just as an increase in the capillary hemoglobin concentration from 34 g/l to 88 g/l, although the characteristic pO$_2$ decrease was obtained at a pO$_2$ of 4.5 kPa, where the slope of the oxygen myoglobin dissociation curve is flat. This is due to the much higher (more than 5 times in resting skeletal muscle of the mixed type) oxygen capacity per tissue volume provided by myoglobin than by hemoglobin.

During stop-flow, CO$_2$ accumulates in the tissue. This does not affect the oxygen myoglobin dissociation curve within the physiological pH range

[Gayeski et al., 1985], but does influence oxygen release from hemoglobin due to the Bohr effect. Assuming a respiratory exchange coefficient of 0.8 and using the dissociation curve determined by Bork et al. (1975) one can calculate that for the mean characteristic pO_2 decrease of 0.44 kPa/s measured in the resting muscle, the slope of the physiological dissociation curve is 13% lower than the slope at constant pH 7.4. However, this reduces the $\dot{V}O_2$ value only by about 6%.

The spatial resolution and accuracy of the method is mainly determined by the spatial resolution and accuracy of the parameter values required for equ. 8. If only mean values from a series of experiments or values from literature are introduced into the equation, then the spatial resolution will be diminished. If, on the other hand, the demands on precision and resolution of the $\dot{V}O_2$ data are high, then the actual values of the parameters have to be determined.

The most simple application of the method is measuring only the pO_2 decrease during stop-flow and determining $\dot{V}O_2$ by taking a mean value for the proportional factor $\dot{V}O_2/\dot{P}_{char}$. For example, F* in the resting muscle is around 200. Applying this value to Figure 3, the proportional factor for the curves a) and e), which are calculated for extreme values of hemoglobin and myoglobin concentrations, ranges between 0.028 and 0.052. Consequently, the maximum error of the $\dot{V}O_2$ data is ± 30%, if a mean proportional factor of 0.04 is used.

For evaluating our experiments the additionally required parameters were measured or taken from literature, with the exception of the hemoglobin and myoglobin concentration which were estimated (Table 3). To calculate the possible error due to the estimations we varied the capillary hematocrit between 10% and 20%, and the myoglobin concentration between 0.5 mg/g (rat white vastus muscle) and 3.65 mg/g (rat red vastus muscle) (Harms and Hickson, 1983). This results in $\dot{V}O_2$ ranging

Table 3. Numerical values of the parameters introduced in equ. 8 for calculating $\dot{V}O_2$ in the resting rat gracilis muscle. Gas volumes are given in STPD

Quantity, Unit	Value	Reference
S_t, 10^{-4} ml O_2/(g kPa)	2.35	Altman & Dittmer (1971)
H, ml O_2/g Hb	1.36	
m_{Hb}, 1/kPa	0.16	measured
C_{Mb}, (con./counter.), mg/g	1.9/2.0	[a]
P_{50Mb}, kPa	0.71	Gayeski et al. (1985)
C_{Hb} (systemic), g/l	150	measured
Hct (systemic), %	45.9	measured
Hct (capillary), %	15	[b]
R_1, μm	1.63	measured
CD (con./counter.), mm^{-2}	561/748	measured

[a] estimated from Harms and Hickson (1983) using the measured muscle fiber composition;
[b] estimated from Schmidt-Schoenbein and Zweifach (1975), and Klitzman and Duling (1979).

between 0.71 and 1.01 ml/(100 g x min) in concurrent perfusion (0.80 and 1.14 in countercurrent perfusion) giving a maximum error of less than ±20%. If, for instance, we had included determinations of the capillary hematocrit, then only the uncertainty of the myoglobin concentration data would persist, reducing the maximum error to about ±12%.

Our experiments demonstrate local differences in the oxygen consumption rate between tissue areas with different perfusion patterns. It is true that these differences are small, but this is probably due to the fact that in spite of an evident difference in the fiber composition between the concurrent and countercurrent type the fraction of fibers with high oxidative capacity is small in both types.

In conclusion, the stop-flow method is suitable for determining $\dot{V}O_2$ of skeletal muscle tissue perfused by blood with physiological pO$_2$. Measurements can be performed at high spatial resolution, if the capillary density, the capillary hematocrit, and the myoglobin concentration are also determined. Since, in contrast to the Fick principle, data on the venous oxygen content are not required, there are no restrictions in the application concerning the architecture of venous drainage and the vessel size. Therefore, the method can also be applied to even the smallest animal, where the Fick principle fails due to technical problems.

Acknowledgements. This study was supported by the Deutsche Forschungsgemeinschaft.

References

1. Altman PL, Ditmer DS (eds) (1971) Biological handbooks: Respiration and circulation. Bethesda, MD, Federation of American Societies for Experimental Biology, p 22
2. Björck A, Dahlquist G (1972) Numerische Methoden. Oldenbourg Verlag, München, p 269
3. Bork R, Vaupel P, Thews G (1975) Atemgas-pH-Nomogramme für das Rattenblut bei 37°C. Anaesthesist 24:84
4. Dubowitz V, Brooke MH (1973) Muscle biopsy: A modern approach. Saunders, London, p 30
5. Gayeski TE, Connet RJ, Honig CR (1985) Oxygen transport in rest-work transition illustrates new functions for myoglobin. Am Physiol 248:H914
6. Harms SJ, Hickson RC (1983) Skeletal muscle mitochondria and myoglobin, endurance, and intensity of training. J Appl Physiol 54:798
7. Henrich HN, Hecke A (1978) A gracilis muscle preparation for quantitative microcirculatory studies in the rat. Microvasc Res 15:349
8. Hill AV (1929) The diffusion of oxygen and lactic acid through tissue. Proc Roy Soc B104:39
9. Honig CR, Frierson JL, Nelson CN (1971) O$_2$ transport and $\dot{V}O_2$ in resting muscle: Significance for tissue-capillary exchange. Am J Physiol 220:357
10. Klitzman B, Duling BR (1979) Microvascular hematocrit and red cell flow in resting and contracting striated muscle. Am J Physiol 237:H481
11. Krogh A (1929) Anatomie und Physiologie der Kapilaren. Springer, Bern, p 224
12. Leninger-Follert E, Lübbers DW (1973) Determination of local myoglobin concentration in the guinea pig heart. Pflügers Arch 341:217

13. Meuer HJ, Baumann R (1988) Oxygen pressure in intra- and extraembryonic blood vessels of early chick embryo. Respir Physiol 73:331
14. Schmidt-Schoenbein GW, Zweifach BW (1975) RBC velocity profiles in arteriols and venules of the rabbit omentum. Microvasc Res 10:153
15. Sillau AH, Banchero N (1977) Visualization of capillaries in skeletal muscle by the ATPase reaction. Pflügers Arch 369:269
16. Theorell H (1934) Kristallinisches Myoglobin. V. Mitteilung: Die Sauerstoffbindungs-kurve des Myoglobins. Biochem Zeitschrift 268:73
17. Thews G (1960) Ein Verfahren zur Bestimmung der O_2-Leitfähigkeit und des O_2-Löslichkeitskoeffizienten im Gehirngewebe. Pflügers Arch 271:227

Myocardial Surface Oxygen Tension is an Indicator of Transmural Tissue Oxygenation of the in vivo Beating Pig Heart

J. Hobbhahn, P. Conzen, E. Hansen, A. Goetz, G. Seidl, P. Gonschior, W. Brendel, K. Peter

Introduction

Measurement of myocardial surface tissue oxygen tension (pO_2) with multiwire surface electrodes is increasingly used with the aim of determining myocardial tissue oxygenation. Previously published studies have shown, however, that mean pO_2 values are approximately twice as high as the coronary venous oxygen [8, 9, 10, 22], which is also considered to be a measure of myocardial tissue oxygenation [4]. In view of this discrepancy, the question arises whether myocardial surface pO_2 is a reliable indicator of transmural tissue oxygenation.

We therefore investigated the relationship between surface pO_2 and other parameters of myocardial tissue oxygenation such as regional blood flow (RBF), coronary venous O_2 saturation, coronary venous pCO_2 and regional myocardial lactate extraction. The study design was based on an experimental model in which the effects of pacing-induced tachycardia on tissue oxygenation of the ischemic and of the normally supplied myocardium were measured. This model was constructed to study worsening tissue oxygenation not only by decreasing O_2 delivery to the poststenotic myocardium but also by increasing O_2 demand.

Methods

6 pigs (mean weight 32.4 kg) were studied in modified neurolept anesthesia. After sternotomy and pericardiotomy a catheter was placed in the left atrium for injection of radioactive labelled microspheres. To induce tachycardia, a pacemaker was inserted into the right atrium via the jugular vein. The proximal part of the left anterior descending coronary artery (LAD) was dissected free and a thin copper wire coated with teflon was placed around it. The copper wire was connected to a micrometer snare to create defined stenosis. The coronary vein accompanying the LAD was cannulated to withdraw blood samples from the area supplied by the LAD. Two multiwire pO_2 electrodes were placed on the myocardium, one on the area supplied by the LAD and the other on the area supplied by the

Clinical Oxygen Pressure Measurement II
A. M. Ehrly et al. (Eds.)
© Blackwell Ueberreuter Wissenschaft Berlin 1990

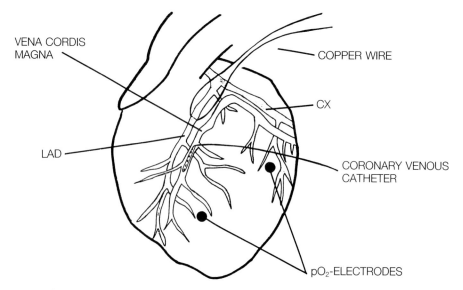

VENA CORDIS MAGNA

COPPER WIRE

CX

LAD

CORONARY VENOUS CATHETER

pO$_2$-ELECTRODES

Fig. 1. Situs of the heart after preparation: two multiwire surface electrodes are fixed on the myocardium, one on the area supplied by the left anterior descending coronary artery (LAD), the other on the area supplied by the left circumflex coronary artery (CX); the copper wire is placed around the proximal part of the LAD; care was taken to insert the coronary venous catheter distal to the constriction of the LAD

left circumflex coronary artery (CX) (Fig. 1). Surface pO$_2$ was measured continuously throughout the experiment, i.e. the electrodes were kept in position. The continuous registration yielded 7 or 8 single pO$_2$ values for each of the samplings.

Baseline

Following these preparations, baseline values of hemodynamics, arterial and coronary venous lactate concentrations, coronary venous O$_2$ saturation and coronary venous pCO$_2$ were determined. Additionally, surface pO$_2$ on the LAD and CX areas were evaluated continuously.

Stenosis

The micrometer snare was tightened to create a stenosis which reduced the surface pO$_2$ to about 50 % of its baseline value. After 20 min of steady state conditions, all measurements were repeated as described above. Additionally, 5 million of 15 μm microspheres were injected into the left atrium to determine RBF.

Stenosis plus pacing

Heart rate (HR) was increased by the pacemaker by 45 beats/min inducing a supraventricular tachycardia. All measurements were repeated after 15 min of tachycardia.

Stenosis

20 min after discontinuation of the pacemaker, all measurements were repeated once more, except for the determination of RBF.

After the end of each experiment the pig was exsanguinated and the heart excised. The left ventricular free wall was divided into 32 pieces, which were in turn subdivided into the endocardial, mediocardial and epicardial layers. All the pieces were weighed and their microsphere content determined by counting the radioactivity in the tissue samples, in the specific microsphere standards, as well as in the arterial reference samples in an auto-gamma scintillation spectrometer type 5650 from Hewlett Packard.

Statistics

Friedman's rank analysis of variance followed by Wilcoxon matched pair signed rank tests were applied to analyze the results. Intragroup comparisons of RBF were performed using the Wilcoxon matched pair signed rank test. The variations in RBF and mean surface pO$_2$ between the LAD and the CX areas were tested by the Fisher-Pitman test. The RBF and surface pO$_2$ data were also calculated as normalized values by expressing both parameters as decimal fractions of the control area (CX area). This permitted a minimization of interindividual differences in the data. Furthermore, normalization was felt to provide an accurate estimate of the severity of ischemia in terms of blood flow and tissue pO$_2$. Differences in the incidence of poststenotic pO$_2$ values in the categories below 5 mmHg and below 15 mmHg were evaluated by Chi-square test. Values of $p<0.05$ were considered significant. The data are given as means $\pm$SD.

Results

The baseline values of mean arterial pressure (MAP) and HR were 97 $\pm$8 mmHg and 94 $\pm$10 beats/min respectively. Left atrial pressure (LAP) was 9 $\pm$2 mmHg and cardiac output (CO) was 113 $\pm$23 ml·kg^{-1}·min^{-1}. The rate-pressure product (RPP, systolic aortic pressure · HR) was 10,690 $\pm$1,980. Arterial and coronary venous blood gas parameters and lactate concentrations are given in Table 1. Mean surface baseline pO$_2$ was 47 $\pm$8 mmHg in the LAD area and 48 $\pm$ 7 in the CX area (Table 1).

Table 1. Myocardial surface oxygen tensions, blood gas values and lactate concentrations, mean values ±SD; mptO$_2$ = mean surface pO$_2$ of the LAD area, calculated from 48 single measurements, mptO$_{2CX}$ = mean surface pO$_2$ of the CX area calculated from 42 single measurements; ptO$_{2LAD\%}$ = incidence of values below 5 and 15 mmHg respectively, p$_a$O$_2$ = arterial pO$_2$, S$_a$O$_2$ = arterial O$_2$ saturation, p$_a$CO$_2$ = arterial pCO$_2$, Lactate$_a$ = arterial lactate concentration; p$_{cv}$O$_{2LAD}$ = coronary venous pO$_2$ of the LAD area; S$_{cv}$O$_{2LAD}$ = coronary venous O$_2$ saturation; p$_{cv}$CO$_{2LAD}$ = coronary venous pCO$_2$, Lactate$_{cvLAD}$ = coronary venous lactate concentration, LE$_{LAD}$ = regional lactate extraction; * = p<0.05 vs corresponding CX value; ° = p<0.05 vs stenosis; § = p<0.05 vs baseline

		Baseline	Stenosis	Stenosis + Pacing	Stenosis
mptO$_{2LAD}$	(mmHg)	47 ± 8	23 ± 7*§	5 ± 5*§°	25 ± 11*§
ptO$_{2LAD\%}$ <5 mmHg	(%)	0	0	71§°	0
ptO$_{2LAD\%}$ <15 mmHg	(%)	0	19	94§°	15
mptO$_{2CX}$	(mmHg)	48 ± 7	46 ± 9	44 ± 8	43 ± 7
p$_a$O$_2$	(mmHg)	93 ± 12	89 ± 13	89 ± 14	95 ± 15
S$_a$O$_2$	(%)	93.2 ± 1.3	93.0 ± 1.8	92.6 ± 2.1	93.7 ± 1.4
p$_a$CO$_2$	(mmHg)	35 ± 2	37 ± 3	38 ± 3	38 ± 4
Lactate$_a$	(mMol x 1^{-1})	1.2 ± 0.3	1.0 ± 0.2	0.9 ± 0.1	0.9 ± 0.3
p$_{cv}$O$_{2LAD}$	(mmHg)	23.6 ± 5.2	20.5 ± 2.5§	22.1 ± 1.5	23.8 ± 2.7
S$_{cv}$O$_{2LAD}$	(%)	22.1 ± 7.7	15.4 ± 4.4§	16.3 ± 4.1	12.4 ± 2.4
p$_{cv}$CO$_{2LAD}$	(mmHg)	46 ± 2	52 ± 3§	59 ± 7§°	50 ± 5
Lactate$_{cvLAD}$	(mMol x 1^{-1})	1.0 ± 0.2	1.5 ± 0.4§	2.9 ± 1.0§°	1.3 ± 0.4
LE$_{LAD}$	(%)	+ 10 ± 9	− 50 ± 48§	− 217 ± 103§°	− 38 ± 58

Stenosis

Creating the stenosis did not alter general hemodynamics and arterial blood gas parameters. Mean surface pO$_2$ in the poststenotic area was reduced to 23 ±7 mmHg. 19 % of all pO$_2$ values were below 15 mmHg, but none were below 5 mmHg (Table 1). Surface pO$_2$ in the CX area remained constant with no values under 30 mmHg. The decrease of surface pO$_2$ in the LAD zone was associated with decreases in coronary venous O$_2$ saturation and pO$_2$, and increases in coronary venous pCO$_2$ and lactate in all the animals (Table 1; Fig. 2). Lactate extraction changed to slight lactate production (Table 1). Total blood flow in the poststenotic area was 20 % lower than in the normally supplied myocardium (Table 2). RBF in the poststenotic area was inhomogeneously distributed, as evidenced by a lower subendocardial to subepicardial ratio (endo/epi-ratio) when compared to the normal endo/epi-ratio in the control area. The more marked hypoperfusion of the subendocardial layer also can be derived from the normalized blood flow data: RBF in the endocardial, mediocardial and epicardial layers was 40, 15 and 10 % lower than in the corresponding layers of the CX area.

Table 2. Total (TBF) and regional blood flow of the subendocardial (ENDO), mediocardial (MID) and subepicardial (EPI) layers of the ischemic (LAD) and non-ischemic (CX) areas during stenosis of the LAD and during stenosis plus pacing (ml · 100g^{-1} · min^{-1}); ENDO/EPI = subendocardial to subepicardial ratio; values are means ±SD; * = p<0.05 vs corresponding CX value; ° = p<0.05 vs stenosis

		Stenosis	Stenosis + Pacing
TBF	LAD	102 ± 22*	94 ± 22*°
	CX	126 ± 32	160 ± 33
ENDO	LAD	80 ± 26*	57 ± 22*°
	CX	128 ± 33	162 ± 34
MID	LAD	101 ± 21*	78 ± 14*°
	CX	118 ± 39	157 ± 43
EPI	LAD	116 ± 29*	130 ± 28*
	CX	129 ± 45	158 ± 47
ENDO/EPI	LAD	0.7 ± 0.2*	0.4 ± 0.2*°
	CX	1.0 ± 0.1	1.0 ± 0.1

Stenosis and pacing

During pacing, HR was 138 ±14 beats/min. MAP, LAP and CO remained constant (Table 1). RPP increased by 45 % to 15,160 ±1,400. Surface pO$_2$ values in the LAD area decreased, approaching or even reaching 0 mmHg: 36 % of all values measured were 0 mmHg, 71 % were below 5 mmHg, 94 % were below 15 mmHg. This means a disproportionate increase of low surface pO$_2$ values under stenosis after pacing compared to values under stenosis before pacing. Surface pO$_2$ in the CX area was not affected by pacing, again with no values under 30 mmHg (Table 1).

The pacing-induced increase in O$_2$ demand was associated with an increase of total flow in the CX area by 27 % (Table 2). In contrast, total flow in the poststenotic area was reduced by 10 %. Furthermore, a redistribution of RBF occurred: RBF in the subepicardial layer increased by 10 %, whereas RBF in the subendocardial layer decreased by 30 %; i.e. the endo/epi-ratio decreased to 0.4 ±0.2. Poststenotic hypoperfusion and redistribution is underscored by the normalized blood flow values: the endocardial, mediocardial and epicardial layers of the LAD area are 65, 50 and 15 % less perfused respectively than the corresponding layers of the control area.

The decrease in surface pO$_2$ and the redistribution of RBF were concomitant with a two to fourfold increase in regional lactate production and an increase in coronary venous pCO$_2$ in each animal. The marked increase in lactate production coincides with the disproportional increase in low surface pO$_2$ values. However, the apparent increase in the severity of ischemia was not associated with an increased O$_2$ extraction, as evidenced by the unchanged coronary venous pO$_2$ and O$_2$ saturation values (Table 1; Figs. 2, 3).

Stenosis

When pacing was discontinued, HR and RPP returned to their baseline values, again with no change in MAP, LAP and CO. Surface pO_2 in the poststenotic area reached prepacing values within a few minutes (Table 1). Lactate extraction and coronary venous pCO_2 corresponded to prepacing values.

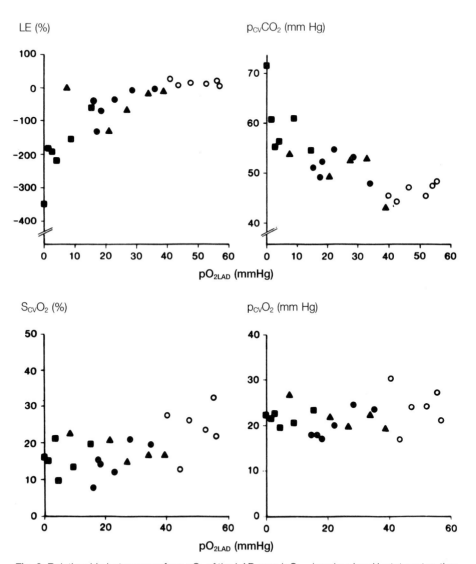

Fig. 2. Relationship between surface pO_2 of the LAD area (pO_{2LAD}) and regional lactate extraction (LE), regional coronary venous pCO_2 ($p_{cv}CO_2$), regional coronary venous O_2 saturation ($S_{cv}O_2$) and regional coronary venous pO_2 ($p_{cv}O_2$); the individual values of each animal are given: $\bigcirc$ = baseline, $\bullet$ = stenosis prior to pacing, $\blacksquare$ = pacing, $\blacktriangle$ = stenosis after pacing

There was a strong dependence of regional lactate extraction and of coronary venous pCO_2 on surface pO_2 (Fig. 2). By contrast, there exists no close relationship between surface pO_2 and coronary venous O_2 saturation and coronary venous pO_2 respectively (Fig. 2).

There is no or only poor correlation between the absolute values of surface pO_2 and the absolute values of subepicardial and subendocardial RBF (Fig. 3). However, there exists a clear and close dependence of the nor-

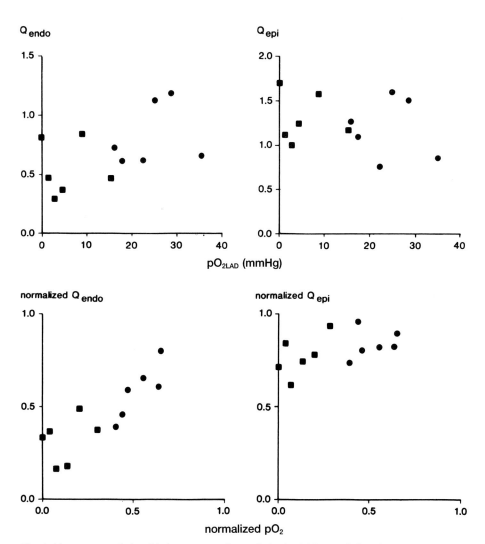

Fig. 3. Upper part: relationship between surface pO_2 in the LAD area (pO_{2LAD}) and the **absolute** values of subendocardial (Q_{endo}) and subepicardial blood flow (Q_{epi}) (ml · g⁻¹ · min⁻¹); at the bottom: relationship between the **normalized** surface pO_2 (normalized pO_2) and the **normalized** subendocardial (normalized Q_{endo}) and subepicardial blood flow (normalized Q_{epi}); pO_2 and blood flow data were normalized by expressing values as decimal fractions of the simultaneously measured parameters in the control area (CX area); for symbols, see Fig. 1

malized subendocardial RBF on the normalized surface pO_2 values (Fig. 3). The distribution of the normalized values (referred to the corresponding RBF and pO_2 values in CX area) indicates a near equivalent course for the decreases of surface pO_2 and subendocardial RBF. The data suggest a 70 – 80 % reduction of subendocardial RBF when creating a degree of stenosis which leads to a surface pO_2 of 0 mmHg. Normalization of subepicardial blood flow results only in a poor association with surface pO_2 (Fig. 3). The plot suggests an approximately 20 % reduction of subepicardial flow when approaching a surface pO_2 of 0 mmHg.

Discussion

Our results show that measurement of surface pO_2 is a sensitive method not only for the determination of regional epicardial tissue oxygenation, but also of transmural oxygenation as evidenced by a clear and close relationship between regional lactate extraction, coronary venous pCO_2 and the normalized subendocardial RBF. Furthermore, it became evident that surface pO_2 is not a parameter for regional O_2 delivery, but actually reflects tissue pO_2, i.e. the net balance of capillary O_2 delivery and cellular consumption. This was shown by the pacing manoeuvre, which led to a slight increase in subepicardial blood flow, whereas surface pO_2 decreased to values near 0 mmHg. The explanation for this finding is that the slight increase in epicardial O_2 delivery was not sufficient to meet the increase in O_2 demand. Consequently, the O_2 balance of the poststenotic myocardium worsened.

It has to be stressed that the measurement of tissue pO_2 by multiwire surface electrodes does not mean that intracellular pO_2 was determined, since the recordings measured are averaged values of several myocardial muscle cells, connective tissue and capillaries. We rather assume that the pO_2 values predominantly reflect extracellular oxygen tension, which nevertheless is of significant impact for the intracellular pO_2.

There is no or only a relatively poor correlation between the absolute values of surface pO_2 and the absolute values of subepicardial and subendocardial RBF, respectively. This can be ascribed to two factors: first, interindividual differences of both parameters and, secondly, the absolute RBF values only reflect O_2 delivery without any relation to actual O_2 demand. In contrast, the normalized subendocardial RBF correlates well with the normalized surface pO_2, since normalizing both parameters eliminates both sources of error: the differences between the animals are minimized and the factor of O_2 demand is included. The rationale for this latter assumption is that the normalized RBF values reflect hypoperfusion (of the poststenotic area) in relation to a given O_2 demand (as reflected by perfusion of the normally supplied area). This conclusion is based on the fact that perfusion of the normally supplied myocardium closely correlates with the myocardial O_2 requirements [4]. Similar considerations apply to the normalized surface pO_2 values: they reflect tissue oxygenation of the ischemic myocardium in relation to that of the normal myocardium. Thus, studying the relationship between the two normalized parameters is equivalent to correlating two measures of the severity of ischemia. And this in fact reveals a clear and close relation between subendocardial RBF and surface pO$_2$ on the one hand, but a poor relation between subepicardial RBF and surface pO$_2$ on the other hand. It is noteworthy that identical findings have been reported when correlating the normalized subendo- and subepicardial RBF values with normalized systolic wall thickening [5], another sensitive indicator of myocardial ischemia.

The missing or only weak correlation between surface pO$_2$ and coronary venous pO$_2$ and O$_2$ saturation, respectively, is poorly understood. Both coronary venous parameters were reduced after stenosis, indicating an increase in O$_2$ extraction due to the reduction of RBF. However, the further deterioration of surface pO$_2$ during pacing was not associated with a further desaturation of hemoglobin. This raises the question whether coronary venous blood samples from an ischemic area of the left ventricle are representative for the myocardial metabolism in that area, or whether dilution by blood from non-ischemic areas has to be considered. A number of studies suggest that blood samples from the coronary vein originate almost completely from the myocardium supplied by the LAD [13, 18, 21]. This particularly applies to a moderate degree of ischemia as used in our experiments [21], where care was taken to place the tip of the catheter in the coronary vein distal to the site of LAD constriction. Furthermore, dilution by blood from non-ischemic areas should be less relevant in pigs with their minimal collateral circulation [16]. Dilution by venous-venous intercommunications [17] cannot be excluded. However, its significance for the assessment of coronary venous parameters from the ischemic LAD zone is unclear, particularly in the pig heart.

The paradoxical finding of a marked deterioration of myocardial tissue oxygenation in the absence of a reduction of coronary venous pO$_2$ or of a further increase in O$_2$ extraction has also been reported by others [2, 7, 15]. Thus, our findings concerning coronary venous pO$_2$ are in accordance with the literature; however, we cannot explain them conclusively. We assume that dilution from non-ischemic areas does play a role. Further studies focusing on distribution of capillary flow, on spatial resolution of coronary venous pO$_2$ and of tissue pO$_2$ values, as well as on the capacity of O$_2$ utilization in the ischemic myocardium might lead to a better understanding of these findings. Regardless of these considerations, the weak correlation between coronary venous O$_2$-saturation and surface pO$_2$ does not invalidate surface pO$_2$ but rather coronary venous O$_2$ saturation as a measure of myocardial oxygenation.

In contrast to the latter parameters, coronary venous pCO$_2$ and regional lactate extraction clearly correlated with pO$_2$. The increase in coronary venous pCO$_2$ with significant myocardial ischemia has been described by others as well [7, 15, 18] and is due to the increased rate of anaerobic glycolysis generating lactic acid. This is associated with an increased production of hydrogen ions, which are buffered by the intracellular bicarbonate buffer system generating carbon dioxide. When analyzing the relation between surface pO_2 and myocardial lactate production, it might be meaningful to focus not only on the mean values of surface pO_2, but also on the incidence of low pO_2 values. The rationale for this is the assumption that it is the low values that reflect myocardial cells at risk to produce lactate. In fact, 20 % of all pO_2 values were below 15 mmHg at the degree of stenosis chosen in our study, and this was associated with a slight lactate production. However, a threefold increase of lactate production occurred during pacing with 92 % of all values below 15 mmHg.

It is of interest that regional myocardial carbon dioxide tension had been considered a more sensitive indicator of the severity of myocardial ischemia than myocardial oxygen tension in a similar experimental model [14]. However, in these experiments pO_2 had been determined by large mass spectrometer probes (22 gauge) which had been inserted in the left ventricular wall. Thus, the lack of major changes in pO_2 in spite of inducing severe ischemia might be predominantly due to the traumatic insertion of the spectrometer probes. Our results show that the atraumatic measurement of surface pO_2 is a very sensitive method for the evalutaion of tissue oxygenation.

Our finding of myocardial lactate production with the lowest surface pO_2 values above $5 - 10$ mmHg and mean surface pO_2 values as high as 25 mmHg (stenosis, prior to and after pacing) has prompted questions concerning

(a) the role of pO_2 as control for metabolic autoregulation,
(b) the transmural pO_2 gradient of the ischemic myocardium and
(c) the pO_2 level below which lactate production occurs.

In our study a 50 % reduction of surface pO_2 occurred in spite of a reserve of vasodilation in the subepicardial layer as evidenced by the 10 % increase of subepicardial RBF during pacing. This questions pO_2 as a primary parameter maintained constant by autoregulatory processes. It has to be considered that other factors becoming effective only at very low pO_2 values are responsible for the adjustment of coronary flow and the activation of coronary reserve. It would lead us too far to discuss the different hypotheses concerning the nature of these factors and how their signals are propagated to the structures regulating capillary perfusion.

With an increasing degree of flow restriction, lactate production at first occurs in the subendocardial layer [4]. Thus, subendocardial pO_2 surely is lower than surface pO_2. Furthermore, according to in vitro studies, the redox state of the respiratory chain in mitochondria is affected only when the pO_2 in the suspension medium is below 1 mmHg [3, 20]. Therefore, one might speculate that subendocardial pO_2 at the degree of stenosis chosen in our experiments is reduced right down to or almost down to 0 mmHg. This would be consistent with an extreme transmural pO_2 gradient under a moderate degree of flow restriction.

On the other hand, there is some evidence of a marked extra- to intra-cellular pO$_2$ gradient [6, 11, 12, 23], suggesting a diffusion barrier for oxygen. Furthermore, onset of lactate production at extracellular pO$_2$ levels as high as 16 mmHg is suggested by studies on cultured chick embryo ventricular cells [1]. This would support the idea of sarcolemma as the main diffusion barrier to oxygen [19]. However, this assumption has been challenged by the suggestion that the capillary is the principal barrier [12]. In any case, there is some evidence for the existence of a marked pO$_2$ gradient between the extracellular and the intracellular space. Thus, sig-nificant subendocardial lactate production might occur in spite of suben-docardial pO$_2$ values distinctly above 0 mmHg. This, however, would point to a less steep transmural pO$_2$ gradient during a moderate degree of stenosis.

In conclusion, our results show that (1) myocardial surface pO$_2$ reflects the net balance between subepicardial capillary O$_2$ delivery and cellular O$_2$ consumption and (2) measurement of myocardial surface pO$_2$ is a sensi-tive method not only for the determination of regional epicardial tissue oxygenation, but also of transmural tissue oxygenation.

References

1. Barry WT, Pober JD, Frankel SR, Smith TW (1980) Effects of graded hypoxia on contraction of cultured chick embryo ventricular cells. Am J Physiol 239:H651
2. Bristow JD, McFalls EO, Anselone CG, Pantley GA (1987) Coronary vasodilator reserve persists despite tachycardia and myocardial ischemia. Am J Physiol 253:H422
3. Chance B, Schoener B, Schindler F (1966) The intracellular oxidation-reduction state. In: Dickens F, Neill E (eds) Oxygen in the animal organism. Pergamon Press, London, p 367
4. Feigl EO (1983) Coronary physiology. Physiol Rev 63:1
5. Gallagher KP, Matsuzaki M, Koziol JA, Kemper WS, Ross J (1984) Regional myocardial perfusion and wall thickening during ischemia in conscious dogs. Am J Physiol 247:H727
6. Gayeski TEJ, Honig CR (1978) Myoglobin saturation and calculated pO$_2$ in single cells of resting gracilis muscles. Adv Exp Med Biol 94:77
7. Griggs DM, Chen CC, Tchokoev VV (1973) Subendocardial anaerobic metabolism in experimental aortic stenosis. Am J Physiol 224:607
8. Hobbhahn J, Conzen P, Goetz A, Habazettl H, Granetzny T, Peter K, Brendel W (1985) Durchblutung und Sauerstoffversorgung des Myokards unter Isoflurane und Enflu-rane. In: Peter K, Brown BR, Martin E, Norlander PO (eds) Inhalationsanästhesie – neue Aspekte. Springer, Berlin, p 178
9. Hobbhahn J, Conzen P, Goetz A, Seidl G, Gonschior P, Brendel W, Peter K (1987) Moderate hypotensive anaesthesia with enflurane and isoflurane – beneficial for the ischemic heart? Anesthesiology 67:A589 (Abstract)
10. Hobbhahn J, Peter K, Goetz A, Conzen P (1987) Influence of the inhalation anesthetics isoflurane and enflurane on the normal and ischemic myocardium. In: Baethmann A, Messmer K (eds) Surgical Research: Recent concepts and results. Springer, Berlin, p 18
11. Honig CR (1977) Hypoxia in skeletal muscle at rest and during the transition to steady work. Microvasc Res 13:377
12. Honig CR, Gayeski TEJ, Federspiel W, Clark A, Clark P (1984) Muscle O$_2$ gradients from hemoglobin to cytochrome: new concepts, new complexities. In: Lübbers DW, Acker H, Leninger-Follert E, Goldstick TK (eds) Oxygen transport to tissue-V. Plenum, New York, p 23

13. Nakazawa HK, Roberts DL, Klocke FJ (1987) Quantification of anterior descending vs. circumflex venous drainage in the canine great cardiac vein and coronary sinus. Am J Physiol 234:H163
14. O'Riardon JB, Flaherty JT, Khuri SF, Brawley RK, Gott VL (1977) Effects of atrial pacing on regional myocardial gas tensions with critical coronary stenosis. Am J Physiol 232:H49
15. Obeid A, Smulyan H, Gilbert R, Eich RH, Syracuse NY (1972) Regional metabolic changes in the myocardium following coronary artery ligation in dogs. Am Heart J 83:189
16. Patterson RE, Kirk ES (1983) Analysis of coronary collateral structure, function, and ischemic border zones in pigs. Am J Physiol 244:H23
17. Roberts DL, Nakazawa HK, Klocke FJ (1976) Origin of great cardiac vein and coronary sinus drainage within the left ventricle. Am J Physiol 230:H486
18. Roberts DL, Nakazawa HK, Nordlicht SM, Sekovski B, Magelil J, Oliveros RA, Orlick AE, Klocke FJ (1979) Evaluation of regional myocardial perfusion and ischemia from coronary venous blood. Am J Physiol 236:H385
19. Rose CP, Goreski CA, Bach GG (1977) The capillary and sarcolemmal barriers in the heart: an exploration of labeled water permeability. Circ Res 41:515
20. Starlinger H, Luebbers DW (1973) Polarographic measurement of the oxygen pressure performed simultaneously with optical measurements of the redox state of the respiratory chain in suspensions of mitochondria under steady-state conditions of low oxygen tensions. Pluegers Arch 341:15
21. Vinten-Johansen J, Johnston WE, Crystal GJ, Mills SA, Santamore WP, Cordell AR (1987) Validation of local venous sampling within the at risk anterior descending artery vascular bed in the canine left ventricle. Cardiovasc Res 21:646
22. Vogel H, Günther H, Harrison DK, Kessler M, Peter K (1984) The influence of isoflurane and enflurane on tissue oxygenation and microcirculation of the dog myocardium. Anesthesiology 61:A5 (Abstract)
23. Whalen WJ, Nair P (1967) Intracellular pO_2 and its regulation in resting skeletal muscle of the guinaea-pig. Circ Res 21:251

Oxygen-Dependent Lysosomal Enzyme Release in Renal Tubular Cells

N. Klause, G. Gronow

Introduction

Microelectrode measurements in the renal cortex in vivo have revealed local oxygen tensions of 10 mmHg and less [Baumgärtl et al., 1972]. This may have been the result of local imbalances due to a high O_2 uptake and an insufficient O_2 supply. On a wet weight basis, for example, oxygen consumption of the renal cortex exceeds that of the brain cortex or the heart (Fig.1, left panel). Additionally, a reduced oxygen delivery by O_2 shunting from descending arterial vasa recta into closely arranged ascending renal veins [Kriz, 1981] may have further reduced local oxygen tension to less than 10 mmHg. At this low pO_2, however, oxygen supply in the renal cortex becomes "critical", the oxygen uptake declines [Leichtweiss et al., 1969], the cytochromes of the mitochondrial respiratory chain are markedly reduced [Balaban et al., 1980], and the cytoplasmatic $ATP/ADP \cdot P_i$-ratio is remarkably low (Wilson et al., 1977, 1979).

The question arises as to what extent mitochondrial generation of ATP had also been a limiting factor for basal ion-pumping activity in renal cortical cells, i.e. whether at an extracellular pO_2 below 10 mmHg the oncotic forces of intracellular macromolecules had been sufficiently counterbalanced by energy consuming outward pumping of diffusible ions. If not, water would have moved into renal cortical cells, a potassium loss in exchange for extracellular sodium would have reduced the cellular membrane potential, chloride, calcium and more water would have entered the cells (MacKnight and Leaf, 1977; Schrier et al., 1987), and the liberation of lysosomal enzymes as well as a disruptive swelling of renal tubular cells would have limited cellular viability (Gronow et al., 1984 a, b; Hochachka, 1986).

To test renal cortical cellular viability at low extracellular oxygen tension we isolated tubular segments of rat kidney cortex and measured ATP-dependent cellular functions (K^+ accumulation, oxygen consumption, gluconeogenesis) as well as the release of cellular marker enzymes at different levels of extracellular pO_2.

Clinical Oxygen Pressure Measurement II
A. M. Ehrly et al. (Eds.)
© Blackwell Ueberreuter Wissenschaft Berlin 1990

Material and Methods

Details of the isolation and purification of isolated tubular segments (ITS) of rat kidney cortex have been reported elsewhere (Bertermann et al., 1975; Gronow et al., 1976, 1984 a,b). Briefly, kidneys of starved male Sprague-Dawley rats (350 – 450g) were cooled and rinsed in situ with ice-cold Krebs-Ringer Bicarbonate solution (KRB). ITS were then isolated by mechanical and Collagenase treatment (0.2g/100 ml CLS II, Worthington, Freehold, N.J., USA), washed twice, incubated at 37°C in KRB (pH 7.4, 10g/l bovine albumine), and gently shaken for 20 min in 50 ml Erlenmeyer flasks.

Different levels of extracellular oxygen tension were adjusted by gassing the surface of the incubation media with a mixture of 95% O_2 : 5% CO_2 and 95% N_2 : 5% CO_2. Extracellular oxygen tension in the incubation medium was registered polarographically with a Clark-type oxygen electrode. Measurements of oxygen consumption were performed in a sealed and thermostatically controlled reaction chamber (Eschweiler, Kiel, FRG). During one series of experiments on the effect of different extracellular oxygen tensions, bath pO_2 in the incubation medium was kept constant at either 1.0, 2.5, 5.0, 10, 40, or 100 mmHg, respectively.

As functional parameters of ITS served a) oxygen consumption ($Q-O_2$), b) formation of glucose from 10 mmol/l lactate (gluconeogenesis = GNG), c) intracellular K^+ accumulation (K^+) and d) loss of marker enzymes (cytoplasmatic lactate dehydrogenase = LDH; γ glutamyl transferase of renal brush borders = γGT; mitochondrial glutamate dehydrogenase = GlDH; and lysosomal acid phosphatase = APase). Assays of enzyme activity and of glucose content in the incubation medium as well as of intracellular K^+ were performed according to standard procedures (Bergmeyer, 1974; Gronow et al., 1984 a, b). A p-value of 0.05 or less (Student's t-Test for unpaired observations) was regarded as indicating a statistically significant difference.

Results and Discussion

Oxygen consumption

According to the observations of others (Harris et al., 1981; Weinberg, 1985), cells of ITS at 37°C and an extracellular pO_2 of 100 mmHg oxygen respired (as calculated in nanomol O_2/mg protein x min) at a rate of 24.4 (endogenous), 30.4 (5 mmol/l lactate), and 33.5 (lactate, glucose, malate, each 5 mmol/l), respectively (Fig. 1, right panel). Obviously, in the range of 100 to 10 mmHg, oxygen consumption of the ITS occurred independently of extracellular pO_2, and it remained constant right down to 10 mmHg. Below 10 mmHg, however, where extracellular pO_2 became "critical" [Leichtweiss et al., 1969], the O_2 uptake declined, especially in the pO_2 range below 5 mmHg (Fig. 1).

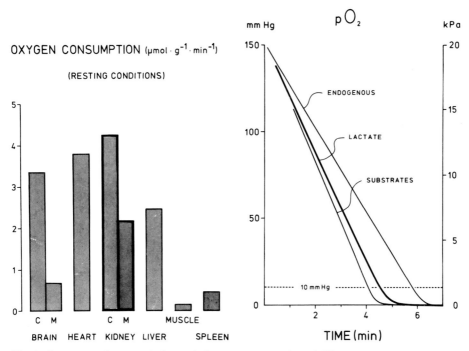

Fig. 1. Oxygen uptake rates. Left panel: Oxygen consumption of different organs of man under resting conditions (wet weight basis); C = cortex, M = medulla. (Modified after several authors according to Grote [1987]). Right panel: Oxygen consumption kinetics of isolated tubular segments of rat kidney cortex (37 °C). Ordinate: oxygen tension in the incubation medium. Endogenous = no substrates added; Substrates = lactate, glucose, malate (each 5 mmol/l); Lactate = 5 mmol/l lactate added (standard in all experiments)

A similar decrease in the oxygen uptake of isolated cells, accompanied by a concomitant reduction of mitochondrial cytochromes in ITS (Balaban et al., 1980), or of the ATP/ADP ratio in isolated hepatocytes (DeGroot and Noll, 1987), has been observed at an extracellular pO_2 of 5 mmHg. To test exclusively aerobic metabolism and to avoid an increase in the anoxic tolerance of ITS by the effect of anaerobic ATP generation via "anaerobic" substrates (Gronow and Cohen, 1984; Gronow et al., 1984 b), 10 mmol/l lactate (heavy line in Fig.1, right panel) served as the only substrate for glucose formation in all of the following experiments.

Gluconeogenesis (GNG)

At a physiological pO_2 (100 mmHg, Fig.2, left panel) GNG of isolated tubular segments remained within the range of earlier observations (Gronow et al., 1984a). At a "mixed venous pO_2" of 40 mmHg (and far above the point where Q-O_2 broke off in Fig.1), the rate of ATP-dependent

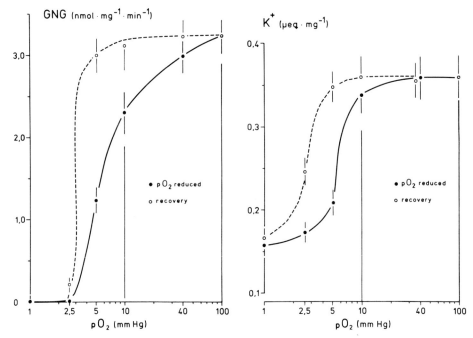

Fig. 2. Cellular functions of isolated tubular segments of rat kidney cortex (37°C) at different levels of extracellular oxygen tension (closed symbols) and after subsequent reoxygenation (open symbols). Left panel: Gluconeogenesis (GNG) from 10 mmol/l lactate. Right panel: Intracellular K^+ content ($\bar{x}$ ±SD, n = 14).

GNG was somewhat smaller (Fig.2, solid circles in left panel); at a pO_2 of 10 mmHg GNG fell significantly to about 75%, and at 5 mmHg GNG was about half of the control value (100 mmHg). At lower oxygen tensions (2.5 and 1 mmHg) no measurable GNG could be detected.

The observed suppression of GNG in the presence of an extracellular pO_2 ranging between 5 and 100 mm Hg, however, was reversible when ITS were reoxygenated by gassing the incubation medium with 95% O_2 : 5% CO_2 (Fig.2, open circles in the left panel). A defect in GNG capacity only persisted when ITS had been incubated for 20 min at a pO_2 of 2.5 mmHg or less, indicating irreversible cellular alterations induced by oxygen deprivation (Gronow et al., 1984 a,b).

Since glucose formation from lactate not only requires consumption of metabolic energy but also the transport of metabolites across intact mitochondrial membranes, an irreversible reduction in GNG at an extracellular pO_2 of 2.5 mmHg or less may indicate irreversible mitochondrial membrane damage as a result of high cytosolic calcium (Schrier et al., 1987) and an increased activity of phospholipases [Hochachka, 1986], which in turn may have liberated mitochondrial GlDH (see below).

Intracellular K+ reaccumulation

When extracellular pO_2 was reduced, K^+ content did not decline as observed for GNG at a pO_2 of 40 mmHg (solid circles in right panel of Fig. 2). Even at a pO_2 of 10 mmHg, the decrease in K^+ was small and insignificant. At 5 mmHg or less, however, K^+ declined to about one third of the aerobic value. This substantial release of intracellular K^+ was similar to the K^+ loss observed previously in anoxic ITS (Harris et al., 1981; Gronow et al., 1984 a,b; Weinberg, 1985).

The observed K^+ loss, however, may have been rather a reflection of active volume regulation than of irreversible cell death (Lang et al., 1988). Thus, only the reduced ability of reoxygenated ITS to reaccumulate K^+ after hypoxic incubation (at an extracellular pO_2 lower than 5 mm Hg, Fig.2, right panel, open circles) indicated an irreversible impairment in ITS monovalent ion homeostasis, which was probably accompanied by a decrease in cellular membrane potential and, in consequence, by a subsequent influx of extracellular calcium (Weinberg, 1985; Schrier et al., 1987). The elevated level of intracellular Ca^{++} may then have accelerated cellular membrane damage by an increased activity of phospholipases (Hochachka, 1986), indicated in the present experiments by a marked loss of cellular constituents.

Loss of cell constituents

Under aerobic conditions, ITS already lost small amounts of intracellular enzymes (in mU/mg protein x min: LDH = 1.1, γGT = 0.80, APase = 0.08, GlDH = 0.01). This small leakage was probably due to the collagenase treatment and the impact of mechanical shaking [Gronow and Weiss, 1976]. Down to a pO_2 of 10 mmHg no further increase in the loss of cell constituents could be observed (Fig. 3). These observations indicated that at this extracellular pO_2 cellular membranes had not become leaky due to anoxic swelling and the liberation of lysosomal enzymes.

At an extracellular pO_2 of 5 mmHg, however, a small but significant leakage of cytoplasm (indicated by LDH loss) and of brush border microvilli (indicated by γGT loss) may have occurred due to membrane deformation (Fig.3, left panel). This loss of cell constituents may have been transient as long as mitochondrial structure was maintained during hypoxia (indicated by no significant loss of mitochondrial GlDH), and as long as a subsequent reoxygenation would have enabled renal mitochondria to form ATP for ion homeostasis, GNG, regeneration of cellular cytoplasm, and brush border microvilli (Herminghuysen et al., 1985; Mills et al., 1986).

However, the significant onset of liberation of lysosomal enzymes at 5 mmHg (as indicated by APase loss), may have already initiated intracellular changes which finally led to the previously described irreversible uncoupling of mitochondrial respiratory function in the hypoxic kidney

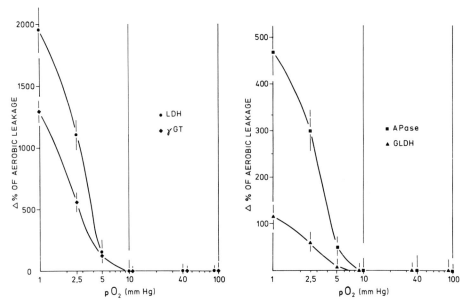

Fig. 3. Enzyme leakage of isolated tubular segments of rat kidney cortex (37°C) at different levels of extracellular oxygen tension. Left panel: loss of cytoplasmatic lactate-dehydrogenase (LDH) and of brush border γ glutamyltransferase (γGT). Right panel: loss of lysosomal acid phosphatase (APase) and of mitochondrial glutamate-dehydrogenase (GlDH). $\bar{x}$ ±SD, n = 14

(Gronow et al., 1986). Lysosomal enzymes, especially phospholipases, may, at this low pO_2, have attacked mitochondrial membranes (Hochachka, 1986), as indicated in the present experiments by a significant loss of the mitochondrial matrix enzyme GlDH.

Finally, at a pO_2 of 1 mmHg, cell death was indicated by the high activity of all 4 marker enzymes (LDH for cytoplasm, γGT for brush border microvilli, APase for lysosomes, GlDH for mitochondria) in the incubation medium (Fig.3) as well as by a negligeble aerobic recovery of GNG and of K^+accumulation (Fig.2). Thus, this low pO_2 may be a sufficient driving force to oxidize respiratory chain cytochromes in isolated heart mitochondria [Chance, 1976], but not in isolated cells where an additional diffusion gradient from cellular surfaces into mitochondria will limit any effective oxidative phosphorylation (Jones and Kennedy, 1982).

Conclusions

A frequency distribution of local oxygen tension including values of 10 mm Hg or less (Baumgärtl et al, 1972), or a "critical" pO_2 of 8 mm Hg estimated for renal cortical tissue (Leichtweiss et al., 1969) does not necessarily imply irreversible hypoxic damage in renal cortical cells. Instead, a broad range of variable extracellular oxygen tension exists in which renal cells can adjust their metabolic activities to compensate for only marginal oxygen supply (Wilson et al., 1979). In the present experiments, limited O_2 availability was indicated at an extracellular pO_2 of 40 mm Hg by a diminution of ATP-dependent glucose formation (which was reversible immediately after reoxygenation), at 10 mm Hg by a decrease in intracellular K^+ (which probably indicated the onset of hypoxic volume regulation, and which was reversible immediately after reoxygenation), at 5 mm Hg by a decline in oxygen uptake (which indicated a decrease in mitochondrial ATP generation) and an increased leakage of cytoplasmatic LDH, lysosomal APase, and brush border γGT (indicating an unphysiological membrane permeability and brush border loss, probably reversible only after a prolonged period of reoxygenation), at 2.5 mm Hg or less by an additional leakage of mitochondrial GlDH. This parameter of oxygen deprivation-induced mitochondrial dysfunction also indicated an irreversible limitation of aerobic recovery, as indicated after subsequent reoxygenation by a reduced intracellular K^+ content (impairment of ion homeostasis and of volume regulation) and a smaller rate of glucose formation (low cellular ATP level and insufficient mitochondrial function). Thus, an extracellular pO_2 below 5 mmHg appeared to be critical with regard to an oxygen deprivation-induced cell injury. In this range, the onset of hypoxic swelling and the release of lysosomal enzymes probably limited cellular function. This process finally became irreversible at an extracellular pO_2 of 2.5 mmHg or less when mitochondrial respiratory dysfunction limited aerobic recovery of tubular cell function (Gronow et al.,1986, 1988).

References

1. Balaban RS, Soltoff SP, Storey JM, Mandel LJ (1980) Am J Physiol 238:F50
2. Baumgärtl H, Leichtweiss HP, Lübbers DW, Weiss Ch, Huland H (1972) Microvasc Res 4:247
3. Bergmeyer HU (ed) (1974) Methoden der enzymatischen Analyse. Chemie, Weinheim
4. Bertermann H, Gronow G, Schirmer A, Weiss Ch (1975) Pflügers Arch 536:9
5. Chance B (1976) Circ Res 38:I
6. DeGroot H, Noll Th (1987) Biochem Soc Trans 15:363
7. Gronow G, Randzio G, Weiss Ch (1976) Curr Probl Clin Biochem 6:40
8. Gronow G, Weiss Ch (1976) In: Tager JM, Söling HD, Williamson JR (eds) Use of isolated liver cells and kidneytubules in metabolic studies. North Holland, Amsterdam
9. Gronow G, Meya F, Weiss Ch (1984b) Adv Exp Biol Med 196:589
10. Gronow GHJ, Benk P, Franke H (1984b) Adv Exp Med Biol 180:403
11. Gronow GHJ, Cohen JJ (1984) Am J Physiol 247:F618
12. Gronow G, Skrezek Ch, Kossmann H (1986) Adv Exp Med Biol 200:515
13. Gronow G, Klause N, Mályusz M (1988) Pflügers Arch 411:R91
14. Grote J (1987) In: Schmidt RF, Thews G (eds) Physiologie des Menschen. Springer, Berlin, 23 ed, p 635
15. Harris SI, Balaban RS, Barret L, Mandel LJ (1981) J Biol Chem 256:10319
16. Herminghuysen D, Welbourne CJ, Welbourne TC (1985) Am J Physiol 248:F804
17. Hochachka PW (1986) Science 231

18. Jones DP, Kennedy FG (1982) Am J Physiol 243:C247
19. Kriz W (1981) Am J Physiol 241:R3
20. Lang F, Völkl P, Paulmichl M (1988) Pflügers Arch 411:R4
21. Leichtweiss H-P, Lübbers DW, Weiss Ch, Baumgärtl H, Reschke W (1969) Pflügers Arch 309
22. MacKnight ADC, Leaf A (1977) Physiol Reviews 57:510
23. Mills JW, Horster M, Wilson P (1986) Cell Biol Int Rep 1:11
24. Schrier RW, Arnold PE, VanPutten VJ, Burke TJ (1987) Kidney Int 32:313
25. Weinberg JM (1985) J Clin Invest 76:1193
26. Wilson DF, Erecinska M, Drown Ch, Silver IA (1977) Am J Physiol 233:C135
27. Wilson DF, Erecinska M, Drown Ch, Silver IA (1979) Arch Biochem Biophys 195:485

Peripheral Ischemia and Epimuscular Oxygenation in Rats: Relevant Factors and Validation of the Method for Experimental Evaluation of Vasoactive Drugs

J. Roux, D. Shelton, E. Costa, E.M. Grandjean, A.-F. Weitsch

Introduction

Ischemic diseases and the associated hypoxia are amongst the major causes of morbidity in industrial countries. This hypoxic state is mainly due to an imbalance between oxygen demand and oxygen delivery which depends on external oxygen supply, lung and cardiac function and red blood cell capacity to fix, transport and deliver oxygen to surrounding tissues. This imbalance is particularly critical in patients suffering from peripheral arterial insufficiency [1-4], where the ischemic events may lead to leg amputation [5]. The management and treatment of such patients has been modified by the development of new methods for evaluating circulatory parameters [6]. Among these techniques, the development of small size sensors for the measurement of signals within and on the surface of the tissues has allowed the monitoring of the local and partial oxygen pressure in various tissues, particularly in muscles [7].

Such sensors may now be used in small laboratory animals such as rats [8], to evaluate the potential usefulness of compounds for the treatment of peripheral arterial occlusive diseases (PAOD). Therefore we studied the epimuscular oxygen partial pressure (pO_2) in an in vivo rat model of peripheral ischemia induced by a ligation technique [8]. We examined its possible changes over time (from 1 hour to 5 weeks after ligation). At an acute stage of peripheral arterial ischemia (1-2 days), we examined the effect of factors known to be critical for the assessment of pO_2, including anesthesia, type and volume of solvent used for the purpose of intravenous injection of vasoactive drugs. Finally, using one vasoactive compound, the advantages and limitations of this animal model and the pO_2 technique were set out.

Material and Methods

Male rats (RAI-f strain from Ciba-Geigy, Basel, Switzerland) with a mean body weight of 250 ±50 g were used in this study. The animals were housed in a temperature-controlled room (21°C) with an alternating 12

Clinical Oxygen Pressure Measurement II
A.M. Ehrly et al. (Eds.)
© Blackwell Ueberreuter Wissenschaft Berlin 1990

hour light/dark cycle. They had free access to food (Standard laboratory diet: Nafag 8905, Gossau, Switzerland) and water, except for the final 16 hours before pO_2 measurement, when the food was withdrawn.

Induction of ischemia

Peripheral ischemia was induced by unilateral (right) ligation of iliac and ilio-femoral arteries under sodium pentobarbital (40 mg/kg, ip) anesthesia. A study at various times (immediately after and 1, 2, 3, 4, 7, 10, 14 days and 5 weeks after ligation) was performed measuring epimuscular oxygenation. The number of animals in each group is indicated in the respective tables or in the text. Following ligation, the animals were put back into their holding cage until pO_2 evaluation.

pO_2 experiments

Local epimuscular oxygenation was measured using multiwire surface electrodes (L.Eschweiler Co, Kiel, FRG), previously described by Kessler and Lübbers [9]. These electrodes (8 channels each) were connected to a recording system (Bruins Instrument, Puchheim, FRG). Each electrode was fitted with Teflon and Cuprophan membranes before use and calibrated with pure nitrogen and a nitgrogen-oxygen gas mixture containing 5 % oxygen. This calibration procedure was applied before and after each rat pO_2 measurement.

Before application of the sensor, the skin was shaved and cleaned with alcohol (ethanol absolute) at the site of measurement. Then, the skin and fascia lata were incised on both legs at the level of the medial head of the gastrocnemius muscle, and a plastic ring was inserted so as to keep the pO_2 electrodes on the surface of this muscle. Then, the two electrodes were fixed, and each animal was maintained at a constant rectal temperature of 36 % ± 0.5°C.

Following a 10-20 min stabilization period, epimuscular pO_2 was measured. So as to obtain a control pO_2 value specific to each animal, the electrodes were rotated 5 to 10 times every 30 sec during the first minutes of the stabilization period. In each rat, pO_2 measurement was performed continuously during 60 min after this stabilization period.

Anesthesia

pO_2 measurements were performed on anesthetized rats using 2 different protocols. A first protocol, used only for normal rats (no ligation, no treatment), consisted of one bolus administration of sodium pentobarbital (50 mg/kg, ip).

A second protocol used for normal and ligated rats, consisted of one bolus administration of sodium pentobarbital (50 mg/kg, ip) followed by a constant perfusion of the same anesthetic (27 mg/hr/kg, ip route) using an automatic pump. This protocol was tested to find stable anesthetic conditions during one pO_2 experiment (1 hour at least), and was finally chosen to measure the effect of time, compounds and solvents on ligated and non-ligated animals.

Solvents and compounds

Rats were studied using different solvent treatments:
- normal rats with saline (NaCl 0.9 %) treatment,
- ligated rats without treatment (immediately, 1, 2, 4, 5, 7, 10, 14 days and 5 weeks after ligation),
- rat ligated for 2 days with vehicule treatment (NaCl 0.9 %, pure PEG 400, diluted PEG 400 : 20 % and pure DMSO) (DMSO = dimethyl sulfoxide, PEG = polyethylene glygol).

We also studied the effect of a known vasodilator: hydralazine (1-hydra-zinophthalazine, Ciba-Geigy, Basel, Switzerland) which was administered in a saline solution (0.5 and 1 mg/kg, iv). Drug and solvents were administered i.v. (0.1 ml/kg), in two days ligated series. The effect of solvents or drugs was recorded during 60 min after their i.v. administration.

Statistics

Results are expressed as mean ±SEM for table and mean ±SD for figures. For statistical analysis, the paired Student's t-test was used. The distribution of the pO_2 values was normal (Gaussian curve).

Results

Effect of anesthesia

The effect of one bolus of sodium pentobarbital in control animals (no ligation, no treatment) is shown in Fig. 1. A significant increase in mean epimuscular pO_2 values on both sides was observed 30 min (+10 %, $p<0.05$) and 60 min (+18 %, $p<0.05$) following the end of the stabilization period. Accordingly, this protocol was abandoned, since no stable pO_2 values were observed. A constant perfusion of anesthetic was used for further studies.

The bolus/perfusion regimen was studied in control (no treatment, no ligation) and ligated rats. Results are shown in Fig. 2 for the control (n=14) and ligated (1 day, n=8) animals. A good stability of pO_2 values

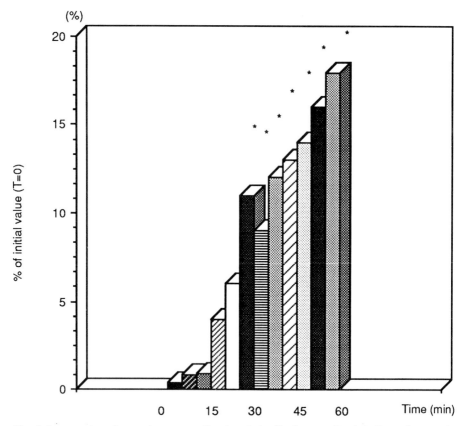

Fig. 1. Increase in epimuscular oxygenation in rats (n=8) after anesthesia with sodium pento-barbital. Anesthesia was given as a bolus administration (50 mg/kg, ip). pO_2 was measured every 5 min for up to 60 min. An asterisk indicates that the pO_2 values (Torr) were significantly different from that of initial (T=0) pO_2 value ($p<0.05$, paired t-test)

was observed on each side during the 60 minute measurement for both series.

In control rats, a significant difference was observed between left and right side. In 70 % of the cases, the mean pO_2 value was lower on the right side than on the left side (-6 %, $p<0.001$). In 1 day ligated rats, a significant difference (-34 %, $p<0.001$) was observed between normal and ligated sides. This difference was fairly constant during the measured period (1 hour). In normal and ligated rats, saline treatment (NaCl 0.9 %) did not modify pO_2 values (data not shown) as compared with non-treated animals. No change was observed that might be related to a possible hemodilution process. These results indicate therefore that such an anesthesia regimen is suitable for evaluating epimuscular pO_2 during 1 hour after the stabilization period.

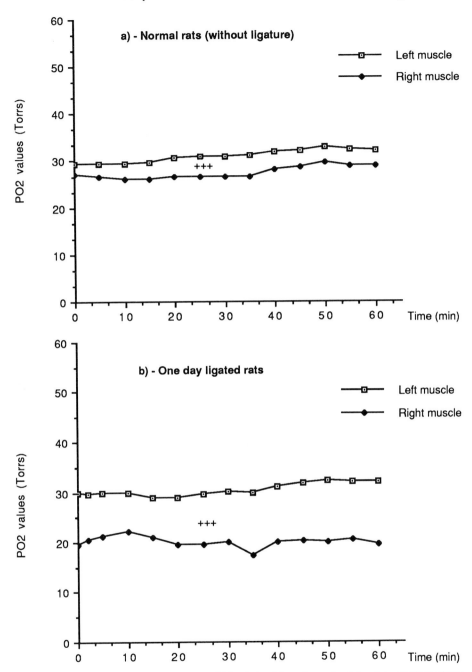

Fig. 2a, b. Evolution of pO$_2$ values in normal **(a)** rats (n=14) and one day **(b)** unilaterally ligated rats (n=8), during one hour after the stabilization period (see text). Anesthesia (sodium pentobarbital) was given as bolus administration (40 mg/kg, ip) followed by a constant perfusion (27 mg/kg/hr, ip). Results are expressed as mean ±SEM. A significative statistical difference (+++:p<0.001, paired Student's t-test) was observed betweeen left and right side during the 60 min measurement for a) and b)

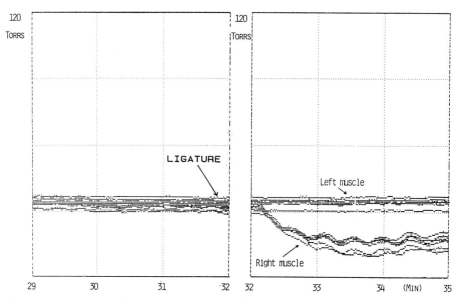

Fig. 3. Example of the effect of a right unilateral ligation on epimuscular pO₂ (Torr) in **one** rat, immediately after the ligation induction. pO₂ values were measured on both left and right gastrocnemius muscles (8 channels measurement for each muscle) during 60 min

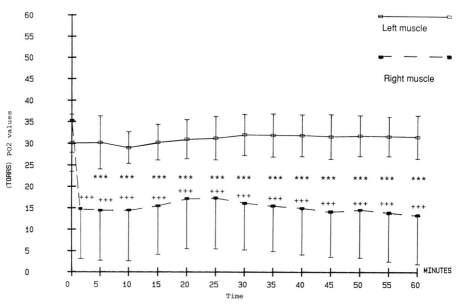

Fig. 4. Effect of a unilateral (right) arterial ligation on epimuscular pO₂ (Torr) in a series of 8 rats, immediately after the ligation induction (T = 2 min). T = before ligation. Results are expressed as mean ± SD. Statistics were performed using a paired Student's t-test: + = versus To, * = left versus right side. (*** = p<0.001, +++ = p<0.001). (——— = normal left muscle, ---- = ischemic right muscle)

Effect of ligation and time

Fig. 4 shows the effect of a right unilateral arterial ligation on epimuscular pO_2 immediately after performing ligation. We observed an important decrease in pO_2 value on the ligated side (-58 %, p<0.001). On the normal (left) side no change in pO_2 value was detected. An individual observation is shown in Fig. 3. Most of the decrease in pO_2 was already observed after 30 sec, while the minimum value was reached 1 to 3 min after ligation. Fig. 5 shows an individual observation in one rat 2 days after ligation. We observed a decrease in pO_2 value of approximately 18 % between normal and ligated sides. The study on a larger series (8 rats) indicated an average 25 % decrease in pO_2 value (p<0.001) measured on the normal side as compared to the ligated one (data not shown).

Comparison of pO_2 values after various periods of time (Table 1), indicated that the pO_2 difference between normal and ligated sides decreased over time. The difference in pO_2 values between normal and ligated sides decreased by 45 % from 1 hour (-58 %) to 5 weeks (-13 %) ligation (Table 1). this difference reached practically the normal range values of control animal (-5 to -10 %) 2 weeks after ligation was induced (-7 to -15 %). This profile observed at rest and under anesthesia was in agreement with the observations of Angersbach et al. [10] in rats, and Sunder-Plassmann [11] in dogs using the same pO_2 technique.

In contrast, Angersbach et al. [10] observed that 4 to 6 weeks after the ligature, an important difference in pO_2 values still remained between normal and ligated rats.

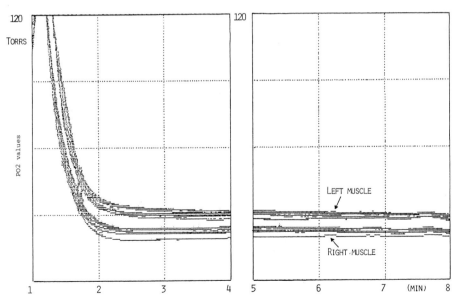

Fig. 5. Example of the effect of a 2 day unilateral (right) arterial ligation on epimuscular pO_2 (Torr) in **one** rat. pO_2 values were measured on both left (normal) and right (ischemic) gastrocnemius muscles (8 channels measurement for each muscle) during 60 min

Table 1. Evolution of epimuscular (gastrocnemius muscle) pO_2 value in rats after a unilateral peripheral arterial ischemia (ligature of right iliac and femoral arteries): time-course study

PO_2 → Series ↓	Normal side (L) (Torrs)	Ligated side (R) (Torrs)	Difference L-R (%)	Statistics (L/R)	n
Control	30.9 ± 0.7	29.2 ± 0.8	− 6%	P<0.01	23
Lig. 1 hour	31.5 ± 1.9	13.2 ± 4.3	− 58%	P<0.001	8
Lig. 1 days	30.8 ± 0.4	21.5 ± 0.5	− 30%	P<0.001	25
Lig. 3 days	32.2 ± 1.3	24.7 ± 1.1	− 23%	P<0.001	18
Lig. 4 days	31.7 ± 1.4	25.6 ± 0.9	− 17%	P<0.001	20
Lig. 7 days	29.4 ± 1.0	24.0 ± 1.1	− 18%	P<0.001	20
Lig. 10 days	32.4 ± 0.8	27.8 ± 0.9	− 14%	P<0.001	20
Lig. 14 days	33.2 ± 0.9	29.1 ± 1.1	− 12%	P<0.001	19
Lig. 5 weeks	28.3 ± 1.1	24.7 ± 1.2	− 13%	P<0.01	15

L and R: Left and right sides. n: number of animal. Results expressed as Mean ± SEM. Statistics: paired Student's t-test.

Our present findings could be due to the development of a collateral vascular bed or to a metabolic adaptation to ischemia.

Using the cast technique, Verheyen [12] has shown that only 5 to 9 days after a unilateral arterial ligation, a new vascular network was observed above and around the rat ligation site giving the image of a vascular "chevelu". Similar results were observed by Sunder-Plassmann [11] in dogs using angiography.

A better utilization of substrates and an improved elimination of catabolic products has been described in human patients with intermittent claudication. These adaptations might occur as a mere physiological adaptation as reported in these patients [13, 14].

The wide inter-individual variability of rat pO_2 values (even in control animals), suggests that it is preferable to compare each leg to the contralateral one for each rat, and not a control group to a ligated group of animals.

The repetition of the experiments 7 and 14 days after ligature (data not shown) confirmed these results with a mean decrease in pO_2 values between normal and ligated sides of 15 to 25 % (7 days) and of 7 to 15 % (14 days), respectively. These results indicated that in rats, only 2 weeks after a unilateral (right) ligature of iliac and ilio-femoral arteries, the partial epimuscular oxygen pressure was practically within the normal range values, at rest.

It appeared that the acute phases (1 to 5 days) in this experimental animal model corresponded to stage III (ischemia at rest) of the clinical classification according to Leriche and Fontaine (stages I to IV). The more chronic phases (2 to 5 weeks ligation) of the model seemed equivalent to stage II (ischemia during muscular exercise). The preliminary results obtained in 2 weeks ligated rats upon muscular electrical stimulation are in agreement with these interpretations (data not shown).

Even taking these considerations into account, we have to keep in mind that the pathophysiological process during which such pO_2 variations were observed, was different in this model (mechanical process by ligature) as compared to the human situation (atherosclerosis). This is particularly true for the acute phases, where the development of the collateral vascular bed is just starting.

Effect of solvents

2 days unilaterally ligated rats were selected for this study. The effect of PEG 400 solutions (20, 50 and 100%) was measured after intravenous administration. The injection of PEG 400 (100 and 50 %) induced significant variations of pO_2 values on both normal and ligated sides, indicating the unsuitability of such a solvent at these two dilutions.

In contrast, i.v. injection of PEG 400 (20 %) showed no effect on epimuscular oxygenatioin as compared with untreated ligated rats. This solvent could be used as vehicle for compound administration. The difference between normal and ligated sides remained constant during the 60 min period following injection.

DMSO solutions (10 to 100 %) were tested using the same protocol. At 10 % and above, a drastic and significant decrease in pO_2 values was observed on both sides, even during the first minutes following intravenous administration (Fig. 6). Solutions below 10 % were not tested. This effect

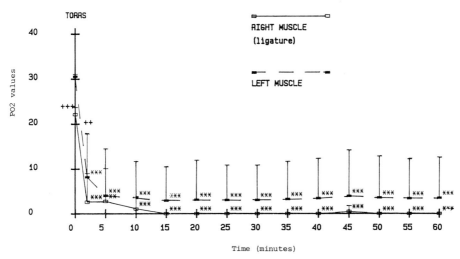

Fig. 6. Effect of DMSO (100 %) on epimuscular pO_2 rats (n=8), 2 days after a unilateral (right) arterial ligation. Results are expressed as mean ±SD. To = before intravenous DMSO injection. Statistics were performed using paired Student's t-test: *** = $p<0.001$ (versus To), +++ = $p<0.001$ (left versus right side)

may be due to a hemolytic effect of DMSO or to an interference with endothelial cells or even to an activity on systemic hemodynamic parameters (cardiac output, stroke volume). A simultaneous measurement of some sytemic hemodynamic parameters (heart rate, blood pressure) could have helped us to evaluate these possibilities.

Effect of Hydralazine

In 2 days unilaterally ligated rats, hydralazine (0.5 and 1 mg/kg, iv) induced a significant increase in pO_2 values in both legs. On the non-ligated side we observed a 43 % (0.5 mg/kg) and 57 % (1 mg/kg)increase in pO_2 values. On the ligated side, the corresponding figures were 15 % and 25 %.

These preliminary results showed the "vasodilating profile" of this compound, with a more marked increase in pO_2 value on the normal side compared to the ligated one.

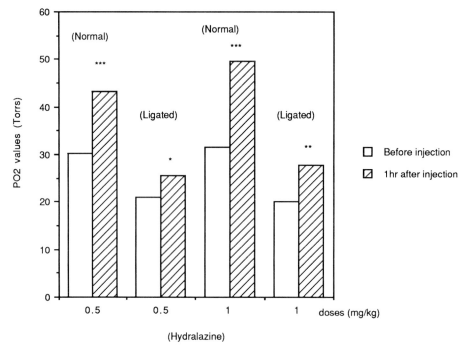

Fig. 7. Effect of hydralazine (0.5 and 1 mg/kg, iv) on rat epimuscular pO_2, study with a two days ligated series (n=8). pO_2 values were recorded up to 60 min after hydralazine injection. pO_2 values measured 1 hr after hydralazine injection were significantly different from that of pO_2 measured before hydralazine injection (* = p<0.05; ** = p<0.01; *** = p<0.001)

Discussion and Conclusion

The results presented in this study suggested that the local and partial oxygen pressure measured at the surface of rat gastrocnemius muscle may be a reliable and sensitive technique to identify different states of muscular hypoxia and possible to evaluate the effect of therapeutic compounds on the local changes in the microcirculation in occlusive vessel disease. However, controlled experimental conditions are of critical importance. Anesthesia (level and stability) plays an important role. Under unstable anesthetic conditions we have shown that the pO_2 values increased with time. A constant perfusion system was then necessary to ensure reproducible results. The nature and the volume of the injected vehicle solvent can also modify pO_2 values in an undesired way. Saline solution (NaCl 0.9 %) or PEG 400 (20 %) seemed to be appropriate solvents for such studies.

The epimuscular pO_2 values observed at various times following ligation are in agreement with what could be expected from published anatomo-histological and angiographic data [11, 12].

This study also illustrated the asymetry in pO_2 values between control non-ligated legs and control ischemic legs, in rats. The effect of one vasoactive compound (hydralazine) in this model suggested that direct measurement of tissue oxygen pressure allows to evaluate effects of drug treatment. In summary, this study suggests that the epimuscular pO_2 measured in ischemic muscle is relevant to the patholological state of peripheral arterial obliterative diseases, where oxygen supply is one of the limiting factors. Although the pathophysiological process was different in this experimental model, the limiting factor was comparable. Therefore, this model micht be a good tool for evaluating drug candidates designed for the aforementioned pathology.

References

1. Bongard O, Krahenbuhl B (1984) Pedal blood flow and transcutaneous pO_2 in normal subjects and in patients suffering from severe arterial disease. Clin Physiol 4:393
2. Franzeck UK, Talke P, Bernstein EF, Golbranson FL, Fronek A (1982) Transcutaneous pO_2 measurements in health and peripheral arterial occlusive disease. Surgery 91:156
3. Salabanzi AM (1986) Mesure de la pression partialle d'oxygène transcutanée. Application à l'étude comparative des effets de l'augmentation de la pression hydrostatique et des effets de l'exercice musculaire chez le sujet sain et l'artériopathe amputé. Thesis, Dijon, France
4. Dowd GSE, Linge K, Bentley R (1983) Measurement of transcutaneous oxygen pressure in normal and ischemic skin. J Bone Joint Surg 65B:79
5. Porters JM, Baur GM, Taylor LM (1981) Lower extremity amputation for ischemia. Arch Surg 116:89
6. Becker F (1983) Exploration de la fonction artérielle dans l'artériopathie chronique oblitérante des membres inférieures par les méthodes non-invasives d'exploration fonctionelle vasculaire. Corrélations avec la classification de Leriche et Fontaine. Lyon Médical, 250, 14:87

7. Hauss J, Spiegel HU, Schönleben K, Bünte H (1987) Monitoring of tissue pO_2 for invasive diagnostics in angiology and vascular surgery. Angiology 38:13

8. Roux J, Gulati O-P (1987) Tissue oxygenation in relation to hemodynamic and biochemical changes in experimental peripheral arterial ischemia in rats. In: Tsuchiya M et al (eds) Microcirculation – an update. Elsevier, Amsterdam, 2:545

9. Kessler M, Lübbers DM (1966) Aufbau und Anwendungsmöglichkeiten verschiedener pO_2-Elektroden. Pflugers Arch Ges Physiol R82:291

10. Angersbach D, Jukna JJ, Nicholson CD, Ochlich P, Wilke R (1987) The effect of short-term and long-term femoral artery ligation on calf muscle oxygen tension, blood flow, metabolism and function. Int J Microcirc Clin Exp 7:15

11. Sunder-Plassmann L, Messmer K, Becker HM (1981) Tissue pO_2 and transcutaneous pO_2 as guidelines in experimental and clinical drug evaluation. Angiology 32:686

12. Verheyen A, Lauwers F, Vlaminckx E, Wouters SL, De Clerck F (1988) Effect of vasoactive agonists on peripheral collateral arteries in *in situ* perfused rat hind quarters. Supersensitivity to serotonin. Int J Microcirc Clin Exp, S132, abst 199

13. Holm J, Bjorntorp P, Schersten T (1972) Metabolic activity in human skeletal muscle. Effect of peripheral arterial insufficiency. Europ J Clin Invest 2, 5:321

14. Bylund AC, Hmmarsten J, Holm J, Schersten T (1976) Enzyme activities in skeletal muscles from patients with peripheral arterial insufficiency. Europ J Clin Invest 6:425

Central Chemosensitivity:
Mechanism, Pathophysiology, and Plasticity

Marianne E. Schlaefke

Introduction

Central chemosensitivity is one of the still not completely understood mechanisms in respiratory physiology, although this important central drive has challenged scientists throughout our century. The concept developed by Winterstein and continued by Loeschcke, based on physiochemical, respiratory, neurophysiological, and morphological data, as well as on a mathematical model, is useful at present in order to interpret experimental findings in basic research as well as clinical observations in patients with central respiratory disorders.

The Mechanism

Winterstein (1911) proposed a unifying theory assuming that pO_2 and pCO_2 act on a single receptor by a single mechanism. He assumed the common denominator to be the hydrogen ion, either dissociated from carbonic acid or from acids formed during oxygen deficiency. After Heymans and Heymans (1927) had discovered the carotid and aortic glomera, Winterstein reformulated his reaction theory accepting that these are two kinds of chemoreceptors, peripheral and central, which had to be considered separately. The central chemoreceptor is not sensitive to hypoxia. The question now is restricted to the alternatives that either hydrogen ion or molecular CO_2 is the adequate stimulus. Experimental and theoretical approaches of Loeschcke et al. (1985) and of Pappenheimer et al. (1965), took into consideration a unique pH sensitive receptor which would be able to signalize both the respiratory and the metabolic acidosis.

In the meantime pH can be measured directly, either within the tissue of the brain or on the ventral medullary surface within the H^+ sensitive areas (Schlaefke et al., 1970). The non-invasive technique is based on the observation that there is free access to the glass electrode from the intercellular compartment (Dermietzel 1976). The time courses of the tissue pH measured with a micro pH electrode within the medulla and of ventilation during CO_2 inhalation are compatible (Cragg et al., 1977). The time

Clinical Oxygen Pressure Measurement II
A. M. Ehrly et al. (Eds.)
© Blackwell Ueberreuter Wissenschaft Berlin 1990

course of ventilation and of brain extracellular pH using the surface technique similarly followed step-changes of inspired CO_2 (Ahmad and Loeschcke, 1982). The tidal volume, especially after denervation of the peripheral chemoreceptors, followed closely the pH. Tidal volume and pH measured on the cortical surface however, were unrelated. Winterstein's and Loeschcke's theory claims that there is a "receptor" in the brain tissue which responds to H^+-ions (Loeschcke, 1982). The transmission from blood to the extracellular fluid is not the same for the three variables of the Henderson-Hasselbalch equation. The choroid plexus and the endothelium of the brain capillaries form the boundaries and have to be passed in parallel. It is to be expected that the a-v CO_2 difference of the plexus blood is low on account of the high blood flow. The CO_2 of the secreted plexus fluid comes into equilibrium with the CO_2 of the brain surface. This partially explains the higher acidity of cerebrospinal fluid (CSF) in comparison to blood plasma. Free exchange between CSF and cerebral extracellular fluid (ECF) reduces the differences in composition between the two fluids. The local extracellular pH is only partly under the influence of the CSF because the tissue is perfused by the blood. Loeschcke assumes that the local pCO_2 is determined by local metabolism, CO_2 binding capacity of the blood, blood flow and the distance to the capillaries. The average tissue pCO_2 in the brain under steady state conditions has been proposed as the algebraic means of venous and arterial pCO_2 of cerebral blood plus 1 Torr (Ponten and Siesjö, 1966; Ahmad et al., 1976).

Bicarbonate in response to acid-base changes in CSF varies by only 40% as much as in blood plasma (Pappenheimer et al., 1965; Mitchell et al., 1965; Kronenberg and Cain, 1968; Fencl, 1971). The HCO_3^- exchange between blood and brain is a fast process occurring simultaneously with an exchange of Cl^- in the opposite direction, (Ahmad et al., 1976; Ahmad and Loeschcke, 1982). The exchange possibly uses a protein carrier through an anion exchange channel of the endothelium of the brain capillaries (Wieth et al., 1980). When CO_2 is inhaled the increase of bicarbonate concentration in ECF is greater than in blood plasma, even if the plasma bicarbonate is kept constant. Ahmad and Loeschcke (1982) used electrochemical methods to demonstrate that HCO_3^- in this case is exchanged for Cl^- in a one to one fashion between ECF and cells. Extracellular pH depends on anion exchange between plasma and extracellular fluid (passing the endothelium) on the one hand, and on anion exchange between brain tissue cells and extracellular fluid on the other hand. In the ECF all five compartments, namely red cells, plasma, endothelium, extracellular fluid, and glia cells must be considered for the pH kinetics (Fig.1). This is true for metabolic as well as respiratory acidosis.

A mathematical model made use of the bicarbonate relation between plasma and CSF (Middendorf and Loeschcke 1976). Hereby was shown that the ventilatory response to respiratory acidosis is much higher than that to metabolic acidosis. The increase of ventilation, however, is more effective in regulating blood pH in metabolic than in respiratory acidosis

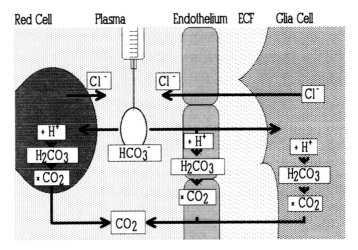

Fig. 1. Diagram (modified) of Loeschcke's five compartment model of exchange processes between red cells, plasma, endothelium, brain extracellular fluid and glia, following i.v. injection of bicarbonate (Loeschcke, 1982)

(Middendorf, 1974; Middendorf and Loeschcke, 1976; 1978). In the light of these experimental and mathematical approaches Loeschcke stated that the extracellular pH in the brain is the main chemical signal determining ventilation. This pH depends on the tissue pCO_2 and the bicarbonate concentration in the tissue. The distribution of bicarbonate between plasma and CSF under given conditions can be experimentally determined. There are processes preventing a full equilibrium and any assessment of the extracellular pH should take account of the exchange processes between the five compartments.

Differences in the ventilatory responses, when comparing mild and severe charges of fixed acids with the responses to CO_2 inhalation, have been reported by Shams (1986). The latter have a much higher slope than during severe metabolic acidosis. Loeschcke assumed that the sensing mechanism resides in a compartment which is initially accessible to H^+, but under the continued application of acid further entrance of H^+ is prevented, whereas the lipid soluble acid CO_2, penetrates as before. A synaptic gap would have been a good model in Loeschcke's eyes. Shams (1985) and Dempsey and Forster (1982) doubted the validity of these assumptions and so also the classic one receptor theory. Their conclusions are substantiated by findings of Teppema et al. (1983), indicating that changes in pH caused by hypercapnia give rise to a greater ventilatory response than the same changes in pH caused by isocapnic changes in arterial pH. Kiwull-Schöne and Kiwull (1983) observed in peripherally chemodenervated cats that the response of ventilation to CO_2 was maintained at any level of medullary pH during hypoxia. However, hypoxia induced decreases in pH had no effect on respiration. Shams directed the interest towards the significance of the intracellular pH for the one receptor theory, since the pH difference between the extracellular and the intracellular compartment might be dependent upon the CO_2 level. So the classic 'one receptor theory' will have to be challenged by new intracellular pH recording techniques.

The responsible chemosensitive site for the respiratory system has been localized within the superficial tissue layer of the ventral medullary surface (Loeschcke and Koepchen, 1958; Mitchell et al., 1965; Schlaefke et al., 1970). Tonically firing neurones within the ventral medullary areas (rostral, intermediate and caudal) change their frequency in correspondence to the pH measured on the ventral medullary surface, whether pH is varied by local superfusion of artificial cerebrospinal fluid, by inhalation of CO_2 or by injection of fixed acid (Schlaefke et al., 1975; Schlaefke, 1976; Prill, 1977; Pokorski, 1976). Blood flow of the ventrolateral surface is CO_2-sensitive as well, and this more than the blood flow in the adjacent white matter, which is comparable to the cortical relations. Hypoxia causes a 70% increase in the flow to the ventrolateral surface, which is again comparable to the conditions of the cortical gray. The central chemoreceptor tissue is more sensitive to hypoxia than the adjacent white matter. The increase in flow with normocapnic hypoxia would lead to a reduction in tissue pCO_2. The extent of this decrease and the amount of consequent respiratory inhibition depends on the normal CO_2 gradient. The possibility that respiratory depression or relative inhibition of ventilation in hypoxia is due to increased ventrolateral surface blood flow cannot be ruled out (Feustel et al., 1984).

In vitro and in vivo experiments with cholinergic drugs on the ventral medullary surface and on H^+ sensitive neurons within the superficial layer resulted in the following conclusion: the chemosensitive mechanism is a cholinergic synapse on which H^+ acts like acetylcholine (ACh) and can be replaced by it. Blockade is possible by mecamylamine, atropine and partly also by hexamethonium, which suggests the presence of both muscarinic and nicotinic receptors (Fukuda and Loeschcke, 1979; Dev and Loeschcke, 1979). The topical distribution of ACh showed two peaks of maximal effect coinciding with the reactions to hydrogen ions. Also nicotine was found to mimic the effect of ACh and physostigmine enhanced its action. The presence of atropine inhibits the ventilatory effect of CSF acidosis and local application of atropine counteracts the stimulating effect of progesterone (Burton et al., 1989; Tok and Loeschcke, 1981). Yamada et al. (1982) localized γ-aminobutyric acid (GABA) receptors with respiratory and cardiovascular functions within the intermediate area. GABA acts on ventral medullary structures especially in relation to inhibitory functions of the sympathetic activity (Mc Gall and Humpphrey, 1985; Keeler et al., 1984; Ruggiero et al., 1985). Cholinoceptive and nicotinoceptive neurons have been mapped systematically (Willenberg et al., 1985). Further neuropeptides and ß-endorphine positive cells were localized within the chemo-sensitive fields. Vasoactive intestinal peptide, substance P and somatostatin were also detected (Leibstein et al., 1985).

Errington and Dashwood (1979) traced interconnections between the ventral medullary surface and the nucleus tractus solitarii (NTS) as well as with the dorsal nucleus of the vagus using horseradish peroxidase. Latencies of 5 - 15 ms were recorded from neurons within the NTS when the caudal area was stimulated (Davies and Loeschcke, 1977). Procaine on the ventral surface was followed by a decrease of the neuronal activity of inspiratory, expiratory and reticular neurons; some nonrespiratory neurons were activated (Schwanghart et al., 1974). Peskow and Piatin (1976) recorded complete cessation of inspiratory activity, brought about by cold block of the intermediate area. The strongest inhibition was observed in the discharge of early and late inspiratory neurons. Expiratory neurons either became silent or continued to exhibit tonic firing with reduced impulse frequency. Functional interconnections between the Bötzinger complex regarding the influence on the respiratory rate and the respiratory motor output and the central chemosensitive mechanism seem to exist (Budzinska et al. 1985).

Tonically firing neurons within the paragigantocellular nucleus respond to H^+ as well as to tibial nerve stimulation (Schlaefke et al. 1979 a). This function coincides with the effect of cold block on the ventral surface (intermediate area), that 'unspecific' stimulation of respiration can be blocked as well as the respiratory response to CO_2 (Schlaefke et al., 1969; Cherniack et al., 1979). Fig.2 describes the converging principle of the central chemosensitive mechanism as a cholinergic system driving respi-

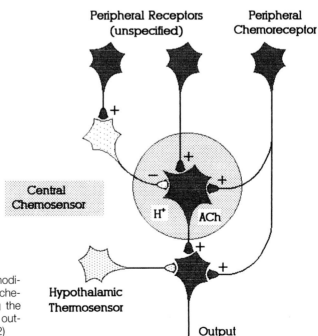

Fig. 2. Loeschcke's diagram (modified) of the cholinergic central chemosensitive mechanism using the principle of convergence on an output neurone (Loeschcke, 1982)

ration in cooperation with peripheral chemoreceptors as well as with other e.g. hypothalamic respiratory afferents (Loeschcke, 1982; Schlaefke et al., 1969; See et al., 1983; See and Schlaefke, 1986).

Pathophysiology

Complete loss of central chemosensitivity is the main symptom of patients suffering from the Ondine's curse syndrome. Strongly reduced CO_2 responses have been observed in infants with an apparent life threatening event (ALTE) during the first month of life. Transiently reduced CO_2 responses were recorded in infants during the first year of life, which were evaluated at risk for the sudden infant death syndrome (Schlaefke et al. 1989). Symptoms like periodic breathing, insensitivity to CO_2, apneas, and irreversible respiratory and circulatory arrest by mild hypoxia were induced by superficial lesion of the intermediate area in chronic nonanaesthetized cats or by local application of glycine in acute experiments (Schlaefke, 1989). The peripheral chemoreceptors in the animal models guarantee the continuation of breathing. However, the ventilatory response to hypoxia is quantitatively reduced (Schlaefke et al., 1979 b; Schlaefke, 1989; Schlaefke et al., 1989). These findings coincide with the observation that the ventral medullary superficial layer in 14 victims of SIDS and Ondine's curse syndrome was impoverished of nerve cells compared with controls (Kille and Schlaefke, 1986).

In 14 infants, aged between 5 weeks and 12 years, we found complete insensitivity to CO_2 measured during NREM-sleep or during sleep onset. The peripheral chemoreceptors were intact in these patients. The degree of respiratory acidosis varies with sleep phases and is severe in NREM- and less severe in REM-sleep. With sleep onset and in light NREM-sleep the peripheral chemoreflex initiated sighs at a $tcpO_2$ of 19 mmHg improving the blood gas situation for a moment. This may occur several times. With further increase of pCO_2, central depression impedes the performance of the peripheral chemoreceptor reflex and arousals. These dangerous phases in infants often remain undiscovered on behalf of 'normal' skin colour, absence of prolonged apneas and brady- or tachycardia, and may precede artificial ventilation during sleep and so contribute to the development of pulmonary hypertension in these patients (Comroe and Botelho 1947).

Plasticity

The neurophysiological organization of the central chemosensitive drive of respiration, its principle of convergence, and the functional interconnections with the peripheral chemoreflex challenged us to ask whether the loss of central chemosensitive function may be reversible by means of a training treatment. Unspecific, as well as chemical respiratory stimuli possibly could be used in analogy to the classical conditioning theory (Pavlov, 1927).

In patients and in the animal model we used pulse oximetry in order to trigger paired stimuli. The aim was 1. to regain the respiratory response to CO_2 and 2. to decrease the O_2 threshold of peripheral chemoreceptors.

We applied a feed back system with transcutaneous pulse oximetry, feeding a computer and so triggering the paired stimulation: an unspecific 'arousing' stimulus, like sound, light, or an air jet blown into the mouth-nose region for 1 sec and a 'specific' chemical stimulus (O_2 or 1.5% CO_2 in O_2) for 1.5 sec after a pause of 0.5 sec. This is repeated every 10 sec and applied in trains of 20 minutes; it is interrupted however, as long as the trigger threshold (e.g. $SaO_2 = 93\%$) is exceeded. In the animal model we used electrical stimulation of the femoral nerve (2V, 20 Hz, 1 ms) as an unspecific stimulus (Burghardt and Schlaefke, 1986; Schlaefke et al., 1981; 1987; 1989).

Fig.3 shows the effect of elimination of central chemosensitivity, by superficial lesions of the intermediate area (Schlaefke et al. 1979 c) in the cat, on the oxygen saturation, and the effect of conditioning using femoral nerve stimulation combined with an increase of $FiCO_2$ as described above. The values were taken 10 minutes after coagulation, and two hours later, when four trains of conditioning had been applied. Fig.4 presents the corresponding CO_2 response curves from the same animal in the control, after coagulation and after conditioning. In control studies we had shown

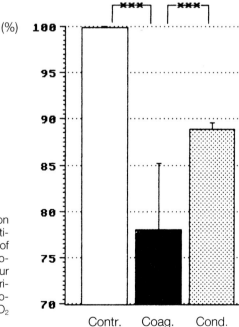

Fig. 3. Average values of oxygen saturation measured by pulse oximetry in the anaesthetized cat before bilateral coagulation (contr.) of the intermediate area (S), 10 minutes after coagulation (coag.) and two hours later after four runs of conditioning (cond.) by pulse oximetrically triggered paired stimulation, using femoral nerve stimulation as unspecific and 2% CO_2 in O_2 as specific respiratory stimulus

Ventilation [ml/min ATPS]

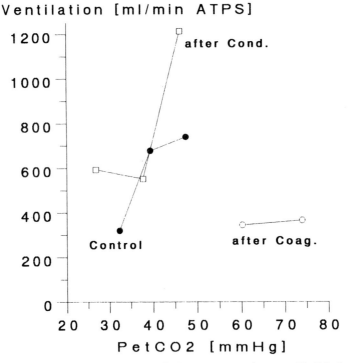

Fig. 4. Respiratory response to CO_2 (the same experiment as Fig.3) before (closed circles) and after coagulation and after conditioning; $PetCO_2$ = endtidal pCO_2

that CO_2 sensitivity does not recover spontaneously. The same could be confirmed in infants, in whom no respiratory response to CO_2 could be found as confirmed a few weeks after birth and eight years later (Schlaefke, unpublished).

In four infants suffering from an Ondine's curse syndrome we applied paired stimulation and obtained effects comparable to those described in the animal model (Schlaefke and Burghardt, 1981; Burghardt and Schlaefke, 1986; Schlaefke et al., 1989). Besides the improvement of the respiratory sensitivity to CO_2, the use of pulse oximetry for triggering the stimulation pursued two aims: 1. to avoid hyperoxia during sleep, and 2. to train the respiratory system processing the chemoreflex within the normal pO_2 range. In two 24 month-old boys with an Ondine's curse syndrome, who were breathing spontaneously during sleep but hypoventilating, we used a trigger threshold of SaO_2 of 93%. In both infants, already after training times of 20 minutes, sighs as a potential sign of 'learning' were elicited just before the SaO_2 came back to the trigger level. Whether this may be evaluated as a reset of the chemoreflex threshold is still an open question. Further studies are necessary in order to decide whether this way of feed back training and of controlled oxygen therapy may be a useful method in overcoming insufficiency of chemosensitive drive as an alternative to artificial ventilation during sleep.

Summary

The central pH sensitive mechanism is an important respiratory drive of a cholinergic type and responsible for the precision of central acid base homeostasis. The mechanism is not the specialization of one neuronal element but a complex system making use of various appropriate morphological, physico-chemical, neurophysiological and neurochemical specifics within the ventral part of the medulla oblongata. Tonically firing neurons could be localized responding to changes in pH of blood and extracellular fluid as well as to different unspecific stimuli. With the loss of the central chemosensitive drive the rhythm generator is dependent upon compensatory functions of the reticular formation, which is possible under waking conditions. During sleep, hypoxia and severe acidosis cause life threatening situations. This pathomechanism also seems to play a role in certain forms of sudden infant death. In Ondine's curse syndrome the excessive increase of pCO_2 with sleep causes a rise of the peripheral chemoreceptor threshold, aggravating the hypoxemia. Making use of the converging principle of the central chemosensitive mechanism for a potential therapeutic purpose, continuous measurement of oxygen saturation was selected as a fast method to replace the lost sensor function. In case the saturation fell below the threshold value, paired stimulation in combination with oxygen supply was triggered. The described method caused a reset of the peripheral chemoreceptor threshold and an increase in respiratory response to CO_2. The first encouraging results should challenge further research on the questioned plasticity of the central chemosensitive drive of respiration for theoretical and practical reasons.

Supported by the SFB 114 'Bionach', Ministerium für Wissenschaft und Forschung NRW: IV A 6 – 401 021 87. In cooperation with Hellige GmbH, D-7800 Freiburg i. Br.

References

1. Ahmad HR, Berndt J, Loeschcke HH (1976) Bicarbonate exchange between blood, brain extracellular fluid and brain cells at maintained pCO_2. In: Loeschcke HH (ed) Acid-base homeostasis of the brain extracellular fluid and the respiratory control system. Thieme, Stuttgart, 19-27
2. Ahmad HR, Loeschcke HH (1982) Transient and steady state response of pulmonary ventilation to the medullary extracellular pH. Pfluegers Arch 395: 285-292
3. Burghardt F, Schlaefke ME (1986) Loss of central chemosensitivity: an animal model to overcome respiratory insufficiency. J Autonom Nerv Syst Suppl 105-109
4. Budzinska K, von Euler C, Kao FF, Pantaleo T, Yamamoto Y (1985) Effects of graded focal cold block in rostral areas of the medulla. Acta Physiol Scand 124: 329-340

5. Comroe JH, Bothelho S (1947) The unreliability of cyanosis in the recognition of arterial anoxemia. Am J Med Sci 214: 1

6. Cragg P, Patterson L, Purves MJ (1977) The pH of brain extracellular fluid in the cat. J Physiol (Lond) 272: 137-166

7. Davies RO, Loeschcke HH (1977) Neural activity evoked by electrical stimulation of the chemosensitive areas on the ventral medullary surface. Proc Int Un Physiol Sci 13: 164

8. Dempsey JA, Forster HV (1982) Mediation of ventilatory adaptations. Physiol Rev 62: 262-346

9. Dermietzel R (1976) Central chemosensitivity, morphological studies. In: Loeschcke HH (ed) Acid-base homeostasis of the brain extracellular fluid and the respiratory control system. Thieme, Stuttgart, 52-66

10. Dev NB, Loeschcke HH (1979) A cholinergic mechanism involved in the respiratory chemosensitivity. Pfluegers Arch 379: 29-36

11. Fencl V (1971) Distribution of H^+ and HCO_3^- in cerebral fluids. In: Siesjoe OK, Sorensen SC (eds) Ion homeostasis of the brain. Munksgaard, Kopenhagen, 175-195

12. Feustel PJ, Stafford MJ, Allen JS, Severinghaus JW (1984) Ventrolateral medullary surface blood flow determined by hydrogen clearance. J Appl Physiol 56: 150-154

13. Fukuda Y, Loeschcke HH (1979) A cholinergic mechanism involved in the neuronal excitation by H^+ in the respiratory chemosensitive structures of the ventral medulla oblongata of rats in vitro. Pfluegers Arch 379: 125-135

14. Errington ML, Dashwood MR (1979) Projections to the ventral surface of the cat brain stem demonstrated by horseradish peroxidase. Neurosci Lett 12: 153-158

15. Heymans JF, Heymans C (1927) Sur les modifications directes et sur la regulation reflexe de l'activite du centre respiratoire de la tete isolee du chien. Arch Int Pharmacodyn Ther 33: 273

16. Keeler JR, Shults CW, Chase TN, Helke CJ (1984) The ventral surface of the medulla in the rat: Pharmacologic and autoradiographic localization of GABA induced cardiovascular effects. Brain Res 297: 217-224

17. Kille JF, Schlaefke ME (1986) Do ventral medullary neurones control the cardiorespiratory system in man? Pfluegers Arch 406: R25

18. Kiwull-Schöne H, Kiwull P (1983) Hypoxic modulation of central chemosensitivity. In: Schlaefke ME, Koepchen HP, See WR (eds) Central neurone environment. Springer, Berlin, 88-95

19. Kronenberg RS, Cain SM (1968) Effects of acetazolamide and hypoxia on cerebrospinal fluid bicarbonate. J Appl Physiol 24: 17-20

20. Leibstein AG, Willenberg IM, Dermietzel R (1981) Morphology of the medullary chemosensitive fields. I. Mapping of the neuronal matrix by a horseradish peroxidase technique. Pfluegers Arch 391: 226-230

21. Loeschcke HH (1982) Central Chemosensitivity and the reaction theory. J Physiol 332: 1-24

22. Loeschcke HH, Koepchen HP (1958) Versuch zur Lokalisation des Angriffsortes der Atmungs- und Kreislaufwirkung von Novocain im Liquor cerebrospinalis. Pfluegers Arch 266: 628-641

23. Loeschcke HH, Koepchen HP, Gertz KH (1958) Über den Einfluß der Wasserstoffionenkonzentration und CO_2-Druck im Liquor cerebrospinalis auf die Atmung. Pfluegers Arch 266: 569-585

24. Mc Gall RB, Humphrey SJ (1985) Evidence for GABA mediation of sympathetic inhibition evoked from midline medullary depressor sites. Brain Res 339: 356-360

25. Middendorf T (1974) Analysis of the efficiency of the respiratory control system. In: Umbach W, Koepchen HP (ed) Central rhythmic and regulation. Hippokrates, Stuttgart, 117-120

26. Middendorf T., Loeschcke HH (1976) Mathematische Simulation des Respirationssystems. J Math Biol 3: 149-177

27. Middendorf T, Loeschcke HH (1978) Cooperation of the peripheral and central chemosensitive mechanisms in the control of the extracellular pH in brain in non-respiratory acidosis. Pfluegers Arch 375: 257-260

28. Mitchell RA, Carman CJ, Severinghaus JW, Richardson BW, Singer MM, Schnider S (1965) Stability of cerebrospinal fluid pH in chronic acid-base disturbances in blood. J Appl Physiol 20: 443-452

29. Pappenheimer JR, Fencl V, Hasey SR, Held D (1965) Role of cerebral fluids in the control of respiration as studied in unanaesthetized goats. Am J Physiol 208: 436-450

30. Peskow BJ, Piatin WF (1976) Reactions of neurons of the respiratory center to local cooling of the ventral surface of the medulla oblongata. Sechenov Physiol J UdSSR 62/7

31. Pokorski M (1976) Neurophysiological studies on central chemosensor in medullary ventrolateral areas. Am J Physiol 230: 1288-1295

32. Ponten U, Siesjö BK (1966) Gradients of CO_2 tension in the brain. Acta Physiol Scand 67: 129-140

33. Prill RK (1977) Das Verhalten von Neuronen des caudalen chemosensiblen Feldes in der Medulla oblongata der Katze gegenüber intravenösen Injektionen von NaHCO₃ und HCl. Dissertation, Ruhr-Universität, Bochum

34. Ruggiero DA, Meeley MP, Anwar M, Reis DJ (1985) Newly identified GABAergic neurons in regions of the ventrolateral medulla which reglulate blood pressure. Brain Res 339: 171-177

35. Schlaefke ME (1976) Central chemosensitivity: Neurophysiology and contribution to regulation. In: Loeschcke HH (ed) Acid-base homeostasis of the brain extracellular fluid and the respiratory control system. Thieme, Stuttgart, 66-80

36. Schlaefke ME (1989) Plötzlicher Kindstod: Klinische Physiologie und Modelle. In: Andler W, Schlaefke ME, Trowitzsch E (eds) Der plötzliche Kindstod. Acron, Berlin

37. Schlaefke ME, Burghardt F (1981) Training of central chemosensitivity in infants with sleep apnea. In: Schlaefke ME, Koepchen HP, See WR (eds) Central neurone environment. Springer, Berlin Heidelberg, 74-81

38. Schlaefke ME, Burghardt F, Mückenhoff K, Heimann J (1981) Technisch unterstütztes Atemtraining bei Säuglingen mit mangelnder COI₂-Empfindlichkeit der Atmung. Biomedizinische Technik, Ergänzungsband 26: 48-29

39. Schlaefke ME, Kille JF, Loeschcke HH (1979 c) Elimination of central chemosensitivity by coagulation of a bilateral area on the ventral medullary surface in awake cats. Pfluegers Arch 379: 231-241

40. Schlaefke ME, Pokorski M, See WR, Prill RK, Kille JF, Loeschcke HH (1975) Chemosensitive neurons on the ventral medullary surface. Bull Physio-Pathol Respir 11: 277-284

41. Schlaefke ME, Schaefer T, Kronberg H, Ullrich GJ, Hopmeier J (1987) Transcutaneous monitoring as trigger for therapy of hypoxemia during sleep. Adv Exp Med Biol 220: 95-100

42. Schlaefke ME, Schaefer T, Nebel B, Schaefer D, Schaefer C (1989) Development, disturbances, and training of respiratory regulation in infants. In: Peter JH, Penzel T, Podszus T, von Wiechert P (eds) Sleep and health risk. Springer, Berlin

43. Schlaefke ME, See WR, Herker-See A, Loeschcke HH (1979 b) Respiratory response to hypoxia and hypercapnia after elimination of central chemosensitivity. Pfluegers Arch 381: 241-248

44. Schlaefke ME, See WR, Kille JF (1979 a) Origin and afferent modification of respiratory drive form ventral medullary areas. Wenner-Gren Cent Int Symp Ser 32: 25-34

45. Schlaefke ME, See WR, Loeschcke HH (1970) Ventilatory response to alterations of H^+-ion concentration in small areas of the ventral medullary surface. Respir Physiol 10: 198-212

46. Schlaefke ME, See WR, Massion WH, Loeschcke HH (1969) Die Rolle "spezifischer" und "unspezifischer" Afferenzen für den Antrieb der Atmung, untersucht durch Reizung und Blockade von Afferenzen an der dezerebrierten Katze. Pfluegers Arch 312: 189-205

47. Schwanghart F, Schroeter R, Klüssendorf D, Koepchen HP (1974) The influence of novocaine block of superficial brain stem structures on discharge pattern of specific

respiratory and unspecific reticular neurons. In: Umbach W, Koepchen HP (eds) Central rhythmic and regulation. Hippokrates, Stuttgart, 104-110

48. See WR, Schlaefke ME, Loeschcke HH (1983) Role of chemical afferents in the maintenance of rhythmic respiratory movements. J Appl Physiol 54: 453-459

49. See WR, Schlaefke ME (1986) The intermediate area of the ventral medullary surface: Point of convergence of respiratory afferents? J Autonom Nerv Syst Suppl 79-85

50. Shams H (1985) Differential effects of CO_2 and H^+ as central stimuli of respiration in the cat. J Appl Physiol 58: 357-364

51. Teppema LJ, Barts PWJA, Folgering HT, Evers JAM (1983) Effects of respiratory and (isocapnic) metabolic arterial acid-base disturbances on medullary extracellular fluid pH and ventilation in cats. Respir Physiol 53: 379-395

52. Tok T, Loeschcke HH (1981) Untersuchung über die zentrale Wirkung von Progesteron auf die Atmung und Vasomotorik bei Katzen. Z Atemwegs- und Lungenkrankheiten 7: 148-153

53. Wieth JO, Brahm J, Funder J (1980) Transport and interactions of anions and protons in the red blood cell membrane. Ann NY Acad Sci 341: 394-418

54. Willenberg IM, Dermietzel R, Leibstein AG, Effenberger M (1985) Mapping of cholinoceptive (nicotinoceptive) neurones in the lower brain stem: with special reference to the ventral surface of the medulla. J Autonom Nerv Syst 14: 299-313

55. Winterstein H (1911) Die Regulierung der Atmung durch das Blut. Pfluegers Arch 138: 167-184

56. Yamada KA, Norman WP, Hamosh P, Gillis RA (1982) Medullary ventral surface GABA receptors affect respiratory and cardiovascular function. Brain Res 248: 71-78

The Effect of Focal Cerebral Ischemia on Tissue Oxygen Tension Distribution in the Brain Cortex

A. Hagendorff, J. Grote, C. Haller, A. Hartmann

Previous investigations on regional or local cerebral blood flow during and after brain ischemia indicate that the brain blood flow regulation is impaired or even abolished following ischemic attacks [Waltz, 1968; Yamaguchi et al., 1972; Haller et al., 1981, 1986; Hartmann et al., 1981; Hossmann, 1982; Strong et al., 1988]. According to these results, subsequent disturbances of local cerebral oxygen supply are to be expected not only in the affected tissue areas but also in nonischemic brain regions. In order to study the influence of the postischemic blood flow alterations on local cerebral oxygen supply, tissue pO_2 measurements were performed in the brain cortex. In a first series of experiments on cats, the effect of a transient brain ischemia, induced by air embolism, was studied, while in a second experimental group the effect of middle cerebral artery occlusion was investigated in baboons.

Methods

The tissue pO_2 measurements were performed using platinum surface microelectrodes as described by Kessler and Grunewald [1969] and Lübbers et al. [1969]. The multiwire electrodes consisted of eight cathodes of 10 μm to 15 μm in diameter each. The electrodes were calibrated in saline solutions equilibrated with three gas mixtures of different pO_2. The calibration was performed at brain surface temperature and at a pCO_2 of 40 mmHg [Söntgerath et al., 1984]. During the measurements, the pO_2 electrodes were fixed to a counterbalancing system so as to minimize the bearing pressure [Grote et al., 1981]. No local blood flow restriction was observed in the brain regions under investigation. The catchment region of a single electrode approximates a hemisphere with a diameter of about 40 μm to 60 μm [Grunewald, 1970; Schneidermann and Goldstick, 1976].

Ischemia experiments on cats

Eight cats weighing 2.2 to 3.4 kg were anesthetized with glucochloralose (40 – 50 mg/kg intravenously). After tracheotomy and relaxation with

Clinical Oxygen Pressure Measurement II
A.M. Ehrly et al. (Eds.)
© Blackwell Ueberreuter Wissenschaft Berlin 1990

pancuronium (0.133 mg/kg per hour), the animals were artificially ventilated by means of a Bird mark 7 Respirator adjusted to yield normal arterial blood gas tensions. Endtidal CO_2 concentration was continuously recorded by an infra-red gas analyser. For serial measurements of arterial pO_2, pCO_2, and pH, the Radiometer BMS blood microsystem was used. One femoral artery and one femoral vein were cannulated with polyethylene catheters for blood sampling, for continuous blood pressure recording and for infusion of Tyrode's solution (2.5 ml/kg per hour). Body temperature was maintained at 37 °C to 38 °C.

Following the fixation of the animal's head in a stereotactic frame, the gyrus suprasylvius of the right hemisphere was exposed by a craniotomy. The dura was opened and the brain surface covered with paraffin oil heated to about 37 °C. Brain ischemia was induced by air embolism according to Fritz and Hossmann [1979]. In order to inject the blood foam, a catheter had to be placed into the innominate artery proximal to the origin of both common carotical arteries via the right axillary artery. The correct placement of the catheter tip was verified by thoracotomy at the end of the experiments. Before and after transient brain ischemia, the tissue pO_2 of the superficial cell layers of the brain cortex and the diameter of the pial arteries in the measuring field were determined simultaneously. The vessels' diameters were measured using an image-shearing device [Haller et al., 1986].

Ischemia experiments on monkeys

Five baboons weighing between 12 and 30 kg were anesthetized with pentobarbital (25 mg/kg i.p. initially). An endotracheal tube was connected to a Schuler respiratory pump (type 2), through which a 3:1 N_2O/O_2 mixture was delivered. Repeated small doses of pentobarbital were given intravenously during the experiments. For application of medication and fluids and for measurement of central venous pressure, the right femoral vein was cannulated. Via one femoral artery a pig-tail catheter was placed into the left ventricle for application of microspheres. To facilitate continuous blood pressure measurements an additional catheter was inserted into one brachial artery. The same catheter allowed intermittent blood sampling for pO_2, pCO_2 and pH analyses as well as for arterial flow measurements. The flow values thus determined served as reference for cerebral blood flow measurements using the microsphere method.

The head of the baboons was mounted in a stereotactic frame. After bilateral craniotomy above the frontal and the parietal brain, the dura was opened. The brain surface was superfused with warm Ringer's solution. The exposed cortical regions are supplied by the middle cerebral artery and the anterior cerebral artery.

Brain infarction was produced using a new technique for embolization of the middle cerebral artery with histacryl-n-butyl-cyanoacrylate as described by Brassel et al. [1988]. Local cerebral blood flow and tissue pO_2

measurements were performed before and one, three, five and seven hours after infarction.

Results and Discussion

Investigations on cats

The results of the tissue pO_2 measurements in the brain cortex of cats are summarized in Fig. 1. Under control conditions with arterial normoxia and normocarbia (p_aO_2 = 109 mmHg; p_aCO_2 = 31 mmHg; pH_a = 7.36) and normal blood pressure (Pm_a = 135 mmHg), the pO_2 histograms ranged from very low values to values near the arterial pO_2. The mean tissue pO_2 was found to be 28.4 mmHg. Comparable tissue pO_2 histograms of the parietal cortex (gyrus suprasylvius) of cats have been recorded by Grote et al. [1981] during pentobarbital anesthesia at normal arterial oxygen and carbon dioxide tensions. Air embolism induced transient blood flow stop in the pial arteries and a decrease in tissue pO_2 of the superficial cells of the brain cortex.

After complete reperfusion, the pO_2 histograms obtained showed a significant shift to higher values with a mean tissue pO_2 of 38.1 mmHg. The

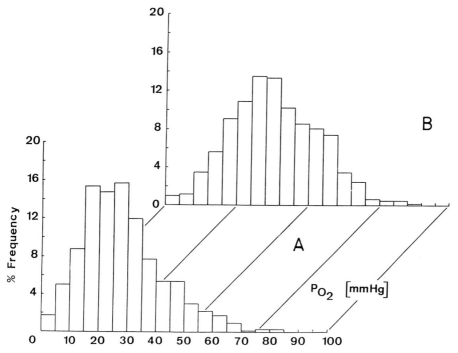

Fig. 1. Tissue pO_2 frequency histograms of the brain cortex (gyrus suprasylvius) of cats during arterial normoxia and normocapnia before (A: n = 639) and after (B: n = 609) transient ischemia

improvement observed in tissue oxygen supply of the brain cortex during the postischemic period seems to be mainly due to hyperemia, since at the same time the diameter of the pial arteries increased from 131 μm to 189 μm. The arterial blood gas tensions determined simultaneously were found to be within the normal range (p_aO_2 = 109 mmHg; p_aCO_2 = 30 mmHg; pH_a = 7.34); the mean arterial blood pressure was 125 mmHg.

During previous investigations in cats, Fritz and Hossmann [1979] and Haller and Kuschinsky [1981] measured a 50 – 70% increase in the pial artery diameter within the first 30 minutes following reperfusion after air embolism. Maximal dilatation of 100 – 200% compared to controls was found after 10 – 15 minutes. In addition, the postischemic increase in brain tissue pO_2 may be due to the improvement in oxygen diffusion from blood to tissue as a consequence of the decrease in hemoglobin oxygen affinity [Hagendorff et al., 1986].

Changes in the oxygen affinity of capillary blood are to be expected as a consequence of the pronounced brain tissue acidosis as demonstrated by simultaneous cortical pH measurements [Fritz and Hossmann, 1979]. The results of the investigations of brain tissue pO_2 as well as of pial artery diameter following transient brain ischemia agree with the concept of "postischemic luxury perfusion" according to Lassen [1966].

Investigations on monkeys

The results of ischemia experiments performed on baboons may be demonstrated by typical examples. Before occlusion of the middle cerebral artery, a normal tissue pO_2 distribution was found in the different measuring fields of all experiments. The pO_2 histograms of the compared cortical regions, however, showed distinct differences, as can be seen in Fig. 2, which shows the pO_2 distributions determined under normal conditions in the parietal (Fig. 2B) and in the frontal (Fig. 2A) cortex of the right hemisphere. In the example described, the difference in the mean tissue pO_2 of the two brain regions was about 13 mmHg (mean pO_2: 21.6 and 35.3 mmHg, respectively). The observed inhomogeneities in regional brain tissue oxygen supply can be attributed to local differences in cerebral blood flow as well as in cerebral metabolism as demonstrated by several investigators using autoradiographic techniques or positron computed tomography [Sokoloff et al., 1977; Sakurada et al., 1978; Phelps et al., 1982; Schröck and Kuschinsky, 1988]. Comparable differences in the regional tissue pO_2 distributions in the cortex and the hippocampus are described for the gerbil brain by Nair et al. [1987].

Embolization of the right or left middle cerebral artery caused a severe brain tissue hypoxia in the supplied territories. Figs. 3 and 4 summarize the results of tissue pO_2 measurements performed in the superficial cell layers of the parietal (suprasylvian and ectosylvian gyri) and frontal brain cortex of the right hemisphere before the occlusion of the right middle

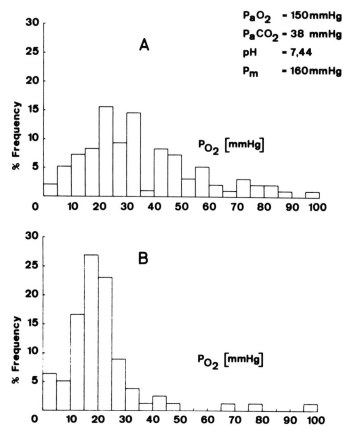

Fig. 2. Tissue pO₂ frequency histograms of the brain cortex of a baboon determined during arterial normoxia and normocapnia in frontal and parietal regions of the brain cortex (A = frontal brain, n = 96; B = parietal brain, n = 78); ph = arterial ph value; P_m = mean arterial blood pressure

cerebral artery as well as one and five hours after occlusion. As demonstrated by the pO₂ frequency histograms during the first five hours following histoacryl injection, pronounced hypoxia was present in the territory of the occluded artery (s. Fig. 3, B and C). The pO₂ values measured five hours after embolization indicate a small improvement in the oxygen supply conditions of the ischemic brain region. The mean tissue pO₂ increased again from 11 to 16 mmHg. These results are in line with the very low local blood flow values (5 – 15 ml 100g⁻¹min⁻¹) determined simultaneously in the upper and deeper layers of the parietal cortex investigated. Both findings suggest that the measuring field was within the core of the ischemic brain area.

The pO₂ measurements performed at the same time in the frontal cerebral cortex (Fig. 4) showed a transient depression in tissue oxygen supply.

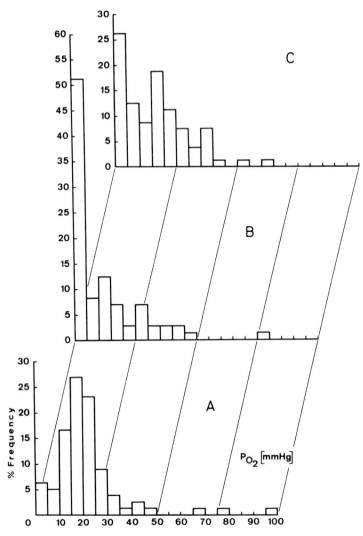

Fig. 3. Tissue pO_2 frequency histograms of the parietal brain cortex of a baboon determined before (A: n = 78), one hour (B: n = 72) and five hours (C: n = 72) after middle cerebral artery occlusion

While the first measurements immediately after middle cerebral artery occlusion resulted in a pO_2 histogram shifted to the left with a significant increase of oxygen tension values between 0 and 5 mmHg, the second measurements performed four hours later showed a near normal tissue pO_2 distribution. The mean tissue oxygen tension decreased from 35 mmHg in the control period to 15 mmHg one hour after infarction, and reached 26 mmHg in the course of the following hours. The arterial

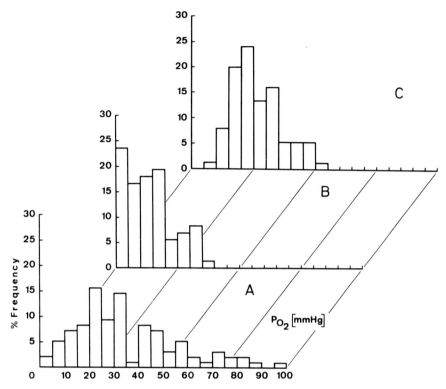

Fig. 4. Tissue pO₂ frequency histograms of the frontal brain cortex of a baboon determined before (A: n = 96), one hour (B: n = 72) and five hours (C: n = 75) after middle cerebral artery occlusion

blood pressure and the arterial oxygen tension remained normal during the entire experiment while the arterial CO₂ tension decreased from normal levels to 34 mmHg and 30 mmHg during the two tissue pO₂ determinations after infarction. The results agree with observations of Strong et al. [1988], who, in experiments performed on cats after middle cerebral artery occlusion, found a comparable transient increase in steady-state NADH fluorescence in the gyrus marginalis indicating temporary ischemia in the border zone of the supplying territory.

The results of the local blood flow determinations in the frontal brain are comparable to those of the tissue pO₂ measurements. The observed improvement in oxygen supply of the border zone of the infarct area may be due to a reincrease in local blood flow through collateral vessels as observed by different authors [Halsey and Clark, 1970; Hossmann, 1982; Coyle and Heistad, 1987; Strong et al., 1988]. The elevation in collateral flow can be explained as a result of the increase in the extracellular activity of potassium and hydrogen and the decrease in the extracellular activity of calcium, which are characteristic features of ischemic brain tissue. Especially the change in extracellular potassium activity is thought to be of great importance for the regulation of collateral flow [Astrup et al., 1977; Branston et al., 1977; Strong et al., 1988].

A decrease of tissue oxygen demand and the effect of arterial hypocapnia have to be discussed as additional factors influencing the tissue pO_2 distribution in the frontal cerebral cortex. Since in the ischemic penumbra a primary suppression of neuronal activity resulting from a loss of normal input to neurons is to be expected [Strong et al., 1988], a subsequent decrease in oxygen consumption should be the consequence. The decrease in arterial carbon dioxide tension induces vasoconstriction in the unaffected brain regions with normal blood flow regulation, which possibly induces a redistribution of local flow in favour of the border zone in the territory of the occluded artery. The latter effect, however, seems to be of minor importance, because in other experiments comparable results of tissue pO_2 measurements were obtained during arterial normocapnia.

References

1. Astrup J, Symon L, Branston NM, Lassen NA (1977) Cortical evoked potential and extracellular K^+ and H^+ at critical levels of brain ischemia. Stroke 8:51
2. Branston NM, Strong, AJ, Symon L (1977) Extracellular potassium activity, evoked potential and tissue blood flow: Relationships during progressive ischaemia in baboon cerebral cortex. J Neurol Sci 32:305
3. Brassel F, Dettmers C, Nierhaus A, Hartmann A, Solymosi L (1988) An intravascular technique to occlude the middle cerebral artery in baboons. In press
4. Coyle P, Heistad DD (1987) Blood flow through cerebral collateral vessels one month after middle cerebral artery occlusion. Stroke 18:407
5. Fritz H, Hossmann KA (1979) Arterial air embolism in the cat brain. Stroke 10:581
6. Grote J, Zimmer K, Schubert R (1981) Effects of severe arterial hypocapnia on regional blood flow regulation, tissue pO_2 and metabolism in the brain cortex of cats. Pflügers Arch. 391:195
7. Grunewald W (1970) Diffusionsfehler und Eigenverbrauch der Pt-Elektrode bei pO_2-Messungen im steady state. Pflügers Arch 320:24
8. Hagendorff A, Haller C, Grote J (1986) Der Einfluß einer postischämischen Hypokapnie auf die cerebrale O_2-Versorgung. In: Funktionsanalyse biologischer Systeme 17:165, Fischer, Stuttgart
9. Haller C,; Kuschinsky W (1981) Reactivity of pial arteries to K^+ and H^+ before and after ischemia induced by air embolism. Microcirculation 1:141
10. Haller C, Kuschinsky W, Reimnitz P (1986) Effect of gammahydroxybutyrate on the reactivity of pial arteries before and after ischemia. J Cer Blood Flow Metabol 6:658
11. Halsey JH, Clark LC (1970) Some regional circulatory abnormalities following experimental cerebral infarction. Neurology 20:238
12. Hartmann A, Menzel J, Buttinger C, Lange D, Alberti E (1981) Die regionale Gehirndurchblutung des Pavians beim ischämischen Hirninfarkt unter Dexamethason-Behandlung. Fortschr Neurol Psychiatr 49:380
13. Hossmann KA (1982) Treatment of experimental cerebral ischemia. J Cer Blood Flow Metabol 2:275
14. Kessler M, Grunewald W (1969) Possibilities of measuring oxygen pressure fields in tissue by multiwire platinum electrodes. Prog Resp Res 3:147

15. Lassen NA (1966) The luxury-perfusion syndrome and its possible relation to acute metabolic acidosis localized within the brain. Lancet II:1113
16. Lübbers DW, Baumgärtl H, Fabel H, Huch A, Kessler M, Kunze K, Riemann H, Seiler D, Schuchardt S (1969) Principles and construction of various platinum electrodes. Prog Resp Res 3:136
17. Nair PK, Buerk DG, Halsey JJ (1987) Comparison of oxygen metabolism and tissue pO₂ in cortex and hippocampus of gerbil brain. Stroke 18:616
18. Phelps ME, Mazziotta JC, Huang SC (1982) Study of cerebral function with positron computed tomography. J Cer Blood Flow Metabol 2:113
19. Sakurada O, Kennedey C, Jehle J, Brown D, Carbin GL, Sokoloff L (1978) Measurement of local cerebral blood flow with iodo (¹⁴C)antipyrine. Am J Physiol 234:H59
20. Schneidermann G, Goldstick TK (1976) Oxygen fields induced by recessed and needle oxygen microelectrodes in homogeneous media. In: Grote J, Reneau D, Thews G (eds) Advances in experimental Medicine and Biology. Vol. 75: Oxygen Transport to Tissue II:9
21. Schröck H, Kuschinsky W (1988) Cerebral blood flow, glucose use and CSF ionic regulation in potassium-depleted rats. Am J Physiol 254:H250
22. Sokoloff L, Reivich M, Kennedey C, Des Rosiers MH, Patlak CS, Pettigrew KD, Sakurada O, Shinohara M (1977) The (¹⁴C)deoxyglucose method for measurement of local cerebral glucose utilization: Theory, procedure and normal values in conscious and anaesthetized albino rats. J Neurochem 28:897
23. Söntgerath C, Steuer K, Grote J (1984) Der Einfluß des pCO₂ auf die Messung des O₂-Partialdruckes mit Platin-Mikroelektroden. In: Grote J, Witzleb E (eds) Atemgaswechsel und O₂-Versorgung der Organe. Funktionsanalyse biologischer Systeme 12:172. Mainz Akad Wiss Literatur. Steiner, Stuttgart
24. Strong AJ, Venables GS, Gibson G (1983) The cortical ischaemic penumbra associated with occlusion of the middle cerebral artery in the cat. 1. Topography of changes in blood flow, potassium ion activity in EEG. J Cer Blood Flow Metabol 3:86
25. Strong AJ, Gibson G, Miller SA, Venables GS (1988) Changes in vascular and metabolic reactivity as indices of ischaemia in the penumbra. J Cer Blood Flow Metabol 8:79
26. Waltz AG (1968) Effect of blood pressure on blood flow in ischemic and nonischemic cerebral cortex. The phenomena of autoregulation and luxury perfusion. Neurology 18:613
27. Yamaguchi T, Regli F, Waltz AG (1972) Effects of hyperventilation with and without carbon dioxide on experimental cerebral ischemia and infarction. Brain 95:123

Oxygen Pressure in Cerebrospinal Fluid

W. Fleckenstein, A.I.R. Maas, G. Nollert, D.A. de Jong

Part 1: Dynamics of Oxygen Transfer at Normal, Increased and Decreased Oxygen Offer

The production, circulation and absorption of cerebrospinal fluid (CSF) and the concentrations of its components have been subjected to physiological and pharmacological studies (reviewed by Cserr 1971; Milhorat 1975 and Wright 1978). It has been proposed that CSF components influence electrical or neurocrine activity of neurons involved in homoeostatic regulations. The mechanisms sensing the concentrations of respective CSF components and transforming the chemical information into regulatory bioelectrical information, are still a matter of controversy. However, H^+, Ca^{++}, neurotransmitter substances, neuropeptides, amino acids and drugs influence circulation and respiration when topically applied to the ventral medullary surface or when injected into the ventricular CSF (Bousquet 1974; Eldrige and Millhorn 1981; Feldberg 1980; Fukuda and Loeschke 1979; Lioy et al. 1981; Trzebski et al. 1980; Wennergren and Öberg 1980).

Respiration, blood pressure, cardiac output and organ blood flow (including cerebral blood flow) can be strongly affected by arterial hypoxia and hyperoxia. Modified reactions of this kind can also be observed if an unphysiological oxygenation of arterial blood is restricted to the intracranial circulation (at normoxic peripheral circulation), and if the afference from carotid body and aortic glome is cut (Cherniak et al. 1971; Chapman et al. 1980; Downing at al. 1963; Miller and Tenney 1975; Santiago and Edelmann 1976; Traystman et al. 1978). From these findings it can be derived that, within intracranial vasculature or tissue, an intracranial oxygen sensing mechanism is present, influencing homoeostatic regulations. This assumption was supported by the demonstration of a modulating effect of changes in pO_2, in vivo and in tissue slices, on the release of neurotransmitters and the neuronal electrical activity (Bingmann et al. 1984; Bingmann et al. 1982; Eldridge and Millhorn 1981; Metzger and Heuber 1977; Speckmann and Caspers 1975). It remains a matter of speculation whether the oxygen pressure within nerve and glial cells, within cerebrospinal fluid or within interstitial cerebrospinal fluid, exerts regulatory influences.

The cerebrospinal fluid (CSF) is in direct and close contact with the brain tissue surfaces and vessels (choroideal, pial, subarachnoideal vasculature);

Clinical Oxygen Pressure Measurement II
A.M. Ehrly et al. (Eds.)
© Blackwell Ueberreuter Wissenschaft Berlin 1990

thus, the pO_2 in CSF is determined by the amount and the direction of diffusive oxygen exchange between tissue and CSF on the one hand, and between vasculature and CSF on the other. In this respect, the $CSFpO_2$ can be regarded as a parameter that reflects the oxygen offer to the brain (Bloor et al. 1961; Jarnum et al. 1964; Skinhøy 1965), the cerebral blood flow (CBF) and the rate of cerebral oxygen metabolism (Bloor et al. 1963; Salaymeh et al. 1971). Hence, $CSFpO_2$ is of clinical interest in cases of disturbed brain oxygen offer and brain oxygen metabolism, e.g. in increased intracranial pressure, in brain edema, in brain acidosis, during hyperventilation therapy and during neurosurgical procedures (Bloor et al. 1961; Gänshirt 1968).

It was demonstrated that the $CSFpO_2$ has a direct and local action on the diameter of pial vessels (Kontos et al. 1978). Taking into account the predominant influence of the pial vessels' flow resistance on brain perfusion, it can be supposed that the pO_2 in the CSF directly contributes to the regulation of cerebral blood flow. It has not yet been examined whether the neurogenic control of the pial vessel diameter (Heistadt et al. 1976; Wahl 1985) is also modulated by the pO_2 in CSF.

Considering a possible role of the $CSFpO_2$ in physiological regulations, we were interested in basal knowledge concerning the statics and dynamics of this parameter.

The question arises whether the $CSFpO_2$ remains at a stable level under physiological conditions. And if so, to what extent do "normal" values within the CSF compartments differ within one species and between different species? Our special interest was focused on speed and extent of $CSFpO_2$ response, after oxygen transfer conditions at the blood brain barrier, and oxygen offer to the brain are changed.

We expected to get a clue from dynamic studies concerning the most effective pathways of oxygen transfer into the ventricular system and of oxygen transport out of the CSF. We were interested to discern which respiratory and circulatory parameters have predominant influence on the level of $CSFpO_2$.

$CSFpO_2$ was continuously recorded with fast responding needle probes, simultaneously in the lateral ventricle and cisterna magna of cats, in the lateral ventricle of dogs and in the subarachnoid space of both species. Intracranial fluid pressure and microvascular flow values were additionally determined. The animals were artificially ventilated under normocanic conditions and subjected to normoxia, hyperoxia and hypoxic hypoxia. In some of the animals, the cranial perfusion pressure was lowered by raising of the intracranial pressure and also by inducing hypotension.

Material and Methods

Abbreviations
ACpO₂D: pO₂-difference of arterial blood and CSF in cisterna magna (read: arterio-cisternal pO₂-difference)

AVpO$_2$D:	pO$_2$-difference of arterial blood and CSF in lateral ventricle (read: arterio-ventricular pO$_2$-difference)
BOFO$_2$:	oxygen offer to the brain
CBF:	cerebral blood flow
CCSF:	cerebrospinal fluid of cisterna magna
CMRO$_2$:	cerebral metabolic rate of oxygen
CPP:	cranial perfusion pressure
CSF:	cerebrospinal fluid
EMBF:	trans-epidural determined microvascular blood flow
FiO$_2$:	fractional volume of inspired oxygen
ICP:	mean intracranial pressure
MAP:	mean arterial blood pressure
paO$_2$, paCO$_2$:	arterial pressures of oxygen and of carbon dioxide resp.
SCSF	cerebrospinal fluid of subarachnoid space
VCSF:	cerebrospinal fluid of lateral ventricle
VFP:	ventricular fluid pressure

In 6 cats (weight 2.5 – 4.0 kg) and 5 beagle dogs (weight 12.3–22.5 kg) intubation narcosis was introduced with Ketamine (40 mg, in cats) or Methohexital (3 mg/kg, in dogs) and maintained by continuous infusing of Fentanyl (0.03 mg/kg h^{-1}, in cats; 0.015 mg/kg h^{-1}, in dogs) and Pancuronium (0.05 mg/kg h^{-1}, in cats; 0.08 mg/kg h^{-1}, in dogs) and an admixture of N$_2$O to the respired gas. Catheters were placed in femoral artery, femoral vein and urinary bladder. Blood pressure was continuously monitored. The endtidal fractional volume of CO$_2$ in expired gas was measured by the infra-red absorption method (device "Binos", mfg. by Leybold-Heraeus, Hanau, FRG). FiO$_2$ was measured by a polarographic sensor (type "oxycom", mfg. by Dräger AG, Lübeck, FRG). Brain temperature and rectal temperature were recorded by thermocouples. The operation table was thermoregulated, so the rectal temperatures lay between 36.4 and 38.2°C. Blood samples were taken at regular intervals for determination of arterial blood gases, acid base status, K$^+$ values, Na$^+$ values, blood hemoglobin concentration and hemotocrit values.

The frontoparietal bones were dissected free in order to install brain sensors and, avoiding CSF leakage, holes were drilled through the skull to the depth of the epidural space. Sensors were introduced for pO$_2$ measurement, temperature recording, intraventricular pressure monitoring and microvascular flow determinations according to the laser doppler method. The intraventricular fluid pressure (VFP) was recorded by a hollow, round-headed steel needle (opened laterally, outer diameter 1 mm) connected by a teflon tube to a Statham pressure transducer, that was positioned at the level of the foramen of Monro. In this study, the ventricular fluid pressure was regarded as the intracranial pressure (ICP). The stereotactic coordinates of the probe tips' positions in lateral ventricles were (with respect to the midpoint of the interaural line) 11 mm towards frontal direction, 3.8 mm laterally and 15–26 mm below the outer surface of skull in cats, and 10 mm towards frontal direction, 8 mm laterally and 20–28 mm below the outer surface of skull in dogs. The pO$_2$ probe was positioned in accordance with the same coordinates but contralaterally to the ventricular drain. Finally, in cats only, the tip of a second pO$_2$ probe was placed in the cisterna magna after operative exposure of the atlanto-occipital membrane.

In order to record "reference" CSFpO$_2$ values, the animals were subjected to the same experimental procedure: measurements were started 1 hour after preparation and, at eucapnia and slightly elevated FiO$_2$ (0.25), "reference" CSFpO$_2$ values were recorded in the parietal subarachnoid space, the lateral ventricle and the cisterna magna (cisternal measurements only in cats).

Subsequently, under eucapnic conditions, mild hyperoxia (FiO$_2$ 0.5, 10 min), strong hyperoxia (FiO$_2$ 0.83, 10 min), mild hypoxic hypoxia (FiO$_2$ 0.15, 10 min) and medium hypoxic hypoxia (FiO$_2$ 0.10, 10 min) were induced. Each of the experiments was ended by a period of eucapnia with slightly elevated FiO$_2$ (0.25) lasting 15 min, thus reference conditions were reinstalled. For simplification, in this study, hypoxic hypoxia is called "hypoxia".

In one of the dogs seven normocapnic hypoxia periods, each lasting between 7 and 9 minutes, and of increasing severity (FiO$_2$ values: 0.16, 0.14, 0.12, 0.1, 0.08, 0.06), were induced. The periods were separated by 30 min under ventilatory reference conditions.

After the ventilation experiments, in four animals (two cats, two dogs), ICP was raised in a stepwise manner by intraventricular injections of CSF which had been collected (slowly and without causing functionally relevant changes of ICP) during the preceding ventilation experiments. After physiological ICP levels were regained, hypotension was induced by infusion of Trimethaphan (a ganglion blocking agent) in increasing doses (beginning with 5 mg/kg min^{-1} up to 12 mg/kg min^{-1}), until MAP reached 0 mmHg irreversibly.

In two of the cats, after the ventilation experiments, a brain cold injury was performed (∅ of kryoprobe was 14 mm; temperature was −40°C for 12 min: method described earlier by Maas [1977]) contralaterally to the ventricular pO$_2$ measuring probe. Measurements were continued during the subsequent 3 h.

Methods of CSFpO₂ measurements

CSFpO$_2$ was determined with polarographic needle probes (low sensitive LICOX probe type, mfg. by G. M. S. mbh., Kiel-Mielkendorf, FRG). The coating tube of the needle probe (outer diameter 0.35 mm, length of needle 60 mm) is made of spring steel which provides flexibility. Hence, the probe cannot be broken. The tip of the probe is ground to a shape similar to that of a hypodermic needle, but the lancet-like cutting edges of the tip are rounded by a polishing process. The pO$_2$ was measured at a polarographic, FEP-membranized, gold microcathode situated within a recess on the ground surface of the probe tip (gold wire diameter: 12.5 μm; gold wire insulation: glass sealing; reaction time T_{90} of the probe current after pO$_2$ change: shorter than 2 s; pO$_2$ sensitivity at 37°C and

−630 mV polarisation voltage: 4 ± 1 pA/mmHg; stirring artifacts smaller than 2%; sensitivity drifting: lower than 2%/h; no measurable pH sensitivity between pH 6.5 and 9.5; non-oxygen-dependent probe current <12 pA). The anodic reference potential was applied by an Ag/AgCl/NaCl-jelly electrode to the shaved and degreased skin of the neck.

Before and after insertion in CSF, the probes were calibrated in buffered physiological saline, saturated by bubbling both with N_2 (purity >99.996%) and with air. The pO_2 probe's current values in the CSF and the corresponding probe temperature values were measured at intervals of 4 s and stored electronically, thus allowing recalibration calculations and determinations of time-histograms and fast fourier transformations (device LICOX, mfg. by G. M. S. mbH, Kiel-Mielkendorf, FRG). By the calibration algorithm, applied onto each single probe current value, the following parameters were considered: barometrical pressure, H_2O partial pressure in the calibration chamber, temperatures of calibration chamber and tissue (brain temperature), temperature coefficient of the probe current (2.44%/°C) and, by time-linear interpolations, the changes in the oxygen-dependent and non-oxygen-dependent probe sensitivities as determined before and after measurements.

Microvascular blood flow measurement by laser doppler signal

In order to record a signal correlated to the cerebral blood flow, a laser doppler device (Tenland [1982]; type "PeriFlux", mfg. by Perimed, Stockholm, Sweden), was applied on the parietal dura of the cats and dogs. The sensor was positioned using a cylindrical perspex holder (∅ 14 mm) mounted into the skull. The plane end of the holder was screwed into an exactly fitting hole in the skull so that the plane end of the holder lay on the surface of the dura without compressing it. The holder had two holes which were parallel to its rotational axis, one to house the cylindrical laser doppler sensor (∅ 6 mm), the other for draining blood that would possibly suffuse from the skull's diploe into the epidural space. After the dura at the bottom of the probe's hole was thoroughly cleaned with physiological saline, the laser doppler sensor was advanced in the holder until the dura was touched and a stable signal was achieved. However, even after careful adjustment of the pressure of the probe on the dura, small changes of the probe's vertical position – with respect to the brain – altered the probe signal. If the compression was too low the flow signal was broken. More compression led to a decline of the signal, probably due to a compression of small vessels. Consequently, it must be assumed that the flow signal was influenced by changes of intracranial pressure.

The method did not provide absolute flow values and no stable readings of the device-defined arbitrary flow units; but for the observation of the trend towards short acting flow variation, the method seems to be useful if short periods (e. g. of 20 min) are evaluated. The laser doppler signal was taken from different compartments (dura, pia, subarachnoid space, arachnoidea, cortical tissue). Due to the inhomogeneity of subdural structures with regard to scattering, reflection and absorption of light, the tissue volume from which the signal reading was influenced could not be exactly determined. Conceivably, the width of the subarachnoid space and the blood flow in dural and subdural vessels varied with the pressure exerted by the probe on the dura. Thus, the relative influence on the laser doppler signal exerted by flow levels in the different compartments may also be varied by the pressure of the probe on the tissue. With respect to the position of the probe in this study, the registered signal is called "epidural determined microvascular blood flow", (EMBF).

Results

Positioning of pO_2 sensor

The probes were fixed in stereotactic drives. When the probe tip for measuring $CSFpO_2$ was driven slowly forward, the pO_2 signal on reaching the upper ventricular wall increased suddenly from a low and variable tissue level to 60–80 mmHg (at reference conditions). In contrast to measuring in tissue, within CSF, the probe signal was not changed if the probe was moved. For the measurements of ventricular $CSFpO_2$, the probe tip was positioned approximately midway between the upper and lower ventricle walls. A probe position was accepted to be "intraventricular" only if the probe signal was stable during the pre-experimental observation period of 1 hour (at unchanged reference conditions), and only if the signal was not altered by upward and downward probe displacements of 2 mm each way. Probes in a definite intraventricular position were fixed with glue (histoacryl) at the skull, thus avoiding CSF leakage and probe displacement.

Reference conditions

Under cardiorespiratory stable reference conditions (normocapnia at FiO_2 of 0.25) in the CSF, only small spontaneous fluctuations of the pO_2 values were observed in cat and dog. During one hour of stable conditions the average of maximal individual fluctuations in ventricular pO_2 lay at 6 ± 3 mmHg in the cats and 5 ± 2 mmHg in the dogs. The average pO_2 value in ventricular CSF ($VCSFpO_2$) obtained from the cats at reference conditions after the ventilation experiments (of 3 hours duration) differed by 0.8 mmHg (1.1%) from values obtained before ventilation experiments. As can be seen from Tab. 1, the average $VCSFpO_2$ of dog and cat, at reference conditions, lay close to each other (73.5 ± 4.5 mmHg in dogs, and 70.8 ± 6.5 mmHg in cats). The average cisternal $CSFpO_2$ ($CCSFpO_2$) of cats was 65.8 ± 9.3 mmHg. The average pO_2 in subarach-

Table 1. CSFpO$_2$ in subarachnoid space, lateral ventricle and cisterna magna under eucapnic conditions at slightly elevated arterial pO$_2$ value, average values from 6 cats and 5 dogs

average pO$_2$ in CSF and arterial blood at reference conditions

	VCSFpO$_2$ [mmHg] ± SD	CCSFpO$_2$ [mmHg] ± SD	SCSFpO$_2$ [mmHg] ± SD	paO$_2$ [mmHg] ± SD
cats (n = 6)	70.8 6.5	65.8 9.3	41.2 4.7	124.7 8.0
dogs (n = 5)	73.5 4.5		47.2 4.9	118.9 7.7

noid CSF (SCSFpO$_2$) in cats and dogs lay at 41.2 ± 4.7 mmHg and 47.2 ± 4.9 mmHg respectively.

Hypoxia

A sharp decline of CSFpO$_2$ was recorded in response to arterial hypoxia, as shown from an individual experiment in Fig. 1A and 1B. Ten minutes after the start of mild hypoxia (FiO$_2$ 0.15) in cats, VCSFpO$_2$ and CCSFpO$_2$ were markedly decreased – and to almost the same extent (Tab. 2). During mild hypoxia, microvascular blood flow (EMBF) and cranial perfusion pressure (CPP) were only slightly increased. However, the most significant effect observed was a decrease in the arterio-ventricular and the arterio-cisternal oxygen pressure differences (AVpO$_2$D and ACpO$_2$D resp.) from 53.9 ± 12.4 mmHg and 58.9 ± 10.3 mmHg resp. at reference conditions, to 18.1 ± 4.3 mmHg and 16.0 ± 8.3 mmHg resp., 10 mins after onset of mild hypoxia.

Ten minutes after inducing medium hypoxia (FiO$_2$ 0.1) in the cats, VCSFpO$_2$ and CCSFpO$_2$ were reduced more than during mild hypoxia. In fact, EMBF was now significantly increased, although CPP was decreased due to an approximate 100% increase in intracranial pressure (ICP), and a decrease in mean arterial blood pressure (MAP). Consequently, the cerebrovascular resistance was decreased. However, it should be noted that the absolute values of the decreases in AVpO$_2$D and ADpO$_2$D during mild and medium hypoxia were not markedly different (Tab. 2). This finding indicates that AVpO$_2$D and ACpO$_2$D are more influenced by arterial pO$_2$ changes at ranges over 60 mmHg; above this level no marked changes of EMBF and CPP were observed.

In order to determine the maximum decrease in AVpO$_2$D that can be induced by hypoxia, a series of hypoxia experiments of increasing severity was performed in one of the dogs (Fig. 1A, 1B and 1C). The VCSFpO$_2$ was zero at an arterial pO$_2$ of 19.2 mmHg. The latter value can be regarded as

Table 2. Effects of normocapnic arterial hypoxia and hyperoxia, average values from 6 cats

average values and standard deviations of data obtained from CSF, arterial blood and circulation of cats (n = 6) at different levels of FiO$_2$

	VCSFpO$_2$ [mmHg] ± SD	AVpO$_2$D [mmHg] ± SD	CCSFpO$_2$ [mmHg] ± SD	ACpO$_2$D [mmHg] ± SD	paO$_2$ [mmHg] ± SD	paCO$_2$ [mmHg] ± SD	art. pH ± SD	EMBF [A.U.] ± SD	ICP [mmHg] ± SD	CPP [mmHg] ± SD	MAP [mmHg] ± SD
reference conditions (FiO$_2$ = 0.25)	70.8 6.5	53.9 12.4	65.8 9.3	58.9 10.3	124.7 8.0	37.8 3.1	7.32 0.05	43.8 13.5	9.2 3.6	118.6 11.1	127.8 10.3
mild hypoxia (FiO$_2$ = 0.15)	44.2 3.2	18.1 4.3	46.3 6.1	16.0 8.3	62.3 6.6	35.4 1.6	7.31 0.05	48.5 14.4	12.0 3.2	119.0 20.9	127.8 22.2
medium hypoxia (FiO$_2$ = 0.1)	20.0 8.7	11.4 5.8	22.3 3.7	9.1 7.1	31.4 5.4	36.0 3.0	7.36 0.04	67.7 23.9	18.8 6.3	96.5 27.5	113.9 25.4
mild hyperoxia (FiO$_2$ = 0.5)	87.3 9.4	194.3 24.2	95.4 17.1	186.2 18.7	281.6 22.0	37.4 1.2	7.37 0.04	38.0 2.0	10.5 3.0	117.4 15.3	127.9 16.3
strong hyperoxia (FiO$_2$ = 0.83)	101.3 10.0	359.7 33.2	138.0 28.5	323.0 21.5	461.0 36.8	34.3 2.8	7.30 0.01	47.3 11.8	12.7 2.9	127.9 5.9	140.6 4.2

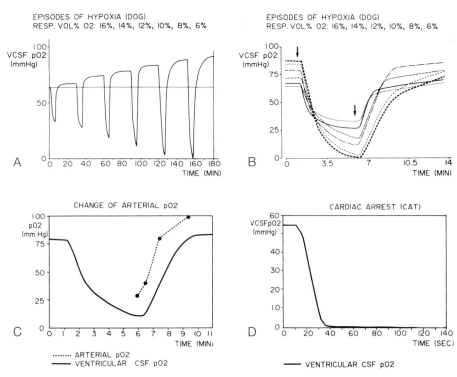

Fig. 1A–D. In all figures (A, B, C and D) swift changes of pO₂ in CSF of lateral ventricle are shown.
A) VCSFpO₂ obtained from a dog subjected to a series of hypoxic episodes induced by reduction of FiO₂. During the intervals ventilatory reference conditions were reinstalled. The FiO₂ values were lowered stepwise (by 0.02) starting with a FiO₂ of 0.16 during the first hypoxia experiment. Post-hypoxic VCSFpO₂ values were higher than pre-hypoxic. **B)** The VCSFpO₂ changes during the hypoxic episodes. Arrows indicate start and stop of hypoxia respectively. After an FiO₂ of 0.08 and 0.06 the late phase of VCSFpO₂ recovery was delayed (ICP exceeded 40 mmHg). **C)** Time course of VCSFpO₂ and paO₂ (broken line) after switching FiO₂ from 0.1 to 0.25. **D)** VCSFpO₂ change after sudden cardiac arrest (time=0) at ongoing artificial ventilation

the dog's lowest possible AVpO₂D under normocapnic hypoxia conditions, if VCSFpO₂ is not zero. After the periods of severe hypoxia the VCSFpO₂ level was higher than before.

Hyperoxia

During the strong hyperoxic periods in the cats (FiO₂ 0.8, applied 10 min), EMBF and CPP were elevated due to an increase in MAP. The increase in arterial pO₂ from 124.7 ± 8.0 mmHg up to 461 ± 36.8 mmHg led to a more or less linear correlated increase in VCSFpO₂ and CCSFpO₂ (Fig. 2A). The same can be said for the AVpO₂D and ACpO₂D (Fig. 2B and Tab. 2). However, VCSFpO₂ is increased less than CCSFpO₂ if the arterial pO₂

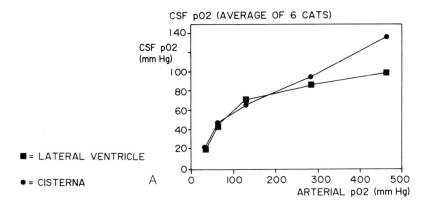

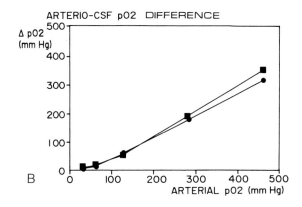

Fig. 2. Effects of arterial hypoxia and hyperoxia on CSFpO₂. **A)** Average ventricular and cisternal CSFpO₂ values of 6 cats are plotted against average arterial pO₂. At arterial normoxia CSFpO₂ lies at about 60 mmHg. **B)** Average of differences between arterial pO₂ and CSFpO₂ in lateral ventricle and cisterna respectively, data obtained from 6 cats

is elevated within the range of non-physiologically high pO₂ values; consequently, AVpO₂D is higher than ACpO₂D at hyperoxia (Fig. 2B). Compared with the alterations of the cats' VCSFpO₂ during hypoxia and hyperoxia, qualitatively analogous results were obtained in the dogs' ventricle. In contrast to the cats, the MAP in dogs was markedly increased during hypoxia.

Time course of respiratory CSFpO₂ changes

In order to study the early phase of response in the cats' CSFpO₂ to variations in the arterial blood gas values, CSFpO₂ (of 4 cats) was averaged during the first 240 s after inspiratory gas concentrations had been switched (Fig. 3A and Fig. 3B). The recording of CSFpO₂ signals was started when, after handling the valves of the respirator, the first deviation of the inspiratory O₂ concentration was observed (time = 0 in Fig. 3A and 3B). The time required to achieve 66% of a new final value of an inspiratory gas concentration after switching it was 23 s, measured at the mouthpiece.

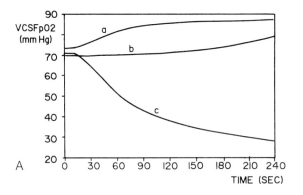

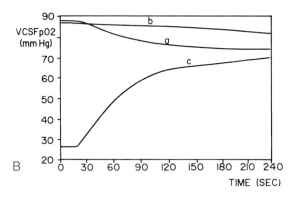

Fig. 3A, B. Slopes in CSFpO$_2$ values after change in ventilatory conditions, curves are averaged from 4 cats. At time=0 first concentration changes of components of inspired gas mixture were measured at the entry of the tubus (66% to full response time of the ventilator was 23 s). **A)** a: switching FiO$_2$ from 0.25 to 0.5, b: admixture of 5% CO$_2$, no change of FiO$_2$ (0.25), c: switching FiO$_2$ from 0.25 to 0.1, **B)** a: switching FiO$_2$ from 0.5 to 0.25, b: stop admixture of CO$_2$, no change of FiO$_2$ (0.25), c: switching FiO$_2$ from 0.1 to 0.25

First changes in CSFpO$_2$ were observed 17.4 ± 2.3 s after the start of recording. After all changes of FiO$_2$ the average maximal slope of CSFpO$_2$ was recorded at 31.4 ± 5.3 s (Fig. 3A [a,c] and Fig. 3B [a,c]).

As Fig. 3A and 3B show, the time courses of CSFpO$_2$ after changes in inspired gas concentrations cannot be sufficiently described as a single-component exponential function. After start and end of medium hypoxia (Fig. 3A [c] and 3B [c]), the initial slope was almost linear. The steepest slope of the averaged CSFpO$_2$ was observed after the end of hypoxia (being on average +0.57 mmHg/s in cats and +0.52 mmHg/s in dogs). In the series of increasingly severe hypoxia applied to dog (Fig. 1A and 1B) almost identical maximal slope values were initially found after the end of each hypoxic period (+0.54 mmHg/s), independent of the extent of hypoxia (Fig. 1B). In one of these experiments arterial blood samples were drawn (4 times) during the first 180 s after the switching of the FiO$_2$ from 0.01 to 0.25, in order to determine the speed of increase in arterial pO$_2$. A maximal slope of paO$_2$ of 0.76 mmHg/s was found (Fig. 1C).

In Tab. 3 the average 66% to full response times CSFpO$_2$ variations after changing ventilatory parameters of cat are shown. The pO$_2$ changes were established faster in ventricular CSF than in cisternal CSF. The fastest

Table 3. Slope of CSFpO$_2$ after change in FiO$_2$ determined as T$_{66}$, the time that is required to reach 66% of the full CSFpO$_2$-response on change of FiO$_2$

	average slope of CSFpO$_2$ after change of FiO$_2$ in cats (n = 6)					
	FiO$_2$ = 0.1		FiO$_2$ = 0.15		FiO$_2$ = 0.5	
	on	off	on	off	on	off
T$_{66}$ [s] in ventricle	142	85	179	75	115	234
T$_{66}$ [s] in cisterna	161	157	257	248	188	318

response was the reattainment of reference values in VCSFpO$_2$ after the end of hypoxia.

Twelve seconds after ending the experiments by means of sudden cardiac arrest (using T 61, Hoechst) at ongoing artificial ventilation, VCSFpO$_2$ began to decrease. The maximal nearly linear slope (-2.8 mmHg/s) was observed 25 s after cardiac arrest; thus, after less than 40 s, VCSFpO$_2$ was below 5 mmHg (Fig. 1D).

Reduction in cranial perfusion pressure

In two cats and two dogs CPP was decreased by (0.2–0.5 ml) injections of previously sampled and air saturated CSF in the ventricle, contralateral to the side of ventricular pO$_2$ measurement. As shown in Fig. 4A and 4B, VCSFpO$_2$ fell with decreasing CPP and increasing ICP. The CCSFpO$_2$ (measured outside the intracranial pressure compartment) was increased (for example, from 64 mmHg to 92 mmHg, in the cat of Fig. 4A) in parallel to a reflex blood pressure elevation (MAP elevation from 132 to 182 mmHg, in the same cat).

In order to override reflex hypertension whilst decreasing CPP by intra-ventricular fluid injections, Trimethaphan was infused into two cats. The procedure took 21 min. The plot of VCSFpO$_2$ against MAP in Fig. 4C shows, below a MAP level of 90 mmHg, the decrease of CSFpO$_2$ during hypotension.

Whilst a cold injury was performed on two cats, ICP and MAP were slightly decreased, resulting in unchanged CPP. The temperature in the grey matter of the contralateral hemisphere (on this side VCSFpO$_2$ was measured) decreased by a maximum of 1.9°C. VCSFpO$_2$ and CCSFpO$_2$ remained unchanged during the cooling procedure.

After cold injury, ICP was raised slowly but gradually during the subse-quent hours. In one of the cats, at an ICP level of 35 mmHg (CPP 95 mmHg), VCSFpO$_2$ began to fall 30 min after the end of cooling. Until the observation was ended 3 h after cooling, VCSFpO$_2$ decreased from 60 to 29 mmHg and CPP from 126 to 48 mmHg. In the other cat CPP was only

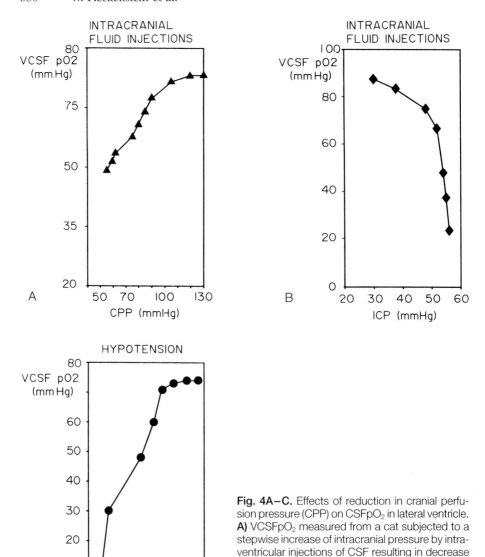

Fig. 4A–C. Effects of reduction in cranial perfusion pressure (CPP) on CSFpO$_2$ in lateral ventricle. A) VCSFpO$_2$ measured from a cat subjected to a stepwise increase of intracranial pressure by intraventricular injections of CSF resulting in decrease of CPP. B) VCSFpO$_2$ measured from a dog subjected to the same procedure as the cat of Fig. 4A. VCSFpO$_2$ is plotted against ICP. C) VCSFpO$_2$ and MAP values are obtained from a cat during pharmacologically (by Trimethaphan) induced hypotension

lowered to a level of 108 mmHg; in this animal no decrease of CSFpO$_2$ was observed.

By withdrawal of 60 ml of arterial blood, in one cat a hemorrhagic hypotension was induced (MAP 65 mmHg). VCSFpO$_2$ and CCSFpO$_2$ were reduced to 24 mmHg and 44 mmHg resp. Obviously VCSFpO$_2$ was, relative to reference values, reduced more than CCSFpO$_2$. The CPP was 58 mmHg. After subsequently infusing 100 ml of a solution of hyperoncotic polypeptides, VCSFpO$_2$ and CCSFpO$_2$ lay at 60 mmHg and 48 mmHg respectively, near reference values.

Discussion

Under conditions of eucapnia and 25% O$_2$ ventilation, the oxygen pressure in CSF of the lateral ventricle in cat and dog lay approximately at the same level (70.8 ± 6.5 mmHg and 73.5 ± 4.5 mmHg resp.). If ventilatory conditions were unchanged, the CSFpO$_2$ was stable and independent of fluctuations in intracranial and arterial pressure levels (within physiological limits). The reproducibility and stability of the CSFpO$_2$ level in different species, even after prolonged experiments, lead to the assumption that the CSFpO$_2$ level is regulated. Since oxygen in CSF is only physically dissolved (resulting in a low oxygen capacity of CSF compared to blood), slight changes in cerebral blood flow (CBF) and oxygen metabolism (CMRO$_2$) should cause marked changes in CSFpO$_2$ in absence of a regulation of CSFpO$_2$. Autoregulation of CBF seems to be influenced by arterial pO$_2$.

As a major influence on CSFpO$_2$ was exerted by the arterial pO$_2$ levels, the CSFpO$_2$ might be a suitable parameter to modulate the regulation of intracerebral gas transport. Only if the brain perfusion is pathologically lowered by an extremely raised ICP (Fig. 4A und 4B), severe arterial hypotension (Fig. 4C) or hemorrhagic shock, is the CSFpO$_2$ level markedly decreased. This indicates that CSFpO$_2$ is not maintainted if CPP and MAP are decreased below autoregulatory levels.

In most studies upon CSFpO$_2$, samples from lumbar, cisternal or ventricular CSF were examined in blood gas analyzers. However, these kind of devices can be unsuitable for O$_2$ measurements from liquids of low oxygen capacity; O$_2$ is dissolved in and transported through the walls of the tubes and samples' chambers that are manufactured from plastic materials in most blood gas analyzers. Using such devices we obtained pO$_2$ readings up to 22 mmHg if physiologic saline saturated with N$_2$ (and transported in a glass syringe) was analyzed. Comparable problems also arise if hyperoxic samples of low oxygen capacity are analyzed.

In order to obtain continuous pO$_2$ readings and in order to circumvent the methodical difficulties of pO$_2$ measurements from CSF samples, polarographic needle probes were applied by Harmsen and Bay (1970) in lumbar CSF, by Jamieson and van den Brenk (1963) in subarachnoid space, by Jarnum et al. (1964) in cisterna magna, and by Bloor et al. (1961) and Schoemaker (1965) in lateral ventricle. A review of available data is given by Nollert (1989). In most of these studies the sensitivity of the probes drifted considerably. Considering different levels of arterial pO$_2$ and pCO$_2$ in different studies, available pO$_2$ data obtained by needle probes lie more or less below our data.

However, our probes drifted less than 2%/h, the probe drift was corrected by recalibration calculations, the effect of temperature on the polarographic probe current was corrected by continuous measurements of brain temperature, the probes were not sensitive to intracranial pressure (due to solid state construction), and probe poisoning by N_2O and protein was ruled out. Hence, we assume that our pO_2 readings correspond to absolute $CSFpO_2$ levels within a range of $\pm$ 0.5 mmHg. Data given by Kazemi et al. (1968) from samples of cisternal and ventricular CSF of dogs (using an Istrum. Lab. device), agree exactly with our data.

As shown in Fig. 2A, at eucapnic arterial normoxia $CSFpO_2$ lies at 60 mmHg. This value is approximately double the mean cerebral tissue pO_2 (Lübbers 1969). In the grey matter only very few of the highest local tissue pO_2 values were observed to be above 60 mmHg. Since there is practically no elevation of tissue pO_2 in superficial regions of brain tissue (Smith et al. 1977), the pO_2-gradient at the fluid-tissue interface is steep, thus providing for an efficient oxygen transport from CSF into tissue. In the surface of cat cortex, superfused with air-saturated physiologic saline, a pO_2-gradient of 70 mmHg (and more) was observed within the superficial tissue layer of a thickness of only 100 μm (Nair et al. 1975). The authors also demonstrated, in accordance with others (Leniger-Follert et al. 1975), that the tissue pO_2 tends towards zero within less than 60 s if arterial oxygen delivery is eliminated by nitrogen breathing. After arterial occlusion, tissue pO_2 of grey matter was below 5 mmHg within less than 10 s (Null and Reneau 1977, Leniger-Follert 1977). Thus, our finding of fast oxygen decay after cardiac arrest (Fig. 1D), demonstrates the effectiveness of the oxygen transfer from CSF into tissue.

The CSF can be regarded as a fluid compartment that is supplied with oxygen by arterialized blood and from which oxygen is removed into tissue and veins. Under steady state conditions, the resulting $CSFpO_2$ values depend on the balance of oxygen flux through the fluid compartment and on the relation of oxygen conductivities at the "O_2-entry" and the "O_2-exit" of the CSF compartment. From this point of view, the differences of pO_2 in ventricle, cisterna and parietal subarachnoid space are not surprising, since the oxygen conductivity of the vascular O_2 exchange most probably differs in different CSF compartments as can be derived from (micro-) vascular anatomy. In the ventricles, the O_2 supply to CSF is most probably provided by the choroid plexus because in this structure of tightly packed and wide capillaries (diameter is 10–15 μm in dog, Gomez and Potts 1981) the blood flow is extremely high (6 ml/g x min in sheep, Page et al. 1980). The tissue layer between arterial blood and ventricular CSF consists only of the capillary endothelium, little connective tissue, a basal membrance and a monolayer of ependymal epithelia. Across this thin "choroid membrane" oxygen can be effectively exchanged between blood and CSF by diffusion, resulting in a diffusional pO_2-gradient perpendicular to the long axis of the choroid capillary ("capillary perpendicular pO_2-gradient"). However, the difference in blood oxygen content between the arterial beginning and the venous end of a choroid plexus capillary ("capillary directional gradient") is caused not only by oxygen transfer into the CSF, but also by the high oxygen consumption of ependymal cells (Quay 1966).

In the cisterna magna a small portion of highly perfused choroid plexus is present, but the pial and arachnoid arterial vasculature may also contribute considerably to the oxygen offer to cisternal CSF.

The 66% to full response times of $CSFpO_2$ on changes in the arterial pO_2 (Table No. 3) lay between 75 s (stop of hypoxia, measured in the ventricle) and 318 s (stop of hyperoxia, measured in cisterna). Considering the volume of ventricles and cisterna with regard to O_2 diffusion times within stationary liquids, the observed swift $CSFpO_2$ changes cannot be explained if oxygen transport within the liquid compartments were provided only by diffusion. An additional highly effective oxygen transport in CSF by convection must be assumed. The observed slopes in $CSFpO_2$ (in response to changes in ventilatory conditions) cannot be explained by the bulk flow in CSF circulation due to liquid production, since its volume flow rate is far too small (CSF production in mammals: 0,3–0,4% of total CSF volume/min). Hence, an alternating (probably multidirectional) movement in CSF must be assumed. The (heartbeat-synchronous and respiration-synchronous) oscillations in intracranial pressure most probably lead to convection in CSF. The assumption of an alternating CSF flow due to the physiological intracranial pressure oscillations seems to be plausible, when one takes into account that the intracranial CSF compartment communicates with the extensible extracranial CSF space. On the other hand, also within the intracranial compartments heartbeat and respiration lead to movements of tissue and fluids since the intracranial veins are considerably compressible. Pulsatile changes of cerebral blood volume between 0,36 and 4,38 ml were calculated in man (Avezaat and Eijndhoven 1986).

At mild and medium hypoxia the pO_2-gradient between the arterial blood and CSF ($AVpO_2D$ and $ACpO_2D$) of cat was decreased (to only 11.4 mmHg and 9.1 mmHg resp.). In order to qualitatively analyze the factors contributing to the arterio-CSF pO_2-gradient, three determinants (I, II and III) can be distinguished: Firstly, (I) the $AVpO_2D$ depends on the amount of oxygen flux through the CSF i.e. oxygen uptake of the tissue surrounding the ventricles; an elevation of its oxygen uptake leads to an increase in $AVpO_2D$ if arterio-ventricular O_2 conductivity is unchanged during the increase of O_2 uptake. Secondly, (II) the $AVpO_2D$ depends on the diffusional oxygen conductivity of the choroid membrane that determines the capillary perpendicular pO_2-gradient. The third factor (III) (by which $AVpO_2D$ is determined) is the capillary directional pO_2-gradient in choroidal capillaries. The latter gradient is reduced at increased choroid perfusion rate, if oxygen flux out of the vessel is not changed as flow increases.

At hypoxia the first factor influencing the $AVpO_2D$, (I) reduction of oxygen flux in CSF, probably contributes to the decrease in $AVpO_2D$, since the pO_2-gradient at the liquid tissue interface is decreased by the fall in

CSFpO$_2$. In severe hypoxia (prolonged FiO$_2$ of 0.1 and below) oxygen flux through CSF is additionally reduced by a decrease in CMRO$_2$ (Leniger-Follert 1977) which persists in the post-ischemic phase (Kintner et al. 1984). This view is supported by our finding that after severe hypoxic episodes (Fig. 1), post-ischemic CSFpO$_2$ was higher than pre-ischemic pO$_2$. Since VCSFpO$_2$ in dog was zero at an arterial pO$_2$ of 19.2 mmHg, oxygen flux at this low arterial pO$_2$ level was eliminated. It was reported, that the threshold of central hypoxic ventilatory depression in dog lies at an arterial pO$_2$ of 18.7 mmHg (Morrill et al. 1975). Obviously hypoxic ventilatory depression at O$_2$ depletion of CSF is induced.

The second factor influencing the AVpO$_2$D, (II) the oxygen conductivity of the choroid membrane, might contribute to the AVpO$_2$D decrease induced by arterial hypoxia, since a dilation of precapillary choroid vessels at hypoxia is most probable (Kontos et al. 1978; Traystman et al. 1978; Heistad et al. 1976); this results in a "blowing up" of the weak tissue of choroid plexus which leads to an enlargement of its surface and a thinning of the choroid membrane.

As can be seen in Tab. 3 and Fig. 1B and 3B, the steepest slope of CSF was observed in the ventricle after stopping hypoxia. The speed of CSFpO$_2$ elevation was only slightly lower than that of arterial blood pO$_2$ (Fig. 1C). This finding indicates – in agreement with the hypoxic AVpO$_2$D reduction – that the oxygen conductivity between blood and CSF is enhanced at arterial hypoxia and this is in turn explained by an increase of choroid blood flow. Thus, we assume that the third factor determining AVpO$_2$D, (III) flow dependency of choroid capillary directional gradient of blood pO$_2$, effectively contributes to the reduction in AVpO$_2$D at hypoxia.

At hyperoxia the AVpO$_2$D and ACpO$_2$D were increased (Fig. 2B). At hyperoxia in the first parts or over the entire length of the choroid capillary, oxygen offer to the CSF is fed from physically dissolved blood O$_2$. Consequently, the directional gradient of oxygen pressure in choroid capillary is larger at arterial hyperoxia (in the flat range of the blood oxygen binding curve) than at normoxia, although the directional capillary gradient of blood oxygen content may be more or less equal in the compared cases. Accordingly, the increase of AVpO$_2$D during arterial hyperoxia is explained by an increase in the directional pO$_2$-gradient in choroid capillary.

No quantitative assumption concerning oxygen flux through ventricular CSF throughout hyperoxia can be made, since no systematic data regarding mean oxygen pressure in peri-ventricular brain tissue at arterial hyperoxia are available. Without such data the pO$_2$-gradient at the ventricular fluid-tissue interface during hyperoxia is unknown. However, as derived from single observations in brain tissue (Nair et al. 1975; Leniger-Follert 1975 and Metzger et al. 1971) and from findings in peripheral tissue, it is unlikely that at eucapnic hyperoxia the mean tissue pO$_2$ was elevated by the same amount as the CSFpO$_2$. So, it can be tentatively assumed that the oxygen flux through CSF is elevated at hyperoxia. This assumption infers an increase of AVpO$_2$D at arterial hyperoxia too.

At the highest arterial pO$_2$ level (average value 461 ± 36.8 mmHg), pO$_2$ was significantly higher in the cisterna magna (138 ± 28.5 mmHg) than in the ventricle (101.3 ± 10 mmHg). This indicates that even at the end of the vessels from which oxygen was delivered to cisterna, blood was entirely saturated and hyperoxic. Consequently, comparing oxygen supply of ventricle and cisterna, the perfusion rate and/or the diameter of vessels supplying cisterna with oxygen might be greater than that of the choroid capillary. This further leads to the assumption that cisternal O$_2$ delivery is fed in most part from precapillary structures of pial and subarachnoid vasculature. The difference in CSFpO$_2$ between ventricle and cisterna, at hyperoxia, can be alternatively explained by a less effective hyperoxic vasoconstriction in pial vessel than in precapillary vessels of choroid plexus, or by the high oxygen consumption of choroid ependymal cells.

For references see part 2 of the study.

Oxygen Pressure in Cerebrospinal Fluid

W. Fleckenstein, A.I.R. Maas, G. Nollert, D.A. de Jong

Part 2: Effects of Hypocapnia and Hypercapnia

Introduction

The arterial pCO_2 level has a pronounced effect on cerebral circulation. In hypercapnia, cerebral resistance vessels are dilated and cerebral blood flow is increased. Hypocapnia causes cerebral vasoconstriction. Severe hypocapnia below $paCO_2$ levels of $20 - 25$ mmHg may even lead to focal cerebral hypoxia. The effect of CO_2 is probably mediated through changes in hydrogen ion concentration of the extracellular fluid in the vicinity of cerebral blood vessels. The transfer conditions at the blood brain barrier for CO_2, bicarbonate, alkali ions and fixed acids were extensively studied (Kazemi and Johnson 1986). As reviewed by Loeschke (1982) and Schlaefke (1981), the acidity of the cerebrospinal and interstitial fluid seems to be the most significant stimulus for respiration; the pH value of CSF also influences cardiovascular regulations. However, the kinetics of CO_2 exchange (and of other constituents of cerebrospinal fluid) between interstitial fluid, cerebrospinal fluid and blood may be modulated by local actions of oxygen on vessel diameter, volume of perivasal space and blood flow. We have already described pO_2 changes of cerebrospinal fluid (CSF) during hyperoxia and hypoxia. It was considered worthwhile to further investigate changes in $CSFpO_2$ secondary to hyper- and hypocapnia.

Materials and methods

For abbreviations see methods of part 1 of the study.
The experimental design has already been described in part 1 of the study. Studies were performed in 6 cats and 3 dogs. The arterial blood pressure, intracranial fluid pressure, $CSFpO_2$ in cisterna magna and lateral ventricle, temperatures of brain and rectum, inspired oxygen concentration, endtidal CO_2 concentration and cerebral microvascular blood flow according to laser doppler technique were continuously measured.
After a one hour stabilization period following operative preparations, the ventilation conditions were changed: under conditions of slightly ele-

Clinical Oxygen Pressure Measurement II
A.M. Ehrly et al. (Eds.)
© Blackwell Ueberreuter Wissenschaft Berlin 1990

vated FiO₂ (0.25), hypoventilation (10 min), hyperventilation (10 min) and hypercarbia (admixture of 5% CO₂ to ventilated gas, 15 min) were induced. Each of the experiments was ended by a period of eucapnia at slightly elevated FiO₂ (0.25) lasting 15 min; thus reference conditions were reinstalled.

Results

As shown in Fig.1, changes in ventilation parameters brought about CSFpO₂ variations. By changes in arterial pCO₂, the pO₂ in VCSF was altered more slowly than by variations in arterial pO₂. In hypercarbia experiments, CSFpO₂ was only slightly changed within the first two minutes. As shown in Figs. 3A[b] and 3B[b] of part 1 of the study, the maximal slope was observed 220 s after admixture of CO₂. In contrast to experiments with changing FiO₂, by alterations in arterial pCO₂, CSFpO₂ was changed faster in cisterna than in lateral ventricle.

Hyperventilation

By hyperventilation the average arterial pCO₂ of the cats was reduced to a hypocapnic value of 21.3 ± 1.3 mmHg within 10 min; CPP, MAP and ICP

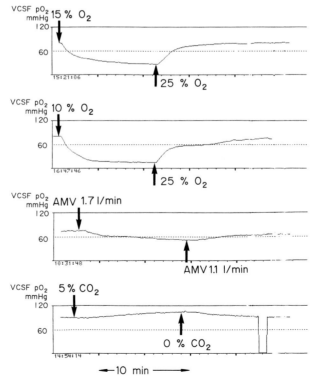

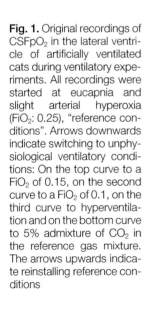

Fig. 1. Original recordings of CSFpO₂ in the lateral ventricle of artificially ventilated cats during ventilatory experiments. All recordings were started at eucapnia and slight arterial hyperoxia (FiO₂: 0.25), "reference conditions". Arrows downwards indicate switching to unphysiological ventilatory conditions: On the top curve to a FiO₂ of 0.15, on the second curve to a FiO₂ of 0.1, on the third curve to hyperventilation and on the bottom curve to 5% admixture of CO₂ in the reference gas mixture. The arrows upwards indicate reinstalling reference conditions

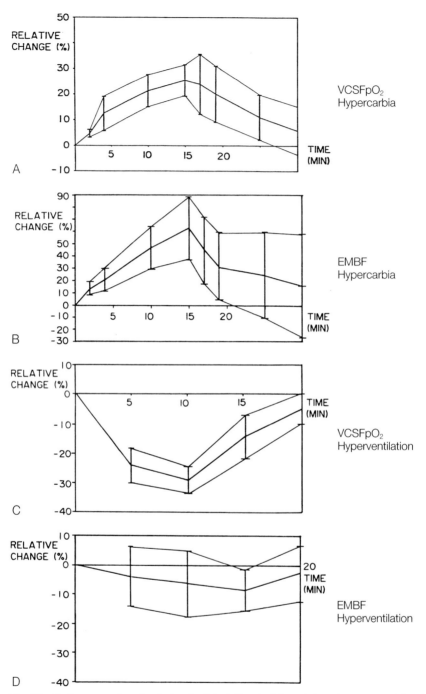

Fig. 2A–D. Average values (and standard deviations) of the relative changes in VCSFpO$_2$ (diagrams A,C) and EMBF (diagrams B,D); average values of 6 cats are plotted against time. **A, B)** Hypercarbia (5% CO$_2$) was started at t=0 and finished at t=15. **C, D)** Hyperventilation was started at t=0 and finished at t=10

were reduced at only slightly reduced EMBF (− 6.3 %). Although the arterial pO_2 was elevated from 124.7 ± 8.0 mmHg to 137.5 ± 17.0 mmHg, the VCSFpO₂ and CCSFpO₂ values were significantly decreased by 20.6 ± 4.3 mmHg (-29%) and 18.5 ± 3.9 mmHg (-28%) respectively (Fig.2C); consequently, the AVpO₂D and the ACpO₂D were increased by 62% and 53% respectively (Table 1, Fig.3).

Hypoventilation

Hypoventilating the cats for 10 min resulted in a hypercapnic average arterial pCO_2 value of 53.4 ± 3.0 mmHg. At decreased CPP and slightly increased MAP, the ICP and the EMBF were markedly increased, indicating a reduction in cerebrovascular resistance. Although the arterial pO_2 was decreased from 124.7 ± 8.0 mmHg (reference level) to 91.4 ± 9.1 mmHg, the CCSFpO₂ was raised and the VCSFpO₂ was only slightly decreased. Consequently, the AVpO₂D and CVpO₂D values were reduced by more than 50% to values of 25.0 ± 8.8 mmHg and 17.0 ± 4.3 mmHg respectively (Table 1 and Fig.3).

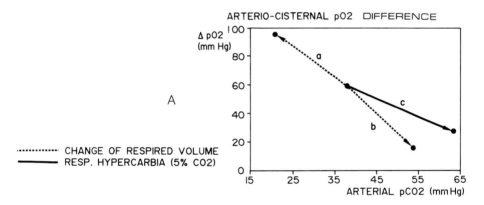

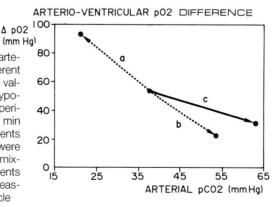

Fig. 3A, B. pO₂-differences between arterial blood and CSF (ordinates) at different pCO₂ levels in arterial blood; average values of 6 cats. Measurements from hypoventilation and hyperventilation experiments (broken lines) were taken 10 min after change of eucapnia. Measurements from hypercarbia (continued lines) were taken 15 min after start of 5% CO₂ admixture to ventilated gas. **A)** Measurements obtained from cisterna magna. **B)** Measurements obtained from lateral ventricle

Table 1. Effects of hypocapnia, hypercapnia and hypercarbia, average values of 6 cats

average values and standard deviations of data obtained from CSF, arterial blood and circulation of cats (n = 6) at different $paCO_2$ levels

	VCSFpO$_2$ [mmHg] ± SD	AVpO$_2$D [mmHg] ± SD	CCSFpO$_2$ [mmHg] ± SD	ACpO$_2$D [mmHg] ± SD	paO$_2$ [mmHg] ± SD	paCO$_2$ [mmHg] ± SD	art. pH ± SD	EMBF [A.U.] ± SD	ICP [mmHg] ± SD	CPP [mmHg] ± SD	MAP [mmHg] ± SD
reference conditions	70.8 6.5	53.9 12.4	65.8 9.3	58.9 10.3	124.7 8.0	37.8 3.1	7.32 0.05	43.8 13.5	9.2 3.6	118.6 11.1	127.8 10.3
hyperventilation	50.2 4.1	87.3 17.5	47.3 10.4	90.2 11.3	137.5 17.0	21.3 1.3	7.50 0.08	41.0 12.1	6.5 1.5	112.7 6.3	114.7 10.5
hypoventilation	66.4 11.1	25.0 8.8	74.4 9.2	17.0 4.3	91.4 9.1	53.4 3.0	7.16 0.06	60.4 14.9	18.5 9.6	113.4 12.9	131.9 13.5
hypercarbia	86.3 12.3	35.4 7.3	95.6 10.2	26.1 5.9	121.7 6.3	63.1 5.4	7.14 0.05	71.4 19.9	17.3 7.6	106.1 6.3	122.0 5.2

Hypercarbic ventilation

Hypercarbic ventilation (15min 5% CO$_2$ admixture) in the cats led to a hypercapnic average arterial pCO$_2$ of 63.1 $\pm$ 5.4 mmHg. While ICP was increased by 89%, MAP remained almost at reference level, resulting in a decrease in CPP, but EMBF was elevated by 63% (Tab.1 and Fig.2B). This was nearly a twofold elevation compared to the EMBF elevation (of 38%) at hypoventilation. At unchanged arterial pO$_2$ – in contrast to hypercapnia by hypoventilation – the VCSFpO$_2$ and CCSFpO$_2$ values were significantly raised (Table 1 and Fig.2A). According to hypercapnia by hypoventilation, in hypercarbic hypercapnia AVpO$_2$D and ACpO$_2$D were reduced. The degree of the reduction was less in comparison to hypoventilation (Table 1, Fig.3).

In three dogs, hypoventilation, hyperventilation and hypercarbia were induced according to the method used on cats. CSFpO$_2$ was measured in the lateral ventricle. In comparison to the cats' VCSFpO$_2$ alterations, qualitatively analogous results were obtained in the dogs' ventricle.

Discussion

A reduction in arterial pCO$_2$ raised the AVpO$_2$D and the ACpO$_2$D, and vice versa arterio-CSF pO$_2$-differences were lowered at elevated paCO$_2$. Hypoventilation was more effective in reducing arterio-CSF pO$_2$-differences than hypercarbia. Within the paCO$_2$ range from 21.3 mmHg to 63.1 mmHg, the average arterio-CSF pO$_2$-differences were shifted in the lateral ventricle from 87.3 to 25.0 mmHg and in the cisterna magna from 90.2 to 17.0 mmHg. Obviously the oxygen transfer into CSF is markedly influenced by the paCO$_2$. Our results correspond to the finding that brain tissue oxygen supply is impaired by hyperventilation (Grote et al. 1985; Wei et al. 1980). Inducing hypoventilation (hyperventilation) in sheep, led to an increase (decrease) of choroidal blood flow of approximately 30% at a paCO$_2$ value of 60 mmHg (25 mmHg) (Page et al. 1980). However, since oxygen transport to CSF and tissue are influenced in the same way by paCO$_2$ changes, pO$_2$ measurements in CSF might be useful in clinical hyperventilation therapy (e.g. treatment of increased ICP), in order to detect unwanted impairments of cerebral oxygen supply.
The CSFpO$_2$ changes in consequence of variations in arterial pCO$_2$, were much slower than those induced by variations in paO$_2$ (see in part 1 of the study Fig.3 and Table 3). Since the perivasal pCO$_2$ and pH are swiftly linked to the intravasal pCO$_2$ (Ahmad and Loeschke 1982; Loeschke and Ahmad 1980; Loeschke 1982; Kuschinsky and Wahl 1979), the delay cannot be explained by a pH equilibration process in perivasal spaces embedded in tissue. The delay in the change of CSFpO$_2$ after a variation in paCO$_2$ can be plausibly interpreted as an equilibration time required to change pH in the whole fluid compartments of ventricle and cisterna,

respectively. The observed course of CSFpO$_2$ in time, after starting inspiratory hypercarbia seems to be similar to a reported time course of CSF pH value decrease after starting hypercarbic ventilation (Bradley et al. 1965). In the latter study, the steepest slopes of pH and pCO$_2$ in CSF were observed later than 3 min after paCO$_2$ increase. This can be interpreted as a "self-favouring" of CO$_2$ transfer into CSF, due to the vasodilation that is induced by CSF acidification in consequence of the increase of pCO$_2$ in CSF. The vasodilation and the increase in blood flow respectively, on the other hand, favour the O$_2$ transfer to the CSF. Thus, in accordance with the conclusions in part 1 of the study, the CSFpO$_2$ increase at hypercarbia can be regarded as a consequence of CSF acidification that leads, due to a direct local effect, to a dilation of choroid and pial vessel (Kuschinsky et al. 1972; Wahl et al. 1970 and Wei et al. 1980).

In contrast to CSFpO$_2$ changes induced by arterial pO$_2$ variations, the CSFpO$_2$ changes induced by starting and ending hypercapnia were faster in cisterna than in ventricle. At hypercapnia, CSF acidification is exerted by CO$_2$ transfer into CSF not only from arterialized blood (Friis et al. 1980), but also from all tissue surfaces and pial vessels including veins. If arterial pO$_2$ is increased, the speed of CSFpO$_2$ change is determined mainly by the oxygen conductivity between the vasculature perfused with arterialized blood and the CSF. These differences between the dynamics of O$_2$ and CO$_2$ transfer into CSF explain in a plausible way that the relation of the time courses of CSFpO$_2$ increases in cisterna and ventricle after onset of hypercapnia is not the same as in the case of onset of hyperoxia (and ending hypoxia).

References

1. Ahmad HR, Loeschke HH (1982) Transient and steady state responses of pulmonary ventilation to the medullary extracellular pH after approximately rectangular changes in alveolar pCO$_2$. Pflügers Archiv 395: 285-292
2. Avezaat CJJ, Eijndhoven JHM (1986) Clinical observations on the relationship between cerebrospinal fluid pulse pressure and intracranial pressure. Acta Neurochirurgica 79: 13-29
3. Bingmann D, Kolde G, Speckmann EJ (1982) Effects of elevated pO$_2$ values in the superfusate on the neural activity in hippocampal slices. In: Klee MR (ed) Physiol Pharm Epeleptogenic Phenomena. Raven Press NY
4. Bingmann D, Kolde G, Lipinski HG (1984) Relations between pO$_2$ and neuronal activity in hippocampal slices. Adv Exp Med Biol 169: 215-225
5. Bloor BM, Fricker J, Hellinger F, Nishioka H, McCutchen J A (1961) Study of cerebrospinal fluid oxygen tension. Preliminary experimental and clinical observations. Arch Neurol 4: 37-46
6. Bloor BM, Neville WE, Hellinger FR, Clowes GHA (1963) Oxygen tension of the brain and its modification with hypothermia. An experimental study. Arch Psychiatr Nevenkr 204: 310-316
7. Bousquet P (1974) Etude des mecanismes de l'action hypotensive de la clonidine. Med Diss, University Louis Pasteur, Strasbourg
8. Bradley RD, Semple JG, Spencer GT (1965) Rate of change of carbon dioxide tension in arterial blood, jugular venous blood and cisternal cerebrospinal fluid on carbon dioxide administration. J Physiol Lond 179: 442-455

9. Chapman RW, Santiago TV, Edelman NH (1980) Brain hypoxia and control of breathing neuromechanical control. J Appl Physiol 49: 497-505

10. Cherniak NS, Edelman NH, Lahiri S (1971) Hypoxia and hypercapnia as respiratory stimulants and depressants. Respir Physiol 11: 113-126

11. Cserr HF (1971) Physiology of the choroid plexus. Physiological Rev 51: 273-331

12. Downing SE, Mitchell JH, Wallace AG (1963) Cardiovascular responses to ischemia, hypoxia and hypercapnia of the central nervous system. Am J Physiol 204 (5): 881-887

13. Eldridge FL, Millhorn DE (1981) Central regulation of respiration by endogenous neurotransmitters and neuromodulators. Ann Rev Physiol 43: 121-135

14. Feldberg W (1980) Cardiovascular effects of drugs acting on the ventral surface of the brain stem. In Koepchen HP, Hilton SM, Trzebski A (eds) Central interaction between respiratory and cardiovascular control systems. Verlag Springer, Berlin Heidelberg New York 45-55

15. Friis ML, Paulson OB, Hertz MM (1980) Carbon Dioxide Permeability of the blood brain barrier in man. Microvasc Res 20: 71-80

16. Fukuda Y, Loeschke HA (1979) A cholinergic mechanism involved in the neuronal excitation by H+ in the respiratory chemosensitive structures of the ventral medulla oblongata of rats in vitro. Pflügers Arch 379: 125-135

17. Gänshirt H (1966) Der Sauerstoffdruck im Liquor cerebrospinalis. Wien Med Woschr 116: 953-954

18. Gänshirt H (1968) Der Sauerstoffdruck der cerebrospinalen Flüssigkeit des Menschen. Seine Physiologische und klinische Bedeutung. Klin Woschr 46: 771-778

19. Gomez DG, Potts DG (1981) The lateral, third and fourth ventricle choroid plexus of the dog: A structural and ultrastructural study. Ann Neurol 10: 333-340

20. Grote J, Zimmer K, Schubert R (1985) Tissue oxygenation in normal and edematous brain cortex during arterial hypocapnia. Adv Exp Med Biol 180: 179-184

21. Harmsen P, Bay J (1970) Cerebrospinal fluid oxygen tension in man during halothane anaesthesia and hyperventilation. Acta Neurol Scand 46: 553-561

22. Heistad DD, Marcus ML, Ehrhardt JC, Abboud FM (1976) Effect of stimulation of carotical chemoreceptors on total and regional cerebral blood flow. Circ Res 38: 20-26

23. Jamieson D, Van den Brenk HAS (1963) Measurements of oxygen tensions in cerebral tissue of rats exposed to high pressures of oxygen. J Appl Physiol 18: 869-876

24. Jarnum S, Lorenzen I, Skinh∅j E (1964) Cisternal fluid oxygen tension in man. Neurology 14: 703-707

25. Kazemi H, Klein RC, Turner FN, Strieder DJ (1968) Dynamics of oxygen transfer in the cerebrospinal fluid. Resp Physiol 4: 24-31

26. Kazemi H, Johnson DC (1986) Regulation of cerebrospinal fluid-acid-base balance. Physiol Rev 66: 953-1037

27. Kintner D, Fitzpatrick JH, Loni JA, Gilboe DD (1984) Cerebral oxygen and energy metabolism during and after 30 minutes of moderate hypoxia. Am J Physiol 247: E475-E482

28. Kontos HA, Wei EP, Raper AJ, Rosenblum WI, Navari RM, Patterson JL (1978) Role of tissue hypoxia in local regulation of cerebral microcirculation. Am J Physiol 234: 582-591

29. Kuschinsky W, Wahl M, Bosse O, Thurau K (1972) Perivascular potassium and pH as determinants of local pial arterial diameter in cats. Circ res 31: 240-247

30. Kuschinsky W, Wahl M (1979) Perivascular pH and pial arterial diameter during bicuculline induced seizures in cats. Pflügers Arch 382: 81-85

31. Leniger-Follert E, Lübbers DW, Wrabetz W (1975) Regulation of local tissue pO$_2$ of the brain cortex at different arterial O$_2$ pressures. Pflügers Arch 359: 81-95

32. Leniger-Follert E (1977) Direct determination of local oxygen consumption of the brain cortex in vivo. Adv Exp Med Biol 94: 325-330

33. Lioy F, Hanna BD, Poiosa C (1981) Cardiovascular control by medullary surface chemoreceptors. J Autonomic Nervous System 3: 1-7

34. Loeschke HH, Ahmand HR (1980) Transient and steady state of chloride-bicarbonate relationship of extracellular fluid. In: Bauer C, Gros G, Bartels H (eds) Biophysics and Physiology of carbon dioxide. Springer, Berlin Heidelberg New York, 439-448

35. Loeschke HH (1982) Central chemosensitivity and the reaction theory. J Physiol 332: 1-24

36. Lübbers DW (1969) Local tissue pO_2 – Its measurement and meaning. In: Kessler et al. (eds) Oxygen Supply. University Park Press, London 151

37. Maas AIR (1977) Cerebrospinal fluid enzymes in acute brain injury. Med Diss Erasmus University, Rotterdam

38. Metzger H, Erdmann W, Thews G (1971) Effect of short periods of hypoxia, hyperoxia and hypercapnia on brain O_2 supply. J Appl Physiol 31: 751-759

39. Metzger H, Heuber S (1977) Local oxygen tension and spike activity of the cerebral grey matter of the rat and its response to short intervals of O_2 deficiency or CO_2 excess. Pflügers Arch 370: 201-209

40. Milhorat TH (1975) The third circulation revised. J Neurosurg 42: 628-645

41. Miller MJ, Tenney SM (1975) Hypoxia induced tachypnea in carotid-deafferentiated cats. Respir Physiol 23: 31-39

42. Morrill CG, Meyer JR, Weil JV (1975) Hypoxic ventilatory depression in dogs. J Appl Physiol 38: 143-146

43. Nair P, Whalen WJ, Burek D (1975) pO_2 of cat cerebral cortex: Response to breathing N2 and 100% O_2. Microvasc Res 9: 158-165

44. Nollert G (1989) Tierexperimentelle Untersuchungen zur Aussagekraft kontinuierlicher pO_2 Messungen in der cerebrospinalen Flüssigkeit. Med Diss Lübeck, submitted

45. Null RE, Reneau DD (1977) A computer analysis of graded ischemia in brain. Adv Exp Med Biol 94: 219-224

46. Page RB, Funsch DJ, Brennau RW, Hernandez MJ (1980) Choroid plexus blood flow in the sheep. Brain Res 197: 532-537

47. Quay WB (1966) Regional differences in metabolism and composition of choroid plexus. Brain Res 2: 378-389

48. Salaymeh MT, Geha AS, Baue AE (1971) Value of the cerebrospinal fluid as an indicator of cerebral metabolic changes. J Surg Res 11: 198-201

49. Santiago TV, Edelman NH (1976) Mechanisms of ventilatory response to carbon monoxide. J Clin Invest 57: 977-986

50. Schlaefke ME (1981) Central chemosensitivity: A respiratory drive. Rev Physiol Biochem Pharmacol 90: 171-244

51. Shoemaker G (1965) Oxygen tension measurements in cerebrospinal fluid during anoxia and ischemia under hyperbaric conditions. In: Ledingham (ed) Hyperbaric Oxygenation. Livingstone, London 213-220

52. Skinhøj E (1965) Cisternal fluid oxygen tension in man. Acta Neurol Scand 41, Sppl 13: 313-317

53. Smith RH, Guilbeau EJ, Reneau DD (1977) The oxygen tension field within a discrete volume of cerebral cortex. Microvasc Res 13: 233-240

54. Speckmann EJ, Caspers H (1975) Responses of spinal and cortical neurons to changes of pO_2 and pCO_2 in blood and tissue. In: Purves MJ (ed) The peripheral arterial chemoreceptors. Cambridge Univerity Press, London

55. Tenland T (1982) On laser doppler flowmeter. Med Diss No 136, Univ Linköping (Sweden)

56. Traystman RJ, Fitzgerald RS, Loscutoff SC (1978) Cerebral circulatory responses to arterial hypoxia in normal and chemodenervated dogs. Circ Res 42: 649-657

57. Trzebski A, Mikulski A, Przybyszewski A (1980) Effects of stimulation of chemosensitive areas by superfusion on ventral medulla and by infusion into vertebral artery of chemical stimuli in non-anaesthetized "encephale isole" preparations in cat. In: Koepchen HP, Hilton S, Trzebski A (eds) Central interaction between respiratory and cardiovascular control systems. Verlag Springer, Berlin Heidelberg New York 65-75

58. Wahl M, Deetjen P, Thurau K, Ingraz DH, Lassen NA (1970) Micropuncture evaluation of the importance of perivascular pH for the arteriolar diameter of the brain surface. Pflügers Arch 316: 152-163

59. Wahl M (1985) Local chemical, neural, and humoral regulation of cerebrovascular resistance vessels. J Cardiovasc Pharm 7 Sppl3: 36-46
60. Wei EP, Kontos HA, Patterson JL (1980) Dependence of pial arteriolar response to hypercapnia on vessel size. Am J Physiol 238: H697-H703
61. Wennergren G, Öberg B (1980) Cardiovascular effects elicited from the ventral surface of medulla oblongata in the cat. Pflügers Arch 387: 189-195
62. Wright EM (1978) Transport processes in the formation of the cerebrospinal fluid. Rev Physiol Biochem Pharmacol 83: 1-34

Determinants of Lung Surface pO_2

H.U. Spiegel, J. Hauss, P. Langhans, J. Höpfner, P.P. Lunkenheimer

Introduction

Sufficient ventilation and perfusion of the lung is a prerequisite for the adequate supply of oxygen for the whole organism. Effects on ventilation due to artificial respiration and pathological changes in the lung are assessed by analysis of arterial blood gas and respiratory gas. The present experimental study aimed at obtaining direct information about gas exchange and microcirculation on the alveolar level by measuring local tissue pO_2 on lung surfaces.

In certain situations quite frequent in clinical practice, the maintenance of oxygen supply requires artificial respiration with physiologically above-normal oxygen concentrations as well as surgical interventions to clean the respiratory tract considerably disturbing ventilation in the short term. So far, the effects of such interventions on microcirculation and therefore on local gas exchange have not been studied experimentally.

In our model, local tissue pO_2 was measured in the presence of physiological as well as of above-normal oxygen concentrations in respiratory gases. The second part of the paper deals with the impact of interrupted ventilation or perfusion on local tissue pO_2 of the pulmonary surface.

Materials and methods

10 mongrel dogs (mean body weight 25 kg) were subjected to left lateral thoracotomy in the fourth intercostal space. On the surface of the left upper pulmonary lobe, local tissue pO_2 was measured with the multiwire surface electrode according to Kessler and Lübbers [8]. Under high-dosage piritramide anesthesia [18, 19], the animals received controlled ventilation with 20.9 % oxygen and with a PEEP of 3 cm H_2O. Catheters were installed in the A. pulmonalis, in the aortic arch, and in the V. cava.

Arterial pressure (Part), pulmonary arterial pressure (Ppulm), cardiac frequency (HF), ECG, and arterial blood temperature (Temp) were measured *continuously*.

Clinical Oxygen Pressure Measurement II
A.M. Ehrly et al. (Eds.)
© Blackwell Ueberreuter Wissenschaft Berlin 1990

Table 1. Mean parameters of blood and circulation during different inspiratory O$_2$ concentrations ($\bar{x}$; n=5); significance: a: $p<0.05$; b: $p<0.01$; c: $p<0.005$)

FIO$_2$	0.21	0.3	0.6	1.0
lung tissue pO$_2$ (in mmHg)	97.7	163.6 (b)	409 (b)	614 (c)
p$_a$O$_2$ mmHg	78	117 (b)	276 (b)	485 (c)
p$_v$O$_2$ mmHg	48	50	57	63
HF/min	107	109	107	112
p$_{art}$ mmHg	101	118	128	124
p$_{pulm}$ mmHg	17	16	17	17
HI l/min/m^2	5.9	5.6	5.1 (b)	5.0 (b)
SI ml/beat/min	55.4	54.3	47.8 (a)	48.1

Cardiac output (CO), pulmonary capillary pressure (Pcap), central venous pressure (CVP), the various respiration parameters, including respiratory rate (RF), tidal volume (VT) and expiratory volume per minute (EMV), as well as arterial and mixed venous pO$_2$, pCO$_2$, pH, CO$_2$, hemoglobin, hematocrit, electrolytes, lactate, pyruvate, and urine production.

5 animals of the *normoxic* group received controlled respiration with 20.9 % O$_2$ for 4 hrs. pO$_2$ histograms were registered at hourly intervals. In the 5 animals of the *hyperoxic* group, the oxygen content of the respiratory gas was increased at hourly intervals, from 20.9 % to 30, 60 and finally 100 %. pO$_2$ histograms were recorded 30 min after each step. Subsequently, total tissue pO$_2$ was recorded during short-term ventilation stops while maintaining perfusion, and during perfusion stops while maintaining ventilation.

Perfusion stops were effected for short terms by the i.v. bolus injection of 10-15 mg acetylcholin, and definitively with the injection of 20 mmol/l potassium chloride.

Ventilation stops were effected by introducing a double tubus into the trachea. Closing the left tubus at the end of inspiration stopped ventilation of the left lung.

Results

Local tissue pO$_2$ was measured with the multiwire surface electrode developed by Kessler and Lübbers [8], which has often been used to study the oxygen supply of various organs [1, 6, 7, 9, 15, 17], and also for therapy monitoring in intensive care. Fig. 1 illustrates the factors affecting local pO$_2$ on the pulmonary surface:

1. alveolar ventilation
2. perfusion and oxygen transport
3. leakage resulting from
   a) oxygen consumption of the tissue
   b) oxygen exchange between uncovered pleura and room air

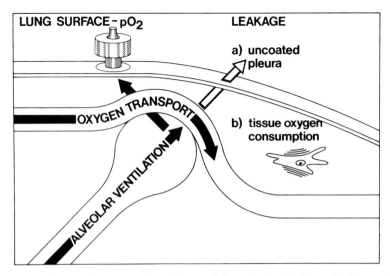

Fig. 1. Schematic presentation of factors influencing local pO$_2$ on the lung surface

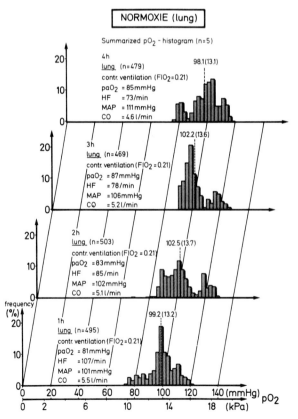

Fig. 2a. pO$_2$ histograms on lung surface under normoxic conditions over 4 hrs

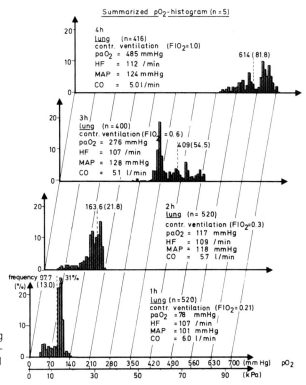

Fig. 2b. pO$_2$ histogram on lung surface under hyperoxia: stepwise increase of FIO$_2$ from 0.21 to 1.0 after 4 hrs

pO$_2$ of the pulmonary surface in normoxia and hyperoxia

Fig. 2a shows comprehensive pO$_2$ histograms of lung surfaces under physiological respiration with 20.9 % O$_2$. Mean values of local tissue pO$_2$ in this *normoxic* group lie around 100 mmHg, and these normal pO$_2$ histograms will serve as control configurations in the following. They remain almost unchanged over the 4 hrs of the assay. Mean parameters of blood and circulation are within the normal range.

In the *hyperoxic* group (Fig. 2b), mean lung tissue pO$_2$ rises parallel to the rising inspiratory oxygen content and arterial pO$_2$ from 98 mmHg to 614 mmHg. The configuration of pO$_2$ histograms is sufficiently normal, but there is a widening of pO$_2$ histograms along with rising FIO$_2$. Mean blood and circulatory parameters change along with changes in inspiratory oxygen concentrations.

Ventilation stop

Ventilation of the left lung was stopped under normoxic and hyperoxic conditions (see Fig. 3). Down to a FIO$_2$ of 0.6, local pO$_2$ shows a linear

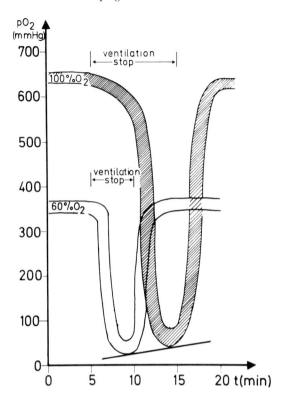

Fig. 3. Continuous measuring of local pO_2 during short-term stop of left lung ventilation at several FIO_2 levels

decrease to a level around 80 mmHg. Subsequently, the FIO_2-dependent slope is less steep until local pO_2 reaches a mean value of 25-35 mmHg.

If inspiratory O_2 is higher than 60 %, the respective curve displays a "shoulder": the initial decrease in local pO_2 is at first delayed, after which follows a very rapid decrease which again slows down at the level of 60 mmHg and finally settles at 40-50 mmHg. After reventilation, local pO_2 resumes the normal level in less than 2 min.

Perfusion stop

Temporary (see Fig. 4) as well as definitive interruption of perfusion (by cardiac failure) causes a rise of pO_2 on the lung surface by 10 to 15 mmHg. It approximates the pO_2 level of respiratory gas, which is about 150 mmHg at an oxygen content of 21 %. When circulation is resumed, pO_2 decreases to about 20 mmHg below the initial level, and then begins to rise again slowly after 90 sec. After a latency of 4 min, local tissue pO_2 is again at the initial level. During definitive perfusion stop, surface pO_2 stays at the 10 mmHg increased level.

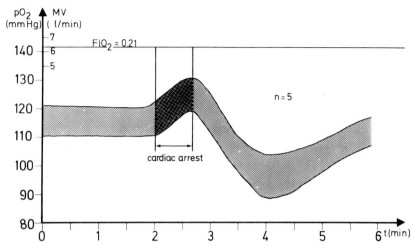

Fig. 4. Effect of temporary stop of perfusion on continually registered pO$_2$ of lung surface under normoxia

The $\dot{V}/\dot{Q}$ concept

The basis for discussion is seen in the concept of ventilation/perfusion developed by Rahn and Fahri (1955), and established as a model for assessing pulmonary function [12, 13]. Assuming equilibration of oxygen between alveolar gas and minicapillary blood, the alveolar pO$_2$ can be closely correlated with the ventilation/perfusion ratio in the alveolar region. In 1955, Rahn and Fenn developed a normogram, based on an idea of Riley et al. [14], which could serve to determine alveolar pO$_2$ as a fundamental factor dominating pulmonary function under physiologic as well as pathologic conditions. The correlation between alveolar pO$_2$ and $\dot{V}/\dot{Q}$ ratio may be characterized by two extremes:
1. from the non-perfused alveole, no oxygen is extracted, and so alveolar pO$_2$ equals inspiratory pO$_2$ ($\dot{V}/= 1$, $\dot{Q} = 0$, $\dot{V}/\dot{Q} = 00$);
2. to the non-ventilated alveole, no O$_2$ is added, so pO$_2$ equals that of mixed venous blood.

Under ideal conditions, characterized by a $\dot{V}/\dot{Q}$ ratio of 1, alveolar pO$_2$ and pCO$_2$ would be 100 mmHg and 40 mmHg respectively. According to this concept, pulmonary function equals the total of alveolar function, i.e., the ideal lung under conditions of optimal coordination of ventilation and perfusion, would have a $\dot{V}/\dot{Q}$ ratio of 1 in all its alveoles.
In reality, hydrostatic pressure is higher in basal than in apical segments, which leads to increased perfusion and a lower $\dot{V}/\dot{Q}$ ratio in basal and a higher $\dot{V}/\dot{Q}$ ratio in apical zones [20]. In addition to this gravity-specific variability of perfusion, right/left shunts and diffusion capacity are in-

volved, under physiological conditions, in the creation of the alveolo-arterial difference in pO_2.

It can be deduced from the above considerations that in equilibrated lung tissue the local tissue pO_2 is an adequate parameter of the $\dot{V}/\dot{Q}$ ratio. The data in this study, however, refer only to the area actually examined with the multiwire pO_2 electrode.

Description of alveolar pO_2 by local tissue pO_2

Canine visceral pleura consists of a layer of mesothelial cells and a comparatively thin layer of connective tissue with small blood and lymph vessels [2]. The rise in local pO_2 parallel to changes in perfusion and ventilation as recorded in this model suggests that surface pO_2 corresponds to alveolar pO_2 and, logically, to capillary pO_2. According to Piiper [11] there is a stable correlation between alveolar pO_2 and the oxygen uptake of the blood. O_2 uptake reduces the O_2 content and therefore the pO_2 in the alveole (see Fig. 5). If pO_2 uptake of the blood is stopped, pO_2 on the lung surface will increase.

These data agree with the $\dot{V}/\dot{Q}$ concept, which – in areas with a high $\dot{V}/\dot{Q}$ ratio resulting for instance from perfusion stop – describes an alveolar pO_2 corresponding to that of inspiratory gas.

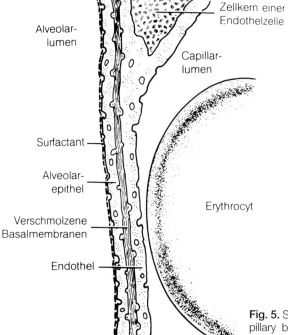

Alveolar-
lumen

Zellkern einer
Endothelzelle

Capillar-
lumen

Surfactant

Alveolar-
epithel

Erythrocyt

Verschmolzene
Basalmembranen

Endothel

Fig. 5. Schematic presentation of the alveolar/capillary borderline (from: Junqueira L (ed) Basic Histology. Lange, Los Altos, 1975)

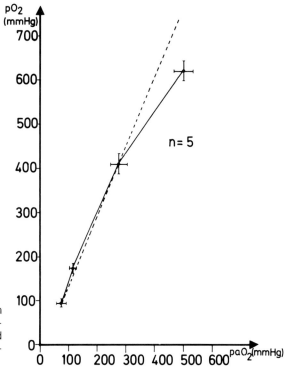

Fig. 6. Correlation of tissue pO$_2$ on lung surface and arterial pO$_2$. Starting at FIO$_2$ = 0.6, there is a marked difference between both parameters

Negative effects of high O$_2$ concentrations

The broader shape of pO$_2$ histograms (see Fig. 2b) and the flattened curve (see Fig. 6) may reflect the increasing instability of the V̇/Q̇ ratio under artificial respiration with 100 % oxygen. This is also suggested by the results of Wagner [21] and Gantzker [3], who reported an increasingly variable alveolar ventilation under hyperoxia. An additional factor may be found in increased diffusion via the leakage from the uncovered pleura. Shepard [16] noted an approximate doubling of O$_2$ diffusion via the pleura under similar conditions of an increase of the O$_2$ gradient between lung and room air.

Increased difference between tissue pO$_2$ and arterial pO$_2$

The increased difference between tissue pO$_2$ and arterial pO$_2$ indicates a rising shunt volume, as described for instance by Thews [20] in the case of hyperoxia. One mechanism contributing to the increasing shunt is the rising number of atelectatic alveoles under 100 % oxygen respiration [4, 10]. The direct measurements related in this study support the idea that raising the inspiratory oxygen content to above 60 % will lead to a distinct increase in arterialisation, but will at the same time augment the alveolar areas with a disturbed ventilation/perfusion ratio.

Oxygen storage in the lung

That oxygen is actually stored in the lung [10] may explain the delayed increase in surface pO_2 (see Fig. 3) when ventilation is stopped altogether. The delay, however, occurs only in the presence of oxygen concentrations above 60 %. Redistribution, for instance from muscle tissue, appears rather unlikely in view of the mixed venous pO_2 levels of 50-60 mmHg recorded in the presence of 100 % O_2 in this study. The curve of O_2 concentration in the myoglobin suggests that release of O_2 is possible only at very low pO_2 levels approaching 0 mmHg [5].

Limited, though quantitatively negligible, oxygen storage in the lung is suggested by the immediate decrease in local tissue pO_2 registered after ventilation stop in the presence of inspiratory oxygen concentrations of 60 %.

Conclusions

The present study confirms the suitability of local pO_2 measurements on the pulmonary surface as a tool for experimental investigation of pulmonary function under physiological and pathological conditions. The results are an encouragement to use this measuring procedure in future studies on the pulmonary function of pathologically altered lungs, and for the experimental testing of various modalities of artificial respiration. Our results further indicate that the use of physiologically abnormally high oxygen concentrations may damage the pulmonary function, independently of the other effects of oxygen toxicity.

References

1. Bünte H (1977) Die Mikrozirkulation – eine entscheidende Kreislaufkomponente für das Überleben kritischer Kranker. In: Schellerer W, Schildberg FW, Straube (eds) Aspekte moderner Chirurgie. Chirurgie Aktuell 4, Erlangen, p 32
2. Daly IB, Hebb C (1966) The architecture of the mammalian lung. In: Pulmonary and bronchial vascular systems. Edward Arnold, London, p 38
3. Dantzker DR, Wagner PD, West JB (1975) Instability of lung units with low $\dot{V}/\dot{Q}$ ratios during O_2 breathing. J Apll Physiol (5) 38:866
4. Duhm J (1984) Physiologie der Lungenfunktion. In: Anästhesiologie und Intensivmedizin (5), Teil I: Ventilation. p 180
5. Farhi LE (1964) Gas stores of the body. In: Handbook of Physiology: Respiration, I. Washington, p 873
6. Hauss J, Schönleben K, Spiegel HU (1982) Therapiekontrolle durch Überwachung des Gewebe-pO_2. Huber, Bern

7. Kessler M, Höper J, Krumme B (1976) Monitoring of tissue perfusion and cellular function. Anaesth 45:184
8. Kessler M, Lübbers DW (1966) Aufbau und Anwendungsmöglichkeiten verschiedener pO₂-Elektroden. Pflügers Arch Ges Physiol R 82:291 .9. Lübbers DW (1966) Methods of measuring oxygen tensions of blood and organ surfaces. In: Payne JP, Hill D (eds) A symposium on oxygen measurement and their significance. Churchill, London, p 103
10. Nunn JF (1977) Applied respiratory physiology. Butterworths, London
11. Piiper J (1981) Bloodgas equilibration in lungs and pulmonary diffusion capacity. Prog Resp Res 16:115
12. Rahn H, Farhi LE (1964) Ventilation, perfusion and gas exchange: the VA/Q-concept. In: Handbook of Physiology Respiration, Vol I. Washington, p 735
13. Rahn H, Fenn WO (1955) A graphical analysis of the respiratory gas exchange. Am Physiol Soc, Washington DC
14. Riley RL, Cournand A (1951) Analysis of factors affecting partial pressure of oxygen and carbon dioxide in gas of blood and lungs: Theory. J Appl Physiol 4:77
15. Schönleben K, Krimme B, Bünte H, Kessler M (1976) Kontrolle der Intensivbehandlung durch Messung von Mikrozirkulation und O₂-Versorgung. In: Junghans H (ed) Chirurgisches Forum 76 für experimentelle und klinische Forschung. p 72
16. Shepard JW jr, Dinh Minh V, Dolan GF (1981) Gas exchange in non perfused dogs lungs. J Appl Physiol (5) 51:1261
17. Spiegel HU, Bünte H (1985) Methodik und klinische Anwendung der lokalen Gewebe-pO₂-Messung mit der Mehrdrahtoberflächenelektrode. In: Ehrly AM, Hauss J, Huch R (eds) Klinische Sauerstoffdruckmessung, Gewebesauerstoffdruck und transcutaner Sauerstoffdruck beim Erwachsenen. Münchner Wissenschaftliche Publikationen, p 40
18. Spiegel HU, Hauss J, Bergermann M, Schönleben K (1983) Die hochdosierte Piritramid-Basisanästhesie als tierexperimentelles Standardmodell bei der Untersuchung von Hämodynamik und Mikrozirkulation. Anästhesist, Suppl 32:143
19. Spiegel HU, Bergermann M, Hauss J, Wendt M, Schönleben K (1983) Die hochdosierte Piritramid-Basisanästhesie in der experimentellen Anästhesie und Chirurgie. Anästhesist 35:36
20. Thews G (1979) Der Einfluß von Ventilation, Perfusion, Diffusion und Distribution auf den pulmonalen Gasaustausch. Steiner, Akademie der Wiss. und Lit. Mainz, p 597
21. Wagner PD, Laravuso RB, Goldzimmer E, Naumann PF, West JB (1975) Distributions of ventilation-perfusion ratios in dogs with normal and abnormal lungs. J Appl Physiol (6) 38:1099

Polarographic Measurement of Conjunctival Oxygen Pressure

G.O. Bastian, U. Beise

Introduction

Adequate oxygen supply to the corneal surface is necessary to prevent corneal edema [1]. Under closed-eye-conditions the palpebral conjunctiva is the main source of oxygen to the cornea [3]. With extended-wear-contact lenses, the oxygen supply is limited by the oxygen transmissibility of the contact lens and by the oxygen tension of the conjunctiva. When oxygen supply is deficient, corneal cells metabolize by anaerobic glycolysis. Lactic acid, the main metabolic product, gives rise to a high osmotic pressure in the corneal stroma [13]. Thus, corneal edema and at times corneal vascularization may develop in contact lens wearers. Although the role of the conjunctiva for oxygen delivery to the cornea is not disputed, the oxygen scores reported in the literature are rather ambiguous [5, 3, 9, 10, 13, 15]. In the majority of these studies, indirect measuring procedures were applied such as investigations on the minimum of oxygen pressure avoiding corneal edema; other studies measuring the oxygen supply to the cornea were restricted only to young age groups. In our study we performed continuous and direct oxygen measurements of the conjunctiva palpebrae in subjects divided in different age groups (Table 1). The probe used has been manufactured by the Orange Medical Instruments (Costa Mesa).

Table 1. Groups of tested subjects

Group	subjects	n	age	number of examinations
1	healthy volunteers I	12	35 ± 7.2	3
2	healthy volunteers II	15	31 ± 9.2	1*
3	diabetic patients	18	54 ± 20	1*
4	nondiabetic patients with cataracts	6	75 ± 5.8	1*
5	pat. with ischemic ophthalmopathy	2		1*

* only partially tested by blood gas analyses

Clinical Oxygen Pressure Measurement II
A.M. Ehrly et al. (Eds.)
© Blackwell Ueberreuter Wissenschaft Berlin 1990

Methods and subjects

The system included a miniaturized Clark-type electrode [3] consisting of a platinum cathode (100 μm in diameter) and a silver/silverchloride anode. A solid state thermistor is incorporated in the electrode body to measure the temperature at the conjunctival surface. The electrodes lie in a small electrolyte chamber. On the side in contact with conjunctiva the system is closed by a polyethylene oxygen-permeable membrane. The probe is mounted in an oval conformer which is molded from polymethylmethacrylate – a material used in the manufacture of hard contact lenses. When the sensor is positioned on the conjunctiva, oxygen diffuses across the membrane and is reduced at the cathode, producing a small (nanoampere) current. Before use, the probe is calibrated at zero and 21% oxygen. In order to test the stability and reproducibility of measurements obtained with the sensor, we carried out 75 investigations involving 51 subjects. pO_2 and temperature were continuously recorded by means of a two-channel printer (Servogor 200, Metrawatt). For comparative purposes we obtained arterial pO_2 scores in 28 subjects (blood gas analyses).

Stability and reproducibility of measurement

In 12 subjects free of any ocular disease, pO_2/t-diagrams from the conjunctiva were determined three times a day. The average was calculated for each diagram (taking values at equal intervals). For evaluation, the shape of the diagrams as well as the differences between the average values were considered (cf. Table 2).

Conjunctival oxygen delivery

In 39 patients and healthy volunteers (group 2 – group 4) of different age (Table 1), pO_2-diagrams were recorded as described above. Using the results of the blood gas analyses, we ascertained the $tcjpO_2$/ a pO_2 (transconjunctival O_2-pressure / arterial O_2-pressure) ratio in 28 subjects. 18 of the subjects tested were diabetics (mean duration of diabetes: 15.6 ± 7.6 years) hospitalized for surgical treatment of diabetes-associated eye-disease (diabetic retinopathy, cataract).

Results

Stability and reproducibility of measurement

The pO_2-diagrams showed an initial decrease since the sensor had to adjust from air to the conjunctival pO_2. The period of adjustment varied

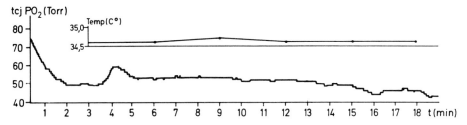

Fig. 1. Continuous measuring of conjunctival pO$_2$ in a young healthy subject. The first 3 minutes have to be neglected as adaptation period after closing eyelids. The curve shows a quite uniform shape with a continuous decrease of about 8 torr

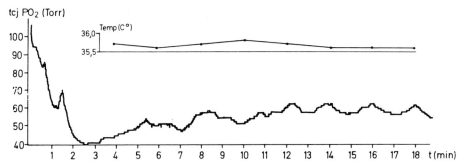

Fig. 2. Continuous measuring of pO$_2$ in a young healthy subject. The curve is characterized by considerable pO$_2$-fluctuations

from 2 – 3 minutes. It was followed by that part of the diagram being characteristic for each subject. The diagram in Fig. 1 shows a quite uniform course with a continuous decrease of about 8 torr. In contrast, the diagram in Fig. 2 is characterized by considerable pO$_2$-fluctuations. In table 2 the values of subjects in group 1 are summarized: For each of the twelve volunteers, pO$_2$-diagrams were determined three times a day. The differences among the three calculated average values are greater than can be accounted for by the inherent error of measurement.

In contrast to the pO$_2$-values, conjunctival temperatures remained fairly constant with a deflexion of maximal 0.2°C in the course of a single measurement period. Repeated measurements yielded, on average, differences of ± 0.3°C.

Conjunctival oxygen delivery

The average pO$_2$ covers a range from 26 to 82 torr. The mean of the averages is 54.0 ± 15.2 torr. The pO$_2$ varies with age (Fig. 3): tcjpO$_2$ is significantly reduced in elder subjects (r = 0.8). For subjects older than 60 years a mean score of 38.6 SD± 6.3 torr was obtained, contrasting to a

Table 2. Mean values calculated from 3 pO_2- and temperature measurements in 12 volunteers. The values listed in this table represent the means and their standard deviations of average values calculated from 3 diagrams drawn from each of the volunteers.

subj	pO_2	sd	temp	sd
1	69.3	1.5	35.7	0.4
2	73.5	4.1	35.8	0.2
3	55.6	3.1	35.1	0.3
4	63.3	4.5	35.8	0.5
5	70.0	4.6	36.1	0.1
6	59.6	1.5	35.2	0.2
7	73.0	3.5	35.0	0.0
8	66.3	2.5	36.3	0.3
9	60.0	7.7	35.7	0.3
10	65.0	1.7	35.7	0.5
11	78.3	3.5	36.2	0,3
12	61.1	4.2	35.6	0.5
means	66.3	3.6	35.7	0.3
SD	6.7	1.7	0.4	0.2

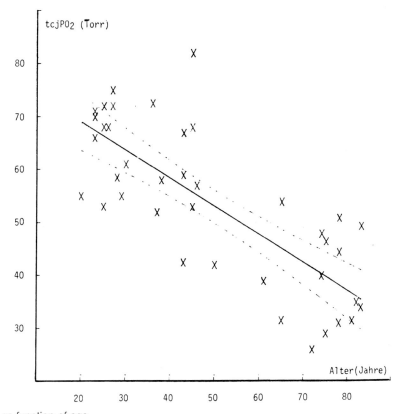

Fig. 3. pO_2 as function of age

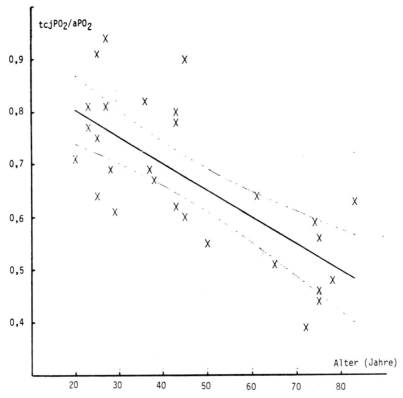

Fig. 4. Ratio conjunctival pO_2 / arterial pO_2 as function of age. The decrease of this ratio with aging suggests a factor in conjunctival vascular bed causing the drop in conjunctival pO_2-delivery

mean score of 64.8 SD± 7.9 torr for subjects 30 years old and younger. The $tcjpO_2$ / paO_2 ratio yields values of 0.4 and 0.9 respectively. It is also dependent on age: The older the patient the lower the ratio (Fig. 4).

Temperature: The temperature values range from 33.5 to 36.8°C. There is a significant negative correlation between age and temperature.

Diabetics: The diabetic patients showed no significant differences compared to other subjects.

Discussion

Stability and reproducibility of measurements

Our results indicate that single pO_2 values taken momentarily, are not representative. In order to get valuable data, averaging pO_2 values is required (Fig. 1 u. 2.). Fluctuations in conjunctival oxygen pressure may be influenced by several factors:

Arterial oxygen pressure: Fabel [4] was able to demonstrate by means of continuous intraarterial measurements that arterial pO_2 varies even during respiration at rest. The average difference between maximal and minimal pO_2 (fluctuation rate) amounted to 14 torr. In comparison we established a mean conjunctival fluctuation range of 16 torr.

Vasomotion: To some extent the $tcjpO_2$ fluctuations we found may indeed reflect the changing pO_2 in the large vessel. However, the special properties of the capillary system constitute an additional set of factors which determine pO_2-fluctuation in the peripheral vasculature and must be taken into account. One of these factors is vasomotion in the small conjunctival vessel: According to Schmid-Schönbein [16] it is responsible for a temporal and spatial heterogeneity of perfusion. The measuring surface of our sensor is about 600 μm^2. It seems to be possible that the pO_2-sensor also keeps track of the temporal heterogeneity of the local perfusion.

Local changes in the sensor probe: Further, it has to be taken into account that the measuring field cannot be assumed to remain constant when measurements are repeated; little displacements cannot be avoided. This means that epithelial thickness of the conjunctiva, which differs from one place to the other, enters the set of conditions responsible for different results in repeated measurements. According to calculations by Fatt [6] an increase in epithelial thickness from 20 μm to 30 μm results in a lowering of the pO_2 by 12 torr.

Irritative effect of the sensor: The circular-shaped conformer has been designed to minimize any disruptive effects on the cornea. Eye movements are possible without displacing the sensor. It may nevertheless give rise to a foreign body sensation in the conjunctival sac. The discomfort so produced could lead to a reflex tic of the eyelid which would be likely to affect the capillary perfusion.

Conjunctival oxygen delivery

Our data indicate that $tcjpO_2$ depends on age. The reduction in the pO_2-values found in older age groups undoubtedly is due in part to a physiological drop in arterial pO_2 with advanced age [18]. As indicated by the ratio $tcjpO_2$ / a pO_2, the $tcjpO_2$ decrease is more pronounced than that of the arterial blood. This suggests the operation of a conjunctival factor as well. This factor may be a reduction of perfusion as observed in age-related arteriosclerotic vascular changes or in congested heart failure. Interesting enough, the lowest pO_2-values were found in two patients suffering from ischemic ophthalmopathy. The assumption of an additional age-related factor is supported by the observation that conjunctival temperature also declines with age. This is probably a phenomenon of vascular bed, because old age does not usually entail reduction of body core temperature [17]. The pO_2 values in the diabetic group did not principally differ from those taken from the non-diabetic groups. This result may not be astonishing because surface oxygen scores are not able to give detailed information about the microcirculation of the underlying vascular bed [7]. The question of whether the oxygen supply of the cornea is sufficient in all situations is relevant for the elderly patient suffering from aphakia. They are usually equipped with extended-wear-contact lenses, which constitute a diffusion barrier. During sleep or with closed eyelids an oxygen deficit can develop.

In the older patients, oxygen supply to the cornea is very critical: according to our findings (39 torr in subjects more than 60 years of age) it is markedly lower than has been assumed so far:

Fatt and Bieber   (1968) 55 torr [5]
Efron and Carney   (1979) 57 torr [3]
Holden and Sweeney   (1985) 61 torr [11]

Moreover, corneal temperature is increased by 1.2 °C in the closed as compared with the open eye conditions (14) involving an increased metabolic rate and hence a raised oxygen demand on the cornea. Altogether these facts may explain why even today's O_2-superpermeable contact lenses lead to metabolic derangement, may lead to corneal edema or in some cases irreversible corneal vascularisation.

Summary

A polarographic sensor measuring the oxygen tension of the conjunctiva palpebrae was tested for its applicability and for the reproducibility of results in 51 subjects. The result suggest, that
1. continuous measuring is required for 15 – 20 minutes to obtain reliable scores.
2. The oxygen tension of the conjunctiva decreases with advancing age presumably due to reduction of lung function and additionally decreased perfusion of the conjunctiva.
3. the O_2-supply of the conjunctiva of elderly people is lower than previously thought.

References

1. Baum, J.L., Martola, E.-L. (1968): Corneal edema and corneal vascularisation. Am J Ophthal 65: 881-884
2. Clark, J.R., Wolf, R. et al. (1953): Continuous recording of blood oxygen tension by polarography. J Apl Physiol 6: 189-193
3. Efron, N., Carney, L.G. (1979): Oxygen levels beneath the closed eyelid. Invest Ophthalmol Vis Sci 18: 93-95
4. Fabel, H. (1968): Die fortlaufende Messung des arteriellen Sauerstoffpartialdruckes beim Menschen. Arch Kreislaufforsch 57: 10-17

5. Fatt, I., Bieber, M.T. (1968): The steady-state distribution of oxygen and carbon dioxide in the in vivo cornea: I. The open eye in air and the closed eyelid. Exp Eye Res 7: 103-112

6. Fatt, I., Deutsch, T.A. (1983): The relation of conjunctival pO_2 to capillary bed pO_2. Crit Care Med 11: 445-448

7. Fleckenstein, W., Weiss, Ch. (1984): Ein neues Gewebe-pO_2- Meßverfahren zum Nachweis von Mikrozirkulationsstörungen. Focus MHL 2: 74-84

8. Grafflin, A.L., Corddry, E.G. (1953): Studies of peripheral blood vascular beds in the bulbar conjunctiva of man. Bull John Hopkins Hosp 93: 275-289

9. Guillon, M. (1983): Der Sauerstoffbedarf der Hornhaut im Lichte des Kontaktlinsentragens. Contactologica 5: 44-48

10. Holden, B.A. et al. (1984): The minimum precorneal oxygen tension to avoid corneal edema. Invest Ophthalmol and Vis Sci 25: 477-480

11. Holden, B.A., Sweeney, F.D. (1985): The oxygen tension and temperature of the superior palpebral conjunctiva. Acta Ophthalmol 63: 100-103

12. Klyce, S.D. (1981): Stromal lactate accumulation can account for corneal edema osmotically following epithelial hypoxia in the rabbit. J Physiol 321: 49-65

13. Mandell, R.B., Farrell, R. (1980): Corneal swelling at low atmospheric oxygen pressures. Invest Ophthalmol Vis Sci 19: 697-702

14. Mapstone, R. (1968): Determination of corneal temperature. Br J Ophthalmol 52: 729-737

15. Polse, K.A., Mandell, R.B. (1970): Critical oxygen tension at corneal surface. Arch Ophthal (Chicago) 84: 505-509

16. Schmid-Schönbein, H. (1986): Rheologie der normalen und pathologischen Blutversorgung der mikroskopischen Conjunctivalgefäße. Fortsch Ophthalmol 83: 377-388

17. Timiras, P.A. (1980): Physiology of aging, in: Mountcastle V.B. (Hrsg.). Medical Physiology Mosby, St. Louis, S. 1988- 1989

18. Ulmer, W.T., Reichel, G. (1963): Untersuchungen über die Altersabhängigkeit der alveolären und arteriellen Sauerstoff- und Kohlensäuredrucke. Klin Wochenschrift 41: 1-9

Arterial and Conjunctival Oxygen Tension in Acute Ischemic Stroke before and after Infusion of 500 ml 10% HAES 200/0.5

U. Staedt, M. Hütt, U. Seufzer, M. Beez

Introduction

Pathophysiological findings [6, 8, 10, 11, 15] and clinical studies [7, 16, 19, 20] lie behind the rationale for hemodilution therapy in patients with acute cerebral infarction. Because of its low incidence rate of allergic side effects [1], superior hemorrheological properties [3, 9, 13, 17, 19] and good clinical results in patients with impaired cerebral [16, 19] or peripheral [3, 4, 13] blood flow, middle-molecular-weight hydroxyethylstarch (HAES 200/0.5) is nowadays used instead of low-molecular-weight dextran (DEXTRAN 40).

Recently, in addition to hemorrheological factors, more interest has been focused on the improvement of microcirculation and oxygen supply in patients suffering from peripheral arterial occlusive disease [3, 12]. Polarographic needle electrodes are used to measure skeletal muxcle oxygen pressure (pO_2), but this invasive technique is not suitable for determination of brain pO_2 in patients with acute ischemic stroke.

A new device for the measurement of conjunctival (cj) pO_2 could be helpful for the obtainment of information on cerebral oxygen supply, since cj pO_2 reflects the oxygen delivery to the areas supplied by the internal carotid artery [5]. Patients with acute ischemic stroke have ipsilaterally, i.e. in the eye on the side where the attack occurred, a low cj pO_2, whereas contralaterally impairment is less pronounced [18].

Patients and methods

The study presents data from 15 patients (9 male, 6 female) with acute cerebral infarction in the territories of one middle cerebral artery as demonstrated by CT scans. Exclusion criteria were coma, myocardial insufficiency, serum creatinine < 2 mg/dl, occlusion or high grade stenosis (< 50 %) of the carotid arteries. Before and after the 3 hour infusion of 500 ml 10 % HAES 200/0.5 (HAES-Steril 10 %, Fresenius AG), hematocrit, red cell aggregation, dynamic whole blood and plasma viscosity, arterial pCO_2 and pO_2 were measured [18, 19].

Clinical Oxygen Pressure Measurement II
A.M. Ehrly et al. (Eds.)
© Blackwell Ueberreuter Wissenschaft Berlin 1990

We used a miniature Clark polarographic electrode embedded in an oval ring-shaped ophthalmic conformer (Orange 1, Orange Medical Instruments, Costa Mesa, USA). One drop of 0.4 % oxybuprocain solution was given into each eye before the upper lid was elevated by gentle traction and the cj O_2 sensor was inserted into the superior cj fornix. It was held in place while the lower lid was retracted to insert the lower part of the conformer into the inferior cj fornix. The patients were lying in their beds and were asked to keep their eyes closed for a few minutes until the display stabilized, which took about 5 minutes. The cornea was not touched, the patients did not suffer any pain and no problems arose.

Measurements of cj pO_2 are of interest, because palpebral conjunctiva gets its principal arterial supply from branches of the ophthalmic artery, and thus cj pO_2 reflects O_2 delivery to the areas supplied by the internal carotid arteries. The cj mucous membrane is only $20 - 30$ µm thick, and therefore no artificial heating procedures are required [5, 18].

Statistical analyses

For comparison of patients' values with age-matched controls Student's t-test was used, and for comparison of data before and after infusion and between ipsilateral and contralateral values Wilcoxon's rank sum test was used [14].

Results

Despite the fact that the patients had hematocrit and fibrinogen values in the normal range, hemorrheological parameters were significantly elevated above the normal range compared to age-matched healthy controls (Table 1). The infusion of HAES 200/0.5 resulted in a fall in hematocrit and fibrinogen concentration and led to a normalization of red cell aggregation and whole blood and plasma viscosity.

Table 1. Hemorrheological parameters in patients with acute ischemic stroke before and after infusion of 500 ml 10 % HAES 200/0.5 within 3 hours, mean (s)

Parameter	Unit	before Inf	after Inf
Hematocrit	vol %	40.2 (3.3)	37.6 (3.1)##
Fibrinogen	g/l	3.32 (.58)	2.85 (.65)#
Red cell aggregation	–	17.6 (3.7)+	13.2 (2.7)##
Plasma viscosity (50/s)	cp	1.64 (.17)+	1.43 (.15)#
Blood viscosity (50/s)	cp	5.47 (.99)+	4.75 (.95)##

p ≤ 0.05 : + vs age-matched healthy controls
p ≤ 0.05 / 0.01 : #/## after vs before infusion

Arterial pCO_2 was in the normal range before and after the infusion, while the initially low arterial pO_2 was slightly but significantly elevated to the reference range by the infusion. Ipsilateral cj pO_2, which all the while remained below the contralateral cj pO_2, reached only 50 % of the expected value for this age group. The infusion of HAES 200/0.5 brought about a marked improvement of cj pO_2, especially on the ipsilateral side, while contralaterally the changes of cj pO_2 were less pronounced though still significant. Nevertheless, ipsilateral cj pO_2 remained below contralateral values in all patients (Table 2).

Table 2. Arterial and conjunctival (cj) pO_2 (torr) in patients with acute ischemic stroke before and after infusion of 500 ml 10 % HAES 200/0.5 in 3 hours (ipsilateral, i.e. cj pO_2 in the eye at the side where attack had occurred, vs contralateral side); mean (s)

Parameter	before Inf.	after Inf.
arterial pCO_2	38.3 (3.8)	37.1 (2.7)
arterial pO_2	71.1 (9.9)+	76.8 (9.6)#
ipsilateral cj pO_2	23.5 (6.4)++	33.0 (7.5)+##
contralateral cj pO_2	34.9 (7.2)+**	38.3 (8.8)+*#

$p \leq 0.05/0.01$: +/++ vs age-matched healthy controls
$p \leq 0.05/0.01$: #/## for after vs before infusion
$p \leq 0.05/0.01$: */** for ipsilateral vs contralateral values

Discussion

Our data confirm the fact that patients suffering from arteriosclerotic vessel lesions like coronary heart disease, peripheral arterial disease and cerebrovascular disease have a disturbed blood fluidity which contributes to impairment of blood and oxygen supply to the afflicted tissues [2, 15]. It is therefore essential under these circumstances to use a solution for hemodilution which improves hemorrheology.

The infusion of HAES 200/0.5 resulted in an improvement of red cell aggregation and whole blood and plasma viscosity by 25 % and 13 % respectively. These results agree with the literature, other groups also having found a marked improvement of blood fluidity after infusions of HAES 200/0.5 [3, 9, 13, 17].

Alongside the improvement of hemorrheological properties, other factors are also involved in the raising of cj pO_2. The administration of a plasma volume expander increases cardiac output [8] and leads to an augmentation of cerebral blood flow in patients with acute ischemic stroke [6, 11]. Due to the disturbed cerebral vascular autoregulation in stroke, perfusion increases especially in the ischemic brain areas [11].

Our data indicate that the infusion of HAES 200/0.5 led, in addition to the normalization of blood fluidity and to the deducible augmentation in cerebral blood flow, to an improvement in impaired microcirculation and oxygen supply in the areas of the internal carotid arteries in patients with acute ischemic stroke.

Summary

Conjunctival oxygen tension and hemorrheological parameters were measured in 15 patients with acute ischemic stroke and compared to values obtained in a reference group. The conjunctival capillary bed is perfused by the ophthalmic artery and thus reflects oxygen delivery to the areas supplied by the internal carotid artery. Measurements of conjunctival oxygen tension are simple and safe. Patients with acute ischemic stroke showed lowered conjunctival oxygen tension especially on the ipsilateral side, i.e. the side where the attack had occurred, and to a lesser extent on the contralateral side too. Furthermore, these patients had pathologically elevated values for red cell aggregation and whole blood and plasma viscosity despite a hematocrit within the normal range.
After the infusion of 500 ml 10 % middle-molecular-weight hydroxyethylstarch, blood fluidity was normalized, whereby the hematocrit was only reduced by 6,5 %. Conjunctival oxygen tension improved by 40 % on the ipsilateral and by 10 % on the contralateral side, the ipsilateral values however remaining all the while significantly lower than the contralateral values.
In addition to the well-known improvement in hemorrheological properties and augmentation of cerebral blood flow following hemodilution in patients with acute ishemic stroke, there seems to be an increase in oxygen supply in the territories of both internal carotic arteries, as indicated by the values of conjunctival oxygen tension.

References

1. Beez M, Dietl H (1979) Retrospektive Betrachtung der Häufigkeit anaphylaktoider Reaktionen nach Plasmasteril und Longasteril. Infustionsther Klin Ernähr 6:3
2. Bruhn HD, Hell K, Balzereit A, Diebold U, Chmiel H (1988) Erhöhte Viskoelastizität des Blutes bei arteriosklerotischen Gefäßveränderungen. Med Welt 39:407
3. Ehrly AM, Landgraf A, Moschner PV, Saeger-Lorenz K (1987) Hydroxyäthylstärke gegen Dextran. Med Welt 39:407
4. Ernst E, Matrai A, Kollar L (1987) Placebo-controlled, double-blind study of haemodilution in peripheral arterial disease. Lancet I:1449
5. Fatt I, Deutsch TA (1983) The relation of conjunctival pO_2 to capillary bed pO_2. Crit Care Med 11:445
6. Gottstein U, Held K (1969) Effekt der Hämodilution nach intravenöser Infusion von niedermolekularen Dextranen auf die Hirnzirkulation des Menschen. Dtsch Med Wschr 94:522
7. Gottstein U, Sedlmeyer I, Heuss A (1976) Behandlung der akuten zerebralen Mangeldurchblutung mit niedermolekularem Dextran. Dtsch Med Wschr 101:223
8. Grotta JC, Pettigrew LC, Allen S, Tonnesen A, Yotsu FM, Gray J (1985) Baseline hemodynamic state and response to hemodilution in patients with acute cerebral ischemia. Stroke 16:790

9. Haass A, Kroemer H, Jäger H, Müller K, Decker I, Schimrigk K (1986) Dextran 40 oder HAES 200/0.5. Dtsch Med Wschr 1681
10. Harrison MGJ, Pollock S, Marshall J (1981) Effect of haematocrit on carotid stenosis and cerebral infarction. Lancet II:114
11. Hartmann A, Tsuda Y, Lagreze H (1987) Effect of hypervolaemic haemodilution on regional cerebral blood flow in patients with acute ischaemic stroke: A controlled study with hydroxyethylstarch. J Neurol 235:34
12. Heinrich R, Günderoth M, Grauer W, Machac N, Dette S, Egberts EH (1987) Gewebe-pO_2 im M. tibialis ant. gesunder Probanden bei
13. Kiesewetter H, Blume J, Bulling B, Gerhards M, Jung F, Radtke H, Frank RP (1984) Mittelmolekulare Hydroxyethylstärke als Volumenersatz. Dtsch Med Wschr 109:1844
14. Sachs L (1984) Angewandte Statistik. Springer, Berlin
15. Schmid-Schönbein H (1982) Physiologie und Pathophysiologie der Mikrozirkulation aus rheologischer Sicht. Internist 23:359
16. Schneider R, Zeumer H, Jung F, Kiesewetter H (1985) Behandlung zerebraler Mikroangiopathien mit 10 % HES 200. Med Welt 36:359
17. Simon J, Jung F, Holbach T, Mrowietz C, Jaksche H, Kiesewetter H (1986) Einfluß verschiedener Volumenersatzmittel auf die Fließfähigkeit des Blutes und den konjunktivalen Sauerstoffpartialdruck. Krankenhausarzt 59:814
18. Staedt U, Holm E, Kortsik CS, Heene DL (1988) Konjunktivaler Sauerstoffdruck von Patienten mit akutem Hirninfarkt. Klin Wschr 66:628
19. Staedt U, Schwarz M, Bayerl JR, Tornow K, Heene DL (1986) Hämodilution bei akuter zerebraler Ischämie. Med Welt 37:695
20. Strand T, Asplund K, Eriksson S, Hägg E, Lithner F, Wester OP (1984) A randomized controlled trial of hemodilution therapy in acute ischemic stroke. Stroke 15:980

Heparin-Coated pO_2 Electrode Compared to Conventional pO_2 Measurement by ABL-Radiometer

R. Tenbrinck, G.J. van Daal, W. Schairer, M.H. Kuypers, G.F.J. Steeghs, B. Lachmann

Introduction

Intensive care units require continuous paO_2 monitoring to enable fast and proper ventilator adjustment according to the patient's needs. Conventional blood sampling techniques followed by blood-gas analysis are not able to monitor sudden changes in oxygen partial pressure. A better solution would be an intravasal paO_2 electrode. Monitoring the arterial and venous oxygen partial pressure simultaneously supplies information about the oxygen extraction rate, and threatening perfusion disturbances and acute changes during spontaneous respiration can be detected immediately. The direct effect of extracorporeal oxygenators during open-heart surgery can be observed, and there is also the possibility of closed-loop feed-back regulation of the respirator for optimal ventilator settings in ARDS patients.

One of the disadvantages of the few available paO_2 catheters is that the surface of the catheter membrane becomes clotted with blood within a short time, which always leads to a decrease in the measured intravasal paO_2. Based on semiconductor technology a heparin-coated intravasal paO_2 electrode was therefore developed by PPG Hellige (Best, Holland). This new electrode was expected to be free of the former disadvantages.

The aim of this study was to investigate the accuracy of this electrode under in-vivo conditions in comparison with normal blood sampling and analysis.

Materials and methods

The pO_2 electrode

The oxygen sensor consists of a chip which can measure pO_2 and temperature, a metal tip with a window-opening for the chip and a lumen for taking blood samples, a flexible polyurethane catheter (F6), a keflar cable for safety and a connector to the calibration resistors for pO_2 and tem-

Clinical Oxygen Pressure Measurement II
A.M. Ehrly et al. (Eds.)
© Blackwell Ueberreuter Wissenschaft Berlin 1990

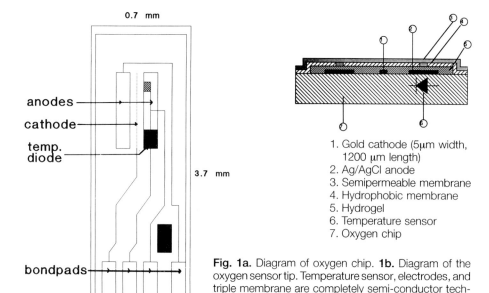

1. Gold cathode (5μm width, 1200 μm length)
2. Ag/AgCl anode
3. Semipermeable membrane
4. Hydrophobic membrane
5. Hydrogel
6. Temperature sensor
7. Oxygen chip

Fig. 1a. Diagram of oxygen chip. **1b.** Diagram of the oxygen sensor tip. Temperature sensor, electrodes, and triple membrane are completely semi-conductor technology

perature (Figs. 1a and 1b). The oxygen chip is based on the Clark cell principle [1, 2] integrated with the chip technology, as described in more detail by Kimmich [2]. Since then some important improvements have been made.

The electrodes, a gold cathode and two silver anodes, are embedded in an electrolyte matrix (hydrogel layer) which in turn is covered with a membrane provided with 10 holes (5 holes above each anode). The holes permit a supply of electrolytes from the blood (Cl⁻) to the hydrogel layer. On top of the membrane, a protein filter is deposited. This layer prevents the proteins from diffusing onto the electrodes. Heparin is also immobilized in this layer to prevent the blood from building a thrombus on the sensing area (Fig. 1b). When the sensor is brought into an arteria and connected to the measuring equipment, a DC voltage of approximately 0.8 Volts with respect to the AG (AgCl) reference electrode is applied to the gold cathode. Thus the oxygen which diffuses through the membrane will be reduced at the cathode, and at the same time the silver of the anode oxidizes to form silver chloride (using the chloride of the blood):

Cathode: $O_2 + 2H_2O + 4e \rightarrow 4OH^-$
Anode: $4Ag + 4Cl^- \rightarrow 4AgCl + 4e$

The result is a current (nano-Amperes) which is proportional to the oxygen pressure of the blood. For clinical purposes it is desirable that allowance is made for temperature differences between patient and blood-gas analyser. This involves a correction of the calculated oxygen solubility (depending on the hemoglobin/oxyhemoglobin equilibrium) and a correction for the sensitivity of the sensor. In order to carry out this correction, the temperature must be measured. This is done by the isolated temperature diode in the chip consisting of an array of anti-parallel couple diodes. This results, according to the manufacturer, in the following characteristics: 95 % response time in 15s; flow dependency (> 8 cm/sec) is 1 %; lifetime is approximately 7 days. For drifting the following specifications were given: First 30 min 4 %; second 30 min 1.5 %; third 30 min 1 %; and for every subsequent hour 0.5 %, provided the catheter is first stabilized.

Method

14 New Zealand white rabbits were anesthetized with pentobarbital (35 mg/kg bw) and trachetomized. They breathed spontaneously while being prepared for ventilation. The electrode (tip diameter 1.2 mm) was inserted into the left arteria carotis. The animals were not heparinized. Blood samples were taken from the left arteria femoralis by means of an intravasal catheter. As amplifier and monitor system a Hellige RM 300 (PPG Hellige, Best, Holland) was used. The values of the electrode were continuously recorded on a Honeywell PM 8221 penrecorder (Honeywell, Best, Holland). During the 8 hour study period, an arterial blood sample was drawn every 30 min from the arteria femoralis catheter and analysed by an ABL 300 blood-gas analyser (Radiometer, Copenhagen, Denmark). Throughout the period of monitoring, there were no efforts made to adapt the electrode values to those obtained by the ABL 300.

Statistics

For statistical analysis of the data we used the Wilcoxon-test for paired measurements and the Student's t-test for paired observations. The outcome of both tests was the same in all cases. $p < 0.05$ was accepted as significant.

Results

The values monitored by the electrode and ABL 300 were combined. The total number of observations was 83. The data were processed in two ways: first, comparison of electrode and ABL value pairs (Fig. 2a); secondly, the differences between ABL 300 and electrode values were plotted over time (Fig. 2b). After 8 hours, the deviation due to drifting had to be less than 10 %; however, in our investigation it was 18 %. During the first 3 hours, there was no significant difference between ABL 300 and electrode data ($p > 5$ %). In the last two hours, these differences became significant ($p < 1.25$ %).

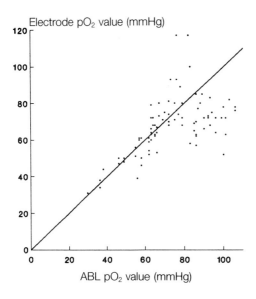

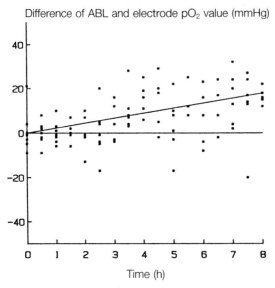

Fig. 2 a, b. Comparison of electrodes and ABL 300 data. X-axis = ABL 300 data in mmHg; Y-axis = electrode data in mmHg. **b.** ABL values minus electrode values over time

Discussion

Similar experiments in beagle dogs and in-vitro experiments using saline solutions showed good correlation and a very acceptable drift in time (Fig. 3; M.H. Kuypers, unpublished results).

During the experiments some problems with the movability of the catheter in the carotic artery occurred. It was assumed that the diameter of the rabbit vessels was not large enough to permit optimal functioning of the

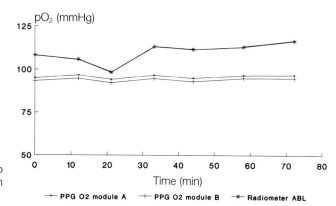

Fig. 3. Results of in-vivo measurements of pO₂ in dogs

catheter. The animals were not heparinized, so as not to conceal any possible clotting effect. Owing to the changed flow pattern, there might have been a precipitation of clotting around the catheter or on the vessel lumen, so that the electrode sensor area had a diminished contact with the blood stream. This finding led us to the conclusion that the vessel diameter was a limiting factor for the electrode, contributing to the deviations in Figs. 2a and 2b as compared to the manufacturer's data.

Another point of interest is that the pO₂ electrode is a very fast-acting device, whilst the ABL is relatively slow. The time lapse between measurements is 15 seconds for the electrode against 3 minutes for the ABL 300. Thus the use of the pO₂ electrode enables visualization of dips in the pO₂ curve that could not be monitored previously (Fig. 4). One example: If one were to take a blood sample in the middle of such a pO₂ dip (without electrode monitoring), this sample would be judged as bad and a new sample would be taken. In the case of a patient being ventilated, this could lead to undesirable alterations in ventilator settings.

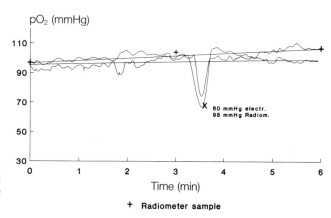

Fig. 4. Electrode pO₂ recording in mmHg revealing a pO₂ dip which could be visualized instantaneously

Conclusion

From these results we conclude that the heparin-coated intravasal pO_2 electrode could be routinely used in intensive care units for continuous pO_2 monitoring, provided it is placed in a vessel that is large enough to allow the electrode membrane to float freely in the blood stream. The use of heparin is, under these circumstances, optional.

References

1. Clark LC (1956) Monitor and control of blood and tissue oxygen tensions. Trans Am Soc Art Int Organs 2:41
2. Kimmich HP, Kuypers MH, Engels JML, Maas HGR (1981) Disposable solid state oxygen sensor. Fifth Intern Symp of the International Soc for Oxygen Transp to Tissue. Detroit, August 1981

Oxygen Supply in an Isolated Lobe of Human Placenta During Dual In-Vitro Perfusion: Experimental Study with Microcoaxial Needle Electrodes

H. Baumgärtl, H. Schneider, R. Huch

Introduction

In order to characterize the oxygen supply in the human placenta during dual in-vitro perfusion, local pO_2 measurements were performed polarographically using microcoaxial needle electrodes. Oxygen supply was investigated experimentally under three different sets of conditions.

Methods and experimental setup

Measurements were done in 12 human placentas weighing 26.8 to 58.0 g. The placentas were from normal, close to term pregnancies and healthy newborns.

Tissue preparation and dual in-vitro perfusion were done according to the technique Schneider and Huch (1985). Fig. 1 shows the experimental perfusion setup and a schematic drawing of an isolated cotyledon of the human placenta in which pO_2 measurements were taken.

The cotyledon was prepared so that the capillary network (6) inside the villi, i.e. the fetal blood flow compartment, was perfused via a catheterized arterial (1) and venous (2) vessel. The maternal blood circulates around the villi in the so-called intervillous space (7), and the perfusate reaches this area via a distributor (3), whereby several arms reach through the decidua plate (5) and penetrate the intervillous space by about 10 mm. At the base, the intervillous space is limited by the chorion plate (4). A homoglobin-free modified Earls buffer was used as perfusate.

Polarographic pO_2 measurements within the placental tissue were done using microcoaxial needle electrodes according to Baumgärtl and Lübbers (1983, 1987). The calibrated needle electrode (8, NE), was fixed to a micromanipulator (MM) movable in x, y, and z directions. A nanostepper (NS) was used to puncture the placenta. Puncturing was performed by stepwise penetration under microscopic control: 6 forward steps of 100 µm each followed immediately by 1 backward step of same length to minimize the pressure effects. Each step was performed in 10 ms and the

Clinical Oxygen Pressure Measurement II
A. M. Ehrly et al. (Eds.)
© Blackwell Ueberreuter Wissenschaft Berlin 1990

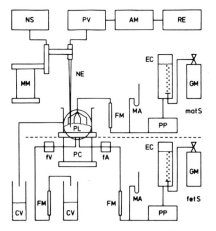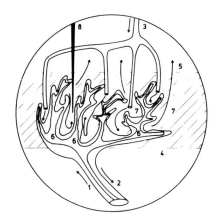

Fig. 1. AM = nanoamperemeter; CV = collecting vessel; EC = equilibrium chamber; FM = flow meter; GM = gas mixture; MA = manometer; MM = micromanipulator; NE = needle electrode; NS = nanostepper; PC = perfusion chamber; PL = placenta; PP = pump; PV = polarisation voltage; RE = recorder; fA = flow through electrode (fetal artery pO_2); fV = flow through electrode (fetal venous pO_2); fet S = fetal perfusion system; mat S = maternal perfusion system.
1 = catheterized arterial vessel; 2 = catheterized venous vessel; 3 = perfusion canulas; 4 = chorion plate; 5 = decidua plate; 6 = capillary network; 7 = intervillous space; 8 = needle electrode

time interval between any two steps amounted to 20 s. The total penetration depth was 23-24 mm, whereby the electrode tip (8) passed the decidua plate (5) and penetrated the intervillous space (7). Withdrawal of the electrode was done in steps of 500 resp. 1000 µm. Response time, t_{90}, of the electrodes was 55-300 ms, depending on recess length and membrane thickness. The response time of the measuring system as a whole was 0.4 to 1.0 s. Oxygen reduction current was recorded continuously using a 2-channel compensation recorder (RE) at a recording speed of 30 mm/min. For conversion of the recorded signals into units of pO_2/Torr the following equation was used:

$$pO_2 = (P_B - P_{H_2O}^T) \cdot \left(\frac{V_F}{100}\right) \cdot \left(\frac{i_t - i_o}{i_c - i_o}\right)$$

pO_2 = oxygen partial pressure
P_B = barometer pressure
$P_{H_2O}^T$ = water vapor pressure at a given measuring temperature
V_F = oxygen concentration of calibration gas mixture in volume percent
i_t = current in tissue
i_c = current in calibration media
i_o = current in nitrogen-equilibrated buffer solution i.e. "zero current"

The pO_2 measurements were done under three different sets of conditions:

1. maternal flow = 11.8 ml/min, perfusion media equilibrated at 95 % O_2 + 5 % CO_2;
   fetal flow = 7.3 ml/min, perfusion media equilibrated at 5 % O_2 + 5 % CO_2 + 90 % N_2;
2. maternal flow = 20.1 ml/min, perfusion media equilibrated at 95 % O_2 + 5 % CO_2;
   fetal flow = 5.9 ml/min, perfusion media equilibrated at 5 % O_2 + 5 % CO_2 + 90 % N_2;
3. maternal flow = 17.1 ml/min, perfusion media equilibrated at 95 % O_2 + 5 % CO_2;
   fetal flow = 5.1 ml/min, perfusion media equilibrated at 95 % O_2 + 5 % CO_2.

Results

pO_2 profiles in the perfused placenta

Local tissue pO_2 in the placenta was measured by puncturing the basal plate perpendicular to the intervillous space using membranized, sharpened pO_2 needle electrodes with an outer diameter of approx. 4-5 μm and a lean shaft.

In Fig. 2 pO_2 profiles are shown corresponding to the different puncture depths. Tissue pO_2 varied considerably within a single puncture channel as well as between the different channels. The pO_2 profiles revealed regions with steep changes in pO_2 and others with fairly constant pO_2. Comparison of the pO_2 profiles obtained under the three different sets of conditions (Fig. 2, I, II and III) revealed similar forms of the pO_2 courses. However, the increase in the maternal blood flow from a mean value of 11.8 ml/min to about 20.1 ml/min also led to an increase of absolute tissue pO_2 (see Fig. 2, II). Increasing oxygen concentration from 5 % to 95 % in the fetal perfusion medium led to even higher tissue pO_2 values (see Fig. 2, III).

Distribution pattern of tissue pO_2 and pO_2 histograms

In order to be able to characterize and compare the pO_2 profiles obtained under the three different sets of experimental conditions, local pO_2 distribution patterns and pO_2 histograms were drawn. In Fig. 3 all the pO_2 values measured under the same set of conditions but in different channels were combined. The resulting pO_2 distribution pattern (Fig. 3, left side) demonstrates clearly that the increase in maternal flow (condition II) and the higher pO_2 in the fetal perfusion medium (condition III) both improved oxygen tissue supply. Under all 3 sets of conditions local mean

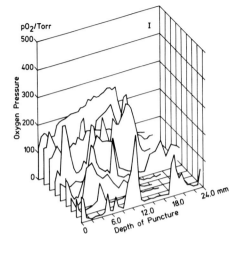

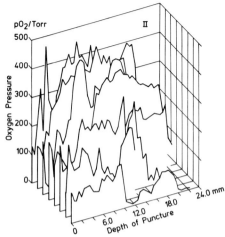

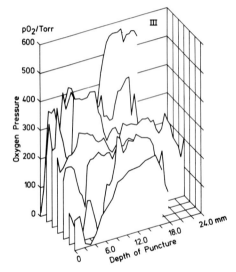

Fig. 2. pO₂ profiles in an isolated cotyledon of the human placenta during dual in-vitro perfusion. I = experimental conditions No 1 (3 placentas, 9 punctures); II = experimental conditions No 2 (4 placentas, 8 punctures); III = experimental conditions No 3 (5 placentas, 7 punctures). All three experimental conditions show that the electrode tip on its way from the decidua through the intervillous space crosses closely connected zones of very high and very low pO₂ values. The absolute oxygen partial pressures tend to be higher when the maternal flow rate (II) and the oxygen supply in the fetal perfusion medium (III) are increased.

pO₂ (solid line) tended to increase up to a depth of 9-12 mm, reaching a local maximum at this level. Deeper down mean pO₂ began to decrease again slowly, so that the largest number of low pO₂ values were found at a depth of 18-23 mm as well as in the surface area. This indicates that O₂ supply is most probably favoured in the region of the perfusion canulas.

On the right side of Fig. 3 all pO₂ values obtained along the total length of the puncture were added together to form column histograms, each column being separated from the next one by 20 Torr. It can be clearly seen that in the dual perfused placenta low pO₂ values between 1-40 Torr are on the decrease, whereas pO₂ values above 300 Torr are on the in-

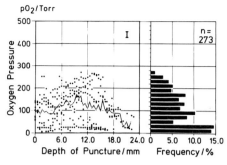

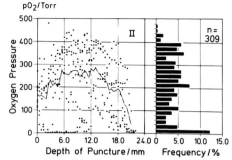

Fig. 3. pO₂ distribution in the human placenta and histograms of dual in-vitro perfusion. I, II and III: same conditions as in Fig. 2.

Left side: Distribution of local tissue pO₂ values corresponding to the puncturing depths. Evaluating the means of all pO₂ values measured in the tissue after 500 µm steps and combining them together we obtained the reconstructed pO₂ profile (solid line). From all three experiments it can be recognized that pO₂ increases between the surface of the placenta down to a depth of 9-12 mm and decreases again in deeper areas. This suggests that O₂ supply is favoured in the region near the tip of the perfusion canulas.

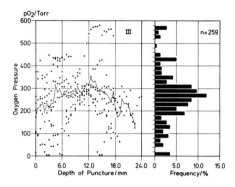

Right side: pO₂ histograms from all pO₂ values measured between 0 and 23 mm; intervals = 20 Torr. It can be clearly seen that in the dually perfused placenta low pO₂ values between 1 and 40 Torr decrease and pO₂ values above 300 Torr increase when the flow rate of the maternal perfusate is increased (II compared to I). This shift is even more pronounced when the oxygen concentration in the perfusate of the fetal system is increased (III). In the latter case an almost bell-shaped distribution results with a maximum between 261 and 280 Torr

crease when the flow rate of the maternal perfusate is increased (II compared to I). This shift is even more pronounced when the oxygen concentration in the perfusate of the fetal system is increased (see III). In the latter case an almost bell-shaped distribution results with a maximum between 261 and 280 Torr.

In order to analyze and compare the three pO₂ histograms, the following values are presented in Table 1: 1) mean tissue pO₂; 2) median; 3) percentage of pO₂ values below 100 Torr; 4) percentage of pO₂ values above 400 Torr.

Table 1

Exp.	mean pO₂ (Torr)	median pO₂ (Torr)	pO₂<100 Torr (%)	pO₂>400 Torr (%)
I	105	97	52.4	0
II	206	213	24.9	3.2
III	261	265	8.7	12.5

By increasing the maternal flow rate from 11.8 ml/min to about 20.1 ml/min the mean pO_2 increased from 105 Torr (I) to 206 Torr (II), whereas median pO_2 increased from 97 Torr to 213 Torr. The percentage of pO_2 values above 400 Torr is zero in case I and 3.2 in case II. The decrease in the number of pO_2 values below 100 Torr was especially marked: 52 % under I compared to only 25 % under II.

Increasing O_2 concentration in the fetal perfusion medium pushed the mean pO_2 up to 261 Torr and median pO_2 up to 265 Torr. Now 12.5 % of the pO_2 values exceeded 400 Torr, and only 8.7 % were below 100 Torr.

These results demonstrate that in the perfusion models presented here it is possible to supply a comparatively large area with sufficient oxygen providing:

1. flow rate is high;
2. oxygen concentration in the perfusion medium is high.

Summary

Local pO_2 measurements were performed polarographically using microcoaxial needle electrodes in order to characterize the oxygen supply in the human placenta during dual in-vitro perfusion. Oxygen supply under three different sets of conditions was investigated experimentally. pO_2 profiles were obtained by forwarding the electrodes stepwise into the tissue up to a depth of 23-24 mm.

The resulting profiles varied considerably both dynamically as well as absolutely, indicating non-homogenous perfusion. In tissue areas of reduced perfusion or no perfusion at all, low pO_2 values were measured. In order to estimate oxygen supply, the pO_2 frequency distributions were determined and illustrated in form of pO_2 histograms.

Under constant equilibration conditions (maternal 95 % O_2 + 5 % CO_2; fetal 5 % O_2 + 5 % CO_2 + 90 % N_2), the histograms show that an increase in maternal flow rate from 11.8 ml/min to 20.1 ml/min results in an increase in oxygen partial pressure from 105 to 206 Torr.

Under conditions of dual perfusion with high oxygen supply (95 % O_2 + 5 % CO_2), pO_2 profiles display a more even course, pO_2 gradients are less steep, and pO_2 values are distinctly higher attaining a mean value of 261 Torr.

Reconstruction of the pO_2 profile from mean local pO_2 values showed that under all sets of conditions the tissues are most optimally supplied close to the tip of the perfusion cannulas.

These experiments demonstrate that in the perfusion model described it is possible to supply a comparatively large area with sufficient oxygen providing

1. flow rate and
2. oxygen concentration in the perfusion medium are high and

3. the catheter transporting the perfusate reaches deep into the placenta.

Acknowledgement. This project was supported by funds of the Schweizerischer Nationalfonds.

References

1. Baumgärtl H (1987) Systematic investigations of needle electrode properties in polarographic measurements of local tissue pO$_2$. In: Ehrly AM, Hauss J, Huch R (eds) Clinical oxygen pressure measurements. Springer, Berlin, p 17
2. Baumgärtl H, Lübbers DW (1983) Microcoaxial needle sensor for polarographic measurement of local O$_2$ pressure in the cellular range of living tissue. Its construction and properties. In: Gnaiger E, Forstner H (eds) Polarographic oxygen sensors. Springer, Berlin, p 37
3. Schneider H, Huch A (1985) Dual in vitro perfusion of an isolated lobe of human placenta: Method and instrumentation. Contrib Gynecol Obstet 13:40

Pyloric-Preserving Longitudinal Resection of the Stomach – an "Ideal" Method of Resection?

J. Hauss, H.U. Spiegel, P. Langhans, G. Heidl, M. Rees, H. Bünte

Introduction

In 1966 Saegesser had proposed the *theoretical* concept for a longitudinal resection of the stomach fundus, corpus and antrum, combined with post-branchial vagotomy and pylorotomy, postulating that this surgical procedure would fulfill all criteria of an "ideal" stomach resection [5].

In our study we aimed to find out whether an extended longitudinal resection alone – without the originally proposed vagotomy and pyloro-plastic – would definitely reduce acid production while preserving stomach motility and pyloric function, and whether the procedure would be suitable for the management of recurrent hyperacid ulcers.

Material and Methods

Under basis anesthesia with high-dose Piritramide (1,5 mg/kg body weight/h plus 0.08 mg/kg/h Pancuronium) in combination with N_2O/O_2 (2/1), a longitudinal stomach resection was performed on 10 dogs (German Shepherds). The major curvature was completely uncovered from cardia to pylorus, the gastrolineal ligament severed, the arteria and vena gastrica brevis and gastroepiploica dextra and sinistra were ligated and severed. The resection limit was chosen to remove about one third of the antral surface and two thirds of the corpus-fundus area on the side of the major curvature (see Fig. 1). For suturing, staplers (LSG 90, Ethicon) were used, the staple line being covered with seroserous sutures. Analyses of gastric secretion were performed pre- and postoperatively (1 and 6 months after surgery) using Pentagastrin in s.c. injections of 6 µg/kg Gastrodiagnost. After 18 hrs of fasting and i.v. sedation with Diazepam, a gastric probe (18 char.) was introduced into the antrum under X-ray monitoring, the gastric juice was sucked off with a Hico-Gastrovac 261 and collected for 15 min with a Fractiomat 283. The samples were cooled down to 4°C, reheated to room temperature before measuring, and titrated to pH 7 with 100 mM NaOH in a Polymetron pH meter. The following parameters were assessed:

Clinical Oxygen Pressure Measurement II
A.M. Ehrly et al. (Eds.)
© Blackwell Ueberreuter Wissenschaft Berlin 1990

PRESERVATION OF:

● PYLORIC FUNCTION
● GASTRO-DUODENAL PASSAGE
● PANKREATICO-BILIARY-GASTRIC
  COORDINATION
● TISSUE PO$_2$

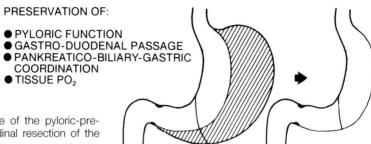

Fig. 1. Principle of the pyloric-preserving longitudinal resection of the stomach

1. Fasting volume and secrete volumes per 15 min;
2. pH values determined with a glass electrode;
3. concentration expressed as mval/l;
4. total amount of H ions (mval), calculated from the concentration and volume of the individual portions.

Basal and stimulated levels of serum gastrin were determined by controlled feeding of 200 g standard diet. After blood sampling at 60 and 30 min and immediately before feeding, further blood samples were taken at 15 min intervals during 2 hrs after feeding to assess serum gastrin, sodium, natrium and blood sugar levels. The blood samples were centrifuged immediately, the serum samples deep frozen. Gastrin values were determined by radioimmunoessay (Beckton-Dickinson kit).
Radiological, encoscopical and histological monitoring was performed pre- and postoperatively at identical intervals.

Results

The overall surface of antum and corpus-fundus was reduced by 64.8 %, which achieved a 72.9 % reduction of basic acid production (BAO) after 4 weeks, and a 71.2 % reduction after 6 months. Stimulated acid production (PAO) was reduced by 66.9 % and 64.7 % respectively (see Table 1). Postoperatively, both basic and stimulated levels of gastrin were found elevated by 45.6 % and 75.9 % after 4 weeks, and by 52.4 % and 80.4 % after 6 months, respectively. Basic and stimulated secrete volumes were reduced by 61 % and 51 %, respectively. After an initial weight loss (about 12 % in 4 weeks), the mean body weight of all dogs returned to normal and exceeded the original body weight half a year later. The dogs' feeding habits were not influenced.
Monitoring of tissue pO$_2$ in the wall areas failed to demonstrate any altered configuration of pO$_2$ histograms. Cumulated pO$_2$ histograms were based on 10 single histograms [3]; the mean values of these cumulated histograms were 36.4 mmHg preoperatively, 35.7 mmHg postoperatively (see Table 2).

Table 1. Influence of the longitudinal resection on body weight, gastrin levels, acid production and secrete volume in the dog (n =10)

		Preop.	4 Weeks Postop.	Changes in %	6 Months Postop.	Changes in %	Unit
Mean Body Weight		23.4	20.6	− 12.0	23.7	+ 1.2	kg
Gastrin	Basic	25.0	36.4	+ 45.6	38.1	+ 52.4	pg/ml
	Stimul.	46.1	81.1	+ 75.9	83.2	+ 80.4	pg/ml
	BAO	5.9	1.6	− 72.9	1.7	− 71.2	meq/h
	PAO	41.9	13.9	− 66.9	14.8	− 64.7	meq/h
	MAO	39.8	11.3	− 71.7	12.5	− 68.6	meq/h
Volume of Basic		43.8	17.2	− 61.8	21.6	− 50.7	ml/h
Secretion (v) Stimul.		201.7	80.2	− 60.3	78.4	− 61.2	ml/h

Table 2. Tissue pO_2 in the intact stomach wall and after longitudinal resection in comparison to B II-resection and SP-vagotomy

	(mean value)	(number of measurements)
Intact Stomach	36.4 mm Hg	(n = 1034)
Longitudinal Resection	35.7 mm Hg	(n = 1040)
B II-Resection	16.8 mm Hg	(n = 1032)
SP-Vagotomy	11.8 mm Hg	(n = 1049)

Endoscopic and X-ray monitoring (see Fig. 2) revealed unimpeded passage, preserved motility and intact pyloric function.

Discussion

The longitudinal resection of the stomach is obviously able to exert a consistent influence on certain factors of ulcer pathophysiology. Excess acid and ferment production is distinctly reduced by diminishing the quantity of chief and parietal cells. Fig. 3 compares several procedures commonly used in ulcer surgery [1]. As opposed to various types of vagotomy and methods of resection, the procedure presented here offers a sufficient reduction in acid production by 73 or 71 % respectively [4]. Preserving the vessels and nerves on the minor curvature safeguards the microcirculation in the essential gastric pathway. A certain storage function of the stomach, the pyloric function, and the duodenal passage are well maintained, and together with them the pancreatocibal synchronism.
Whilst applying all the necessary caution indicated for transferring experimental results to human conditions, we feel that current hyperacid

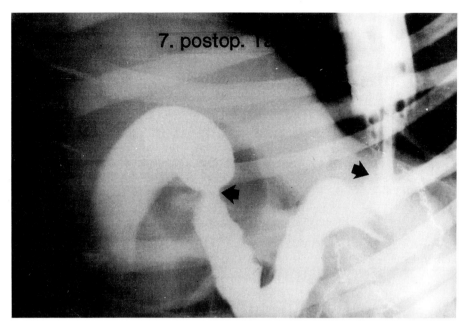

Fig. 2. Postoperative X-ray control after one week. Cardia and pylorus are marked (->)

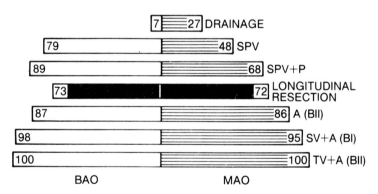

Fig. 3. Influence of acid reduction induced by different procedures which are used in ulcer surgery

ulcer may present an indication for longitudinal resection. Our results suggest that the procedure might find its place in the concept of surgical ulcer therapy.

Summary

The effects of a longitudinal stomach resection – as proposed by Saegesser in 1966 – on acid secretion, basic and stimulated gastrin levels, and on the microcirculation of the stomach wall was studied in 10 German Shepherds. The aim of the resection was to eliminate about one third of the antrum surface and two thirds of the fundus-corpus surface. The basic acid output (BAO) was distinctly lowered (72.9 %), and the peak acid output (PAO) was also reduced (66.9 %). The basic and stimulated serum levels of gastrin increased after the resection (45.6 % and 75.9 % respectively). The tissue pO_2 was not altered by the operation, and microcirculation remained intact. It seems possible that this procedure might be suitable for the treatment of recurrent duodenal ulcer.

References

1. Bauer H (1978) Therapeutisches Prinzip: Vagotomie. In: Blum AL, Siewert JR (eds) Ulcus-Therapie. Springer, Berlin, p 159
2. Ehrly AM, Hauss J, Huch R (1986) Clinical Oxygen Pressure Measurement. Springer, Berlin
3. Hauss J, Schönleben K, Spiegel HU (1982) Therapiekontrolle durch Überwachung des Gewebe-pO_2. Huber, Bern
4. Langhans P, Bünte H (1987) Operationsindikation und Verfahrenswahl beim Gastroduodenalulkus. In: Bünte H, Demling L, Domschke L, Langhans P (eds) Folgeerkrankungen in der Ulkuschirurgie. Medizin, Weinheim
5. Saegesser M (1966) Der Ulkus-Magen. Huber, Bern, p 70